THE SEVEN AGES
OF A
MEDICAL SCIENTIST

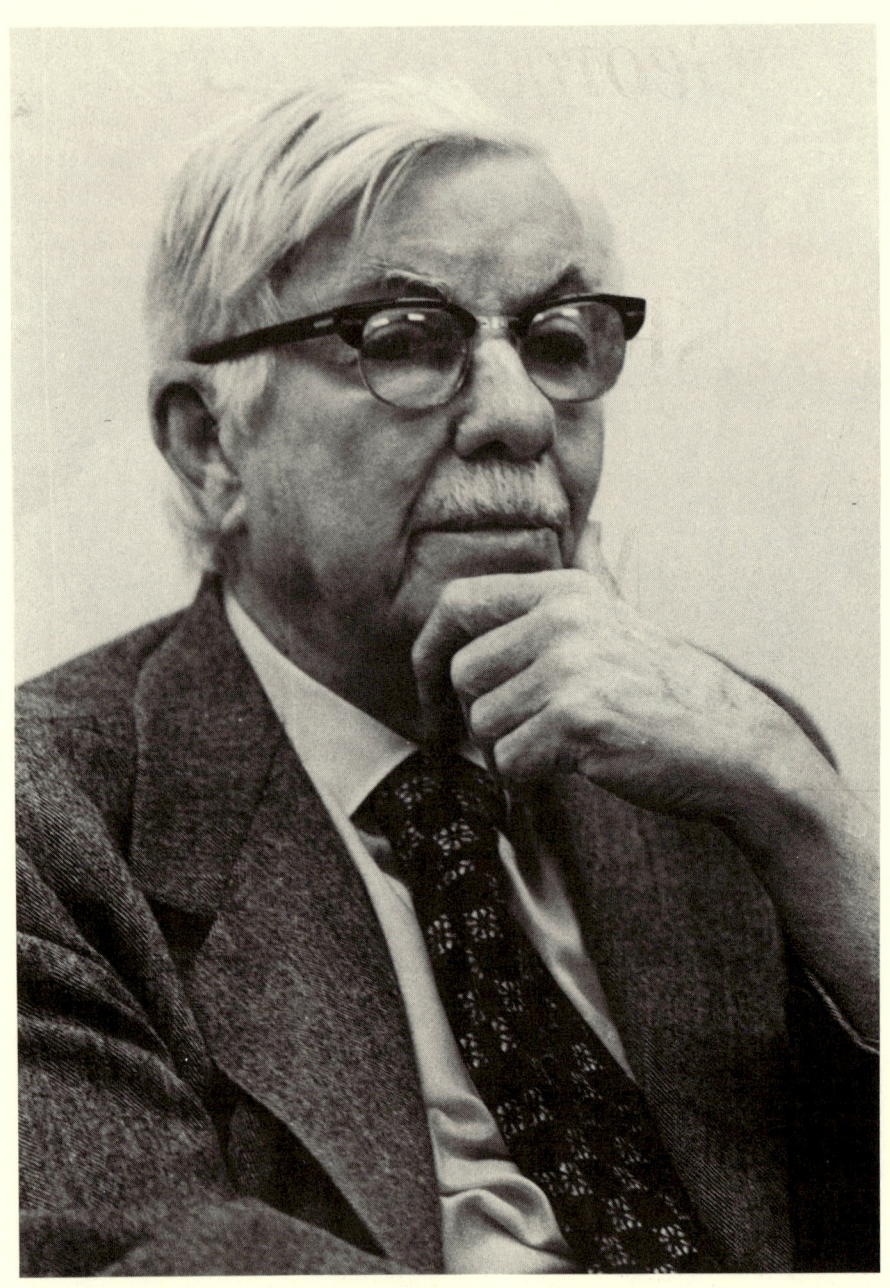

George W. Corner

George W. Corner

THE SEVEN AGES OF A MEDICAL SCIENTIST

An Autobiography

UNIVERSITY OF PENNSYLVANIA PRESS

Philadelphia · 1981

Publication of this book has been aided by a grant from the Macy
Foundation

Frontispiece: George W. Corner
Photograph by William McCormick. Courtesy of the *Huntsville* (Ala.) *Times*.
Portions of "City Child and Schoolboy"
were published in the *Baltimore Sun*, May 2, 1978.
Portions of "Collegian" are reprinted
by permission from *Johns Hopkins Magazine*, May 1978.
Portions of "The Preclinical Years" and "At Home and on the Road"
were published in *Perspectives in Biology and Medicine*,
vol. 21, no. 3. Copyright © 1978 by the University of Chicago Press.
Reprinted by permission.

Designed by Adrianne Onderdonk Dudden

Library of Congress Cataloging in Publication Data

Corner, George Washington, 1889–
The seven ages of a medical scientist.

"Publications of George W. Corner": p.
Includes index.
1. Corner, George Washington, 1889–
2. Anatomists—United States—Biography. 3. Embryologists—United States—Biography. 4. Medical
historians—United States—Biography. I. Title.
[DNLM: 1. Physicians—United States—Personal
narratives. WZ 100 C816s]
QM16.C66A37   610′.92′4 [B]   81–51143
ISBN 0-8122-7811-9   AACR2

Printed in the United States of America

For Thomas and Christopher
and little Jason

CONTENTS

ILLUSTRATIONS

ACKNOWLEDGMENTS

Chapter 1 of this book was first published, in large part, in the *Baltimore Sun*'s Sunday magazine for May 2, 1978. Most of chapter 2 appeared in the *Johns Hopkins Magazine* for May 1978.

Some of the anecdotes in chapters 3 to 12 were published in *Perspectives in Biology and Medicine,* vol. 21, no. 3 (Spring 1978), under the title "Doctors Limited: Notes for an Autobiography." Dr. Willard M. Allen and S. Karger AG, Basel, publisher of *Gynecological Investigations,* have kindly permitted the use of passages from Allen's "Recollections of My Life with Progesterone." A few excerpts from other periodicals have been acknowledged in the text or footnotes.

The following friends of the author have supplemented his memory with names and dates: Edward F. Adolf, Roberta Yerkes Blanshard, Caryl P. Haskins, and Gordon M. Meade. George L. Erikson supplied names and dates from the archives of the American Association of Anatomists.

Graham Weddell read the Oxford chapter, and two scholarly friends, R. Stewart Rauch, lawyer and banker, and Kenneth M. Setton, medieval historian, read chapter 11 to test its intelligibility for lay readers.

Special help was kindly given by Thomas R. Forbes, Yale University; Philip S. Weimerskirch, the University of Rochester Medical Library; and Nancy McCall, archives of the Johns Hopkins Medical Institutions. Roy Goodman, reference librarian at the American Philosophical Society, was a constant adviser.

The late E. Kent Kane of Kane, Pennsylvania, persistently and persuasively urged the author to venture upon this book, as did Theodore G. Duncan, M.D., who generously provided the assistance of Mrs. Susan Kircher. Miss Julia Noonan of the American Philosophical Society's staff read the manuscript and supplied facts and dates that had escaped the author's memory. Mrs. Susan Kircher and Miss Susan Hersker Rubinstein, typists, did well to decipher the author's scribbled drafts.

GROWING UP

1

CITY CHILD AND SCHOOLBOY

When I was born, at 24 North Broadway, Baltimore, Maryland, on December 12, 1889, Benjamin Harrison was president of the United States, Victoria was Queen of England, and Lord Salisbury was her prime minister. The Spanish flag flew over Cuba and Puerto Rico. Arizona, New Mexico, Oklahoma, Utah, and Wyoming were not yet states of the Union. Alfred Tennyson and Walt Whitman were alive and writing poetry.

Baltimore was less than half its present size, having a population of about 400,000. Like all large cities it was a collection of villages, more so than today because people did not get around the city as easily as now. Urban transport was by horse-drawn vehicles and cable cars. Electric streetcars were just coming in. So the citizens were divided into Baltimoreans of the east and west, north and south sections, fringed by Highlandtown, Waverly, Walbrook, and other still semidetached suburban villages. Some kinfolk of ours who lived on what is now Erdman Avenue, in Orangeville, were considered by us to be country cousins.

The family business, the shipping firm of James Corner and Sons, had been for almost a century in East Baltimore, on Corner's Wharf, near the foot of Central Avenue. My father had not joined that business; he was a member of a wholesale firm a mile uptown, Rouse, Hempstone, and Company, dealing in men's furnishings, but he continued to live close to his parents and to my mother's and to the family home, which was his birthplace and mine. Until I was about fourteen, East Baltimore was my home town. My urban orbit was bounded, roughly speaking, by the harbor, Howard Street, Patterson Park, and North Avenue (which latter in my early childhood the old folks called Boundary Avenue), making an area about a mile and a half in length and breadth. I knew that there were other parts of the city, some of them more elegant than ours, for I had cousins in the region of Eutaw Place and Lanvale Street, but I seldom saw them. To go to Druid Hill Park for a picnic was a special undertaking; the trip took almost an hour by the Madison Avenue cable cars.

My parents were Methodists and teetotalers. I never saw a stage play or an opera until I was past twenty-one, and I was well into my thirties before I took to alcoholic refreshment. The Corners had not always been puritans, however. The first of the line to whom I can surely trace my ancestry, Solomon Corner, kept the village inn at colonial Easton, Talbot County, on Maryland's Eastern Shore. He certainly had a taproom, and at one time he owned a racehorse. Family tradition says that Solomon's son, my great-grandfather, James Coleman Corner, 1783–1842, was converted to Methodism and, being unwilling to serve liquor at the inn, moved to Baltimore. There he founded the firm of James Corner and Sons, which owned several large sailing vessels, among them the full-rigged ship *James Corner* and the beautiful bark *Serene*, trading first with Mediterranean ports, later with South America, and finally with Savannah in the tar and turpentine trade. James's son, my grandfather, George W. Corner, Sr., 1821–1904, joined the firm when he was a youth and never left it.

My maternal grandfather, Henry Evans, was brought to America from Somerset, England, as a little boy. He became a pioneer in the food-packing industry, especially the canning of oysters, for which he designed machinery for large-scale production. He smoked tobacco but (I believe) was restrained from indulgence in alcohol by his wife, my grandmother, née Hester Ann King, daughter of a Baltimore merchant, a Methodist so rigidly puritanical that he would not even allow his family to eat pork because of the Mosaic law against it.

My first home was my grandfather Corner's large house at 24 North Broadway, on the southwest corner of Broadway and Fairmount Avenue, just south of the Church Home hospital, but my parents moved far out Broadway when I was about three years old. A year later they came back and settled at No. 113

Jackson Place, only a half-block east of Broadway, and so I did most of my growing up just off Broadway. I was always welcome at No. 24. We went there for dinner every Sunday, and my grandfather's garden, almost an acre of greenery in that region of close-set brick houses, was always open as a playground to me, my brother, Harry, and our cousins Donald Fenhagen and Willie Lambdin.

Not long ago I went to East Baltimore to see what had happened to those places I remember so happily. My grandfather's house has been replaced by a modern business building, and Jackson Place, too, is gone, alas. It was a neat little square, just one block long, between Fairmount Avenue and Fayette Street, lined by brick houses with white marble steps along both sides of the block. Cobblestoned roadways ran along the front of both the east and west rows of houses. In the middle was a little park with green lawns, formal pathways, and flower beds, centered on an ornamental iron fountain surrounded by a basin in which a school of goldfish spent their summer days.

The permanent residents of Jackson Place, of varied races and religions, were lifetime Baltimoreans, but there was an exotic, transient element of our population, the medical students. The Johns Hopkins Medical School opened just about the time we moved to Jackson Place, and a score of students, attracted by the quiet of the square, had found lodgings with some of the local families. They were such an interesting novelty that Jackson Place was sometimes called the Latin Quarter of East Baltimore, though there was no such gaiety or philandering as in Paris. These students were incipient professionals, serious and hard-working. The gas lights in their third-floor rooms could be seen burning far into the night. I remember two of them by name. One was a plain-looking, plainly dressed young woman. My aunt pointed her out to me one day, saying in muted voice, "That's a woman medical student," as if she had just escaped from a zoo. This was Florence Sabin from Colorado, destined to be the first woman professor in the Johns Hopkins University and the first female member of the National Academy of Sciences. I gazed at her with wide open eyes, little knowing that in a few years I would be her pupil, later her teaching assistant, and her lifelong friend. Another, more conspicuous student was Frank Lynch, nicknamed "Heavy" by his fellows because of his stout frame and slow movements. He became professor of obstetrics at the University of California and presided at the birth of my first child.

I said that the medical students were not lighthearted people, but I can remember just once seeing some of them cut loose with a wild display of exuberant spirits. Perhaps a final examination had gone well. Whatever the cause, while the neighbors were sitting on their front stoops making the best of a hot summer evening about the first of June, a dozen of the medics came roaring out of a house near the fountains, dressed only in abbreviated underwear, climbed into the fishpond, and had a hilarious time splashing and dunking each other, all the while filling the square with raucous laughter. Some of the neighbors were amused, others were scandalized. I didn't know any of those revelers by name, but a half-century later I learned that one of them was George Whipple, later my teacher in medical school and my dean at Rochester, winner of the Nobel Prize for Medicine in 1934.

At the foot of the square, looking north, was a Lutheran church, and a half-block away at Broadway and Fairmount Avenue was another church, of another variety of Lutherans, whose pastor's voice could be heard on Sundays booming out his sermons in *echt Deutsch.*

Over the housetops to the north we could see the cupola of the Johns Hopkins Hospital. To balance, so to speak, the churches there was narrow little Mullikin Street, hardly more than an alley, off the west side of Broadway between Fayette and Orleans streets, lined with two-story houses that according to some of my more sophisticated playmates were whorehouses. When I was about fourteen, a slightly younger playmate explained their function to me. He said he had learned where babies come from. "Your father," he said, "goes up to Mullikin Street and does something or other with a whore. She produces a baby and he brings it home to your mother." The memory of that conversation haunted me until I had growing children of my own, and led me to write for them two little books on sex and reproduction.

People who grew up in the suburbs or the country may wonder what games we boys could play on cobblestoned streets in a built-up city, but we did not feel deprived on that score. In infancy we stayed on the sidewalks and played hide-and-seek and ring-around-a-rosy. Later we had hoops and marbles (a game of marbles can be quite sporting, played on cobblestones). Among my playmates at that age was a gentle, mannerly little boy whose handsome mother was a soloist in the choir of a church somewhere uptown. His name was Otto Ortmann. He grew up to be director of the Peabody Conservatory of Music.

As we grew older we could ride bicycles and roller skate on Broadway, which was smoothly paved with asphalt. When there was no cop in sight we could even play hockey on roller skates; the traffic was light enough for that. When a cart or carriage came along, we simply adjourned to the sidewalk for a few moments. In winter there was often good coasting on Broadway downhill northward from Monument Street—not on sophisticated steel Flexible Flyers; they had not yet been invented—but on low wooden sleds, belly-whopper style. Sometimes four to six boys sat on a high, heavy "cheese box" sled, or up to eight or ten on a majestic "patent" built of two sleds connected by a long plank, the front sled steered by the pilot's feet on a crossbar or even with a wheel. My cousin, G. Corner Fenhagen, architect of the Baltimore City College, when he was sixteen years old designed and built the handsomest and most admired "patent" on the hill.

In summer there were vacant lots big enough for a small boy's kind of baseball. And of course we Corner boys and our cousins had Grandfather Corner's garden and lawn for a playground—too often, I fear, to the detriment of the flower beds. Enjoying as we did this luxury of a private playground, we left to the less privileged class of East Baltimore urchins their favorite sport of chasing stray cats on the run down side streets and alleys, armed with old brooms, all the while shouting "Skinner, skinner"—a derogatory term, in the East Baltimore language, for homeless, half-starved felines. I don't remember ever seeing one of these hunts end in a kill; a skinner could always find a hole in a backyard fence through which to escape his tormentors. In the heat of summer these juvenile huntsmen turned their attention to the large grasshoppers that lived on the lawns in the middle of Broadway and on the weeds that sprang up between the cobblestones of the side streets—an even more sporting kind of prey than skinners, for they buzzed away from under the descending broom only to settle down a dozen yards away, awaiting another onslaught.

Of course our leisure was not all devoted to play. There were always books to read, and I was a constant user of the Pratt Library branch on the west side of Broadway, north of the Johns Hopkins Hospital. There were no children's librarians in those days to protect us from literary trash. The library had all of the Horatio Alger books and all of G. A. Henty's juvenile historical stories. I read these, every one, and I am here to say that they did me no harm whatever. But that little branch library also held Sidney Lanier's edition of Malory's *Morte d'Arthur*, and so at the age of twelve or thirteen I struggled through the King Arthur tales in diluted Middle English, and that did me a lot of good.

In the eighth grade I had my first formal instruction in natural science. Our elderly teacher had probably taken a course in mineralogy. She brought to school lots of stones—quartz, feldspar, slate, and sandstone—explained them to us, and encouraged us to look for other kinds of rock. With one of my schoolmates I once or twice explored the roadsides and footpaths in Clifton Park, filling my pockets with pebbles to be exhibited to Miss Porter. I also began, prematurely, my career as a student of animal reproduction in my grandfather's backyard, where the gardener's son and I kept a few rabbits in a homemade pen until their numbers increased so undesirably that we were ordered to discontinue the enterprise. At one point during this period I told my mother's sisters (one an old maid, the other not yet married) about the sex of our rabbits, that we had "two he's and five she's." Father, embarrassed, took me aside and told me that gentlemen do not mention such matters before ladies.

I have said that our part of East Baltimore was like a village. A good part of our food was brought by street vendors— Mr. Immel, the baker's man, who always gave me a doughnut or a cruller when he left my mother's order of bread or pastry —the meat man, the fish man, each with his horse-drawn cart— the hucksters, called "Arabs" in the East Baltimore language, with their street cries: "Red ripe tomatoses, Annie Rannel tomatoses" or "crab, crab, crabby—get your live soft cra-abs, crabby, crabby." The knife grinder had a dinner bell to call attention to his arrival in the square. The Italian hurdy-gurdy man's monkey in a little red vest never failed to attract a juvenile audience.

In midsummer came the watermelon vendors, their carts heaped high with the handsome fruit direct from Anne Arundel's sandy fields, and the hokey-pokey boy, pushing his handcart filled with ice to preserve his five-cent blocks of hokey-pokey ice cream, dear to the small boy's heart. Another summer treat, the snowball, so-called, was generally sold by a local juvenile entrepreneur who set up a stand, a box on four legs, holding a big cake of ice from which with a scraper he produced a glassful of mushy shavings, over which he poured a richly colored and oh, how tasty syrup. You half ate, half drank this poor relation of a sherbet.

The most exciting event in my eleven years on Jackson Place was the great Baltimore fire of February 1904, when I was fourteen years old. While we were in church on a Sunday morning we heard the fire engines running, and when, after the last Amen, we came out on the street, the air was heavily tinged with smoke, for there was already a tremendous blaze in the business district, three-quarters of a mile to the west of Broadway.

Jackson Place was on rising ground. We then lived on the west side of the square at No. 100. From the rear of our house we had a full view of the blazing business section. All afternoon and far into the night we watched the flames creep southward and northward until the western skyline from the harbor to Saratoga Street was a mile-long wall of fire and smoke. We saw the brick and stone sheathing of tall buildings peel off and fall away until only the red-hot steel frames were left standing. Smaller brick buildings just blazed up and crumbled to the ground. We heard the explosions as the fire fighters dynamited buildings to create a fire break along Lexington and Saratoga streets. The fire spread eastward to Jones's Falls, then an open stream. My father told us that if it crossed the falls he would abandon our house and take us to our country cousins at Orangeville. How he could have managed that I can't imagine. There were five of us, parents and children. We had no carriage or cart. Over at 24 North Broadway my grandfather, eighty-three years old, was lying mortally ill. Fortunately for us, the wind changed and the homes of East Baltimore were saved. I remember that seven nights after the fire began, the glow from the smoldering ruins was so bright that sitting on our back steps I could read the *Sun* paper by the light from the burned area.

If seldom exciting, school days were happy and interesting. I was first tutored by a young aunt, who got me into the third grade at the age of eight. Then I went to Grammar School No. 11, later renumbered 71, on McElderry Street, a block or two west of Broadway. The Baltimore public schools must have been excellent in those days, or else I was lucky. I liked all my teachers, and they were all competent. The last of them, in the eighth grade, spotted and encouraged my budding scientific interests and observed that I was getting by without much work. She advised my parents to send me to a private school.

I entered the Boys' Latin School of Baltimore in the autumn of 1903, in my fourteenth year. The school then occupied a plain but well-planned building on Brevard Street, looking down a grassy slope toward the handsome Mt. Royal Station of the Baltimore and Ohio Railroad, now used by the Maryland Institute art school. "Dunham's," as our school was often called from the name of the headmaster, Mr. James A. Dunham, followed English preparatory school traditions. The teachers were called masters, the classes were known as forms, and the curriculum emphasized Latin, English, and mathematics. It was tacitly assumed that all the boys, mostly sons of upper-middle-class families in comfortable financial circumstances, were to be prepared for college, especially Princeton and Johns Hopkins.

The fourth form, to which I was admitted, was roughly equivalent to the first year of the city's two public high schools for boys, the City College and the Polytechnic Institute. I was qualified to begin the fourth form work in mathematics and English but not Latin, which at Dunham's was begun in the first form. This difficulty was solved by my Aunt Rena, my mother's younger sister, who had attended Goucher College for a year or two. During the summer of 1903 she led me lovingly and efficiently through the declensions and conjugations and a book of easy readings, covering in three months the work of three years in the school. We even took a peek at Caesar so that I should not be overwhelmed by "Omnis Gallia in partes tres divisa est." This sound preparation was fortunate, for neither my aunt nor I foresaw that at Dunham's I was to go on with Latin under a superb but exacting teacher.

Edward Lucas White was thirty-seven years of age in 1903, but to us boys he was clothed in authority not measured in years. He had hidden himself behind a black square-cut beard, above which his dark eyes, sometimes sparkling with humor, sometimes dauntingly intense, looked out over his roomful of pupils. Since he seated us alphabetically, with the A's, B's, and C's at the front, in my three years with him I got the full range of his glances. Whiskers White's health was not robust, and he had become something of a hypochondriac. Whenever his classroom was a bit cool, he wrapped a scarf around his neck. We noticed, however, that his throat was not so weak as to prevent him from roaring at anybody who looked inattentive or committed a stupid error. Every now and then he would pull out of his desk drawer a chocolate bar and nibble at it, explaining that it helped his poor digestion. We were amused by this habit, so boyish of him but not permitted to us in class. At the school's Christmas party in 1905, a jolly occasion held in the large study room, at which the pupils presented gifts to the masters, when Mr. White's turn came the whole upper school rose, stormed to the front of the room and, cackling with laughter, each boy thrust into his hands a ten-cent chocolate bar.

Another master at Dunham's as competent as Mr. White, though without such endearing personal quirks, was William Wilhelm. He was teacher of mathematics for the upper school, and he made algebra, geometry, and trigonometry clear and interesting. Shortly after our form finished school, Mr. Wilhelm went to the Baltimore Polytechnic Institute to head its mathematics department. Dr. George Shipley (he was a Ph.D.) taught English to the upper forms. He was also a night city editor of the *Baltimore American.* He could not have gotten much sleep, and I think he was often tired, considering how many themes he had to grade, but he was clear and careful—and humorless. Foreign languages, French and German, were introduced in the fourth form by a tall, dark young man named Downes.

Since the school had no provision for teaching science, I picked up at home what scientific information I could get from electrical toys such as a little battery-operated motor my grandfather Corner gave me, from amateur photography, the *Na-*

tional Geographic, and the old Munn and Company *Scientific American,* a subscription to which my father gave me as a Christmas gift, and from constant reading in *Johnson's Universal Encyclopedia,* at hand in our library–sitting room.

My school work went quite well during all three years at the Boys' Latin School. Mr. Dunham did not announce numerical grades or list our relative standings, but at graduation he awarded honorable mention to the boys who had done well in various courses. I received honorable mention in English, history, geometry, analytic geometry, Latin, and German. Only two other boys in the sixth form of 1906 received as many as six honorable mentions. One of them was John King. The other, Matthew Gault, had seven honorable mentions and was designated, English fashion, as head boy. He became a lawyer in Baltimore.

I have not yet spoken at all about one facet of growing up in East Baltimore that deeply channeled my boyish thoughts and opened my eyes to the wide world outside. That was the nearness of Baltimore harbor, barely a half-mile away. In the quiet hours of dawn and dusk one could hear the whistles of the bay steamboats entering or leaving the Basin, and now and then the deeper horn of an ocean freighter docking at Locust Point. From the corner of Broadway and Fairmount Avenue we could look down Broadway past one side or the other of the Fells Point market and could see through that narrow slot a slice of a passing steamboat or schooner. When, years afterward, I read Henry Mencken's story of his boyhood on Hollins Street, I was struck by the absence of any hint that he grew up in a maritime city, whereas from early childhood I knew and was proud to know that I lived in a major seaport from which my great-grandfather's ships had sailed to the Mediterranean and to Rio and which might some day be a port of departure for me on the voyage of life.

After the death of my grandfather Corner in 1904, which broke our last ancestral ties to East Baltimore, my parents felt free to give their three children the advantages of suburban life. My father's partnership in the mercantile firm of Rouse, Hempstone, and Company was giving him a comfortable income, and both he and my mother had legacies from their parents that would help to finance building a house. After a summer's trial in a rented cottage in Roland Park, a northern suburb of Baltimore, they bought a lot there at 212 Ridgewood Road and employed a leading architectural firm, Wyatt and Nolting, to design a home to their liking.

Roland Park had been planned by the renowned New York landscape architect Frederick Law Olmsted, who laid out through wooded hillsides a network of curving roads that provided charming vistas. Our house stood on the rim of the suburb overlooking toward the west a wide view of green country in the valley of Jones's Falls, partly farm land, partly the golf course of the Baltimore Country Club. At the foot of the hill on the Falls Road below our house was a little village still rural in aspect that must have taken its odd name, Cross Keys, from a tavern sign in colonial days. A much-traveled friend of my parents, admiring the view from our rear porch, said that the green valley and distant hills reminded him of Ireland. The whole area is built over now, and the Falls Road is a modern major highway.

Our house still stands, looking as homelike as when we moved there, covered with brown shingles set off by white columns at the front doorway and white railings over the wide porches my father insisted upon. Here I lived from 1904 to the autumn of 1914 with my parents, my brother, Henry ("Harry") Evans Corner, three years younger than I, and my sister Hester, eight years my junior—a family with thoughtfully devoted parents and happy, intelligent, and dutiful children. I had a comfortable bedroom with a roomy desk and bookshelves, and I shared a bathroom with my brother.

Downstairs there was a parlor, stiffly furnished and used only to receive formal visitors, and a large library–sitting room with a fireplace, whose bookcases housed a stock of sound literature—sets of Dickens and Washington Irving; the favorite poets of my parents' day, including Tennyson, Longfellow, Whittier, and Bryant (but not Walt Whitman), current novels of the more serious kind, and many travel books. We took the *National Geographic*, the *Saturday Evening Post*, the *Christian Advocate*, and one or two literary magazines—*Harper's* or the *Atlantic Monthly*.

I spent many hours in the library, generally sprawled in a large leather-covered chair, reading anything and everything, very often educating myself from *Johnson's Encyclopedia*. My brother and I taught ourselves to play chess from an article in that excellent work. On winter evenings, after we children had done our homework, Father would often clear the large round table that stood under a Tiffany-style chandelier in the center of the room. Then he would play dominoes with us or one of those games that were played on a marked board with little round pieces that you pushed or flicked with your forefinger; the family's favorite of this sort was called "Crokinole." In summer we had family games of croquet on the back lawn, which had a gentle slope that made one's aim sportingly uncertain.

My mother, quietly efficient administrator of the household, had two black servants, a cook and a man to care for the lawn and hedges, do the heavier kind of housework, wait on table, and wash dishes. These servants did not "live in." The cook, Emma Grant, née Banks, plump and warm-hearted, came several miles by trolley seven days a week with Thursday afternoons and alternate Sundays off, arriving at seven in the morning to get breakfast and staying until evening dinner was over and the dishes washed. Emma kept alive in some ways a bit of the old black mammy tradition. She loved the whole family and enjoyed cooking for us but felt free to comment on our doings and our ways. She talked in a delightful vernacular of her own about which I used to tease her. On a warm summer day when lemonade was to be served, I asked her, "Emma, is the lemons squoze?" to which she replied, "Oh, Mr. George, do you say squoze? I says squizzen." Once when my parents returned from a trip abroad with tales of meeting some of our distant English relatives, Emma said, "When I get the time, I'm going to Africa to look up the Bankses"—an idea that does not seem surprising as I write in 1978, considering Alex Haley and his *Roots*.

When my father acquired an automobile, the black handyman added chauffeuring to his other duties, but as long as I lived with the family we went to town by streetcar, Father to business and I to school. On Sundays this meant for him a long ride to East Baltimore, where he continued to be the Sunday school superintendent at Broadway Methodist Church, a post that his father had once held and my brother later took over for several years.

Father was a really devout Methodist and long kept up the

custom of daily family prayers, generally held in his little den just off the library. Each of us read in turn a passage from the Bible and then, on our knees, heard Father pray extemporaneously for the good of the nation and our household. His petitions to the Almighty were eloquent, deeply sincere, and moderate. I should have become accustomed to them, but some temperamental quirk had subjected me from childhood to embarrassment by religious talk and observances by other than the official clergy. When, as happened a few times, I was called on to pray at meetings of the Epworth League (the Methodist religious society for young people) I was completely tongue-tied. I was, therefore, not comfortable at family prayers, and though I never openly rebelled, my brother, my sister, and I must have shown —by tacit reluctance or tardiness in coming to prayers—a latent unwillingness to participate. When I was about seventeen Father wistfully discontinued prayers because, he said, he could see that we were not really interested.

We children, however, accepted without demur the Methodist ban on the theater, horse racing, gambling, smoking, and alcoholic drinks. My mother was not altogether happy about the restriction on theatergoing. I once overheard her complain to Father that if he could take his boys to a professional baseball game, she thought it unfair that she could not see a play. Surely there must be decent plays, she said, and they would be more elevating than a ball game. Oratorios were the nearest available substitutes for secular drama. I heard with rapt enjoyment performances of *The Messiah* and Haydn's *Creation* by the excellent Baltimore Oratorio Society. Our parents occasionally attended symphony concerts but did not take us children. We were not really a musical family.

An outdoor activity—in which my father often joined us— was fishing, of a simple kind. On a Saturday afternoon in spring he would take us by the Baltimore and Ohio Railroad to Relay station on the Patapsco River above the fall line, where it is a running stream, to fish for what were locally called gudgeons, small shiny fish coming annually in great numbers, I suppose to spawn in fresh water. They took the hook so readily that small boys could catch them by dozens—no tedious wait for a bite.

Another sport for boys was crabbing. For that our handiest place was on the Patapsco below Baltimore where the river is a wide tidal estuary. You operate from a flat-bottomed skiff in shallow water near shore. The bait is small chunks of meat, all the better if it is a bit spoiled and smelly. You tie two or three chunks of it along a string with a weight on the end. You drop the line overboard, wait a few minutes, and slowly haul it in. The chances are that a crab will have grasped the bait with its strong claws and will greedily hang onto it, to be taken aboard with a hand net and put in a sack. The only really sporting element in crabbing is to avoid being nipped by those fierce claws.

Once or twice Father arranged a party for us and a few of his friends to go fishing for bluefish in Chesapeake Bay. That meant rising in the small hours and getting to Annapolis before dawn. A fisherman took us in his boat out into the bay to troll with hook and line among a school of the handsome fish. The Chesapeake at dawn has a calm beauty all its own, enhanced by the sight of the big fish greedily racing through the water in search of food, often splashing above the calm surface. When one of them takes the bait there is a tug of war, and when it is pulled over the gunwale of the boat, you have a delicious dinner for a whole family.

Indoors at home, my hobbies included woodwork and especially construction of model sailboats, not the elegant ones that boys now put together from a prefabricated kit, but simple sturdy craft for sailing in the bathtub or a pond—sloops and schooners designed by myself with hulls carved out of wood and leaden keels that I cast in wooden molds. Once Harry and I made a crude collapsible canoe of laths and painted canvas which we tested successfully on Jones's Falls. I often worked with self-constructed electrical apparatus, making electromagnets, induction coils, and a voltmeter calibrated with dry batteries—simple things, but they helped me understand the basic principles of electricity: voltage, amperage, resistance, induction. I bought a good camera and did my own developing and printing, learning a little chemistry and something about artistic composition. Thus I made up, to some extent, for the lack of physics and chemistry at school.

One winter when I was fifteen or sixteen years old I wanted to construct a static electrical machine of the Wimshurst type but, lacking equipment for precise woodwork, asked my cousin Donald Fenhagen to join me because at his school, the Baltimore

Polytechnic Institute, he had access to a lathe. I had a glazier cut the circular glass plates, and Donald turned the two hubs from hardwood. At that stage of the project the season for outdoor sports set in. The electrical machine languished, and I could never get Donald to resume it. The plates and hubs lay around my workshop for years, producing in me a resolve never again to start a project unless I could see my way to complete it.

My budding intellectual life was greatly stimulated by guests who came to our dinner table. Father was active in church and in philanthropic affairs. Methodist ministers often dined with us, always ready talkers and often with something worth a boy's listening. Our pastor at Broadway Church, a frequent guest while we lived in East Baltimore, sometimes came to dinner on Ridgewood Road and, being a good Latinist, enjoyed going over with me Whiskers White's homework assignments. Now and then a Methodist bishop stayed overnight when presiding over the Baltimore annual conference. Those were impressive men with wide practical interests. One of the professors of English at Goucher College became a close and stimulating friend of the family, and I recall particularly an evening with Herman Harrell Horne, then professor of philosophy at Dartmouth College, in town on some church business, whose cultivated and interesting conversation made me think that I wanted to be a professor like him.

Most of all, my boyhood was enriched by the love of my mother's two sisters. Aunt Laura Evans, eldest of the three, never married. Irene, the youngest, married a veterinary surgeon named Dickinson Gorsuch, son of a prosperous Baltimore County farmer. The wedding was held at our house soon after we moved to Roland Park—a great occasion for us young people. Uncle Dick and Aunt Rena settled on a small farm at Glencoe, about twenty-five miles north of Baltimore. Aunt Laura lived with them. The two women, city born and city bred, took to country life with remarkable zest. The Gorsuches to their endless regret had no children, and Aunt Laura was as reluctant to accept a country swain as she had been when courted by several eligible bachelors in East Baltimore. Those two good women therefore lavished their maternal affections upon the Corner children. As the eldest, I was the special recipient of their loving kindness. I was always welcome to stay at the Glencoe farm. Aunt Rena had taught me to read and introduced me to Latin; Aunt Laura watched me grow up with gentle solicitude for my health and happiness, encouraging me in my studies and my hobbies. As I grew older she was concerned about my social life, delicately indicating which girls in our vicinity were worthy of my attention and which I should shun because they attended cocktail parties and played cards.

I really had very little practical experience with girls. There were no female cousins nearby of my own age. My sister's friends, years younger than I, were children to be kindly patronized, though I confess that I enjoyed being Hester's admired big brother. Grammar school classes were mixed, but the girls and boys did not socialize. We played separate games in the school yard during recess and did not walk home together. The Boys' Latin School was a masculine enclave. Even in Sunday school the sexes were largely segregated. At parties in Roland Park I was a wallflower because I did not dance. As it happened, there were no girls of my age in our immediate neighborhood with whom I might have had a round of tennis at the country club or whom I could have treated to an icecream soda on a summer afternoon.

Among all the girls whom I met during my adolescence, among our family and acquaintances, in church, at parties and elsewhere, there were three who awoke in me strong romantic feelings. The first was a little girl of about thirteen years with whom I was enamored for a while when I was fourteen, just before we moved to Roland Park. I never really met her. Her first name, I believe, was Edna; if I ever knew her last name I have forgotten it. I noticed her first on the platform at a Sunday school entertainment, singing the chorus of a cantata. She had a squarish face, a snub nose, and dull brown hair, but something in her manner, some grace of movement, made her stand out from her companions, and I thought her charming.

Edna was soon replaced in my regard, during the trial summer we spent that year in Roland Park, by the very pretty youngest daughter of a large family who lived near our temporary home. I thought Annette beautiful beyond words. We occasionally met on the streetcar going to or from our respective schools. On one such occasion she coyly remarked that I was a very bright boy, much brighter than herself. I didn't care how bright she was as long as she was so beautiful. But there was a gap between us that prevented a deepening friendship—her family was Roman Catholic; she was free to enjoy dancing and card games and the theater. I could never share her social ambience. When I was in college I saw her even less often, and our acquaintance diminished. *Tempora mutantur;* I have lived to see one of my grandsons marry a Catholic and another marry a Jewish girl.

The third girl who attracted my attention in those adolescent years was the daughter of our minister at Broadway Methodist Church. I had known Martha (as I shall call her) since in our childhood her father was first assigned to the pastorate there. Her parents and mine became close friends, and while we lived in East Baltimore I was often in her company. We went to each other's birthday parties and met at other social affairs. She was a nice-looking girl but not a beauty like Annette. I was more at ease with Martha than with other girls, but she really had no enduring appeal for me. I think she was too much like a member of our family. I was inclined to exotic rather than domestic inamoratas—the intangible Edna, the Catholic Annette. When I finally married another minister's daughter, I found her in a faraway land, under another flag than ours; she came from a distant part of our nation and spoke with a different accent. Her father's pulpit was by no means Wesleyan. But I did not meet her until after I had almost finished my university studies.

2

COLLEGIAN

When I enrolled at Johns Hopkins in the fall of 1906, an awe-struck freshman three months short of my seventeenth birthday, the university was only thirty years old. I was to see three famous survivors of the original senior faculty—Daniel Coit Gilman, when he came over from Washington to attend commemoration days and commencements, Basil Lanneau Gildersleeve in all his bearded dignity, on his way to the Latin seminar, and Ira Remsen, in my day president of the university.

We entering students were welcomed and briefed by Dean Edward H. Griffin in the Donovan Room of McCoy Hall. I recall not a word of what was said on that occasion. All I remember is a room full of students and two faces—the schoolmasterly visage of the dean, whose shrewd eyes and thin pointed nose were surrounded by Victorian muttonchop whiskers, and behind him, in bronze on a pedestal, the noble head and meditative features of the poet-professor Sidney Lanier.

More new students than usual were being welcomed that day, for two freshman classes were entering at once. The curriculum and requirements for admission had been changed that year. About forty of us had met the stiff requirements for the old three-year college course. We were the last class that would have no sophomore year. The rest would constitute the class of 1910. We were nearly all Baltimoreans, mostly from City College, but I was not to be lonesome among those strangers, for five of us came from the Boys' Latin School, among them my closest school friend, Samuel Clagett Chew.

The university's buildings, like those of its European proto-
types, were crowded together on city streets. There were eight
unimposing brick halls and laboratories just off the west side of
Howard Street. McCoy Hall, the largest, containing the library
and classrooms, faced two ways, north on Monument Street and
south on Little Ross Street. On the south side of that narrow
way stood a small administration building and a row of three
laboratories for geology, chemistry, and biology. The university
YMCA building, Levering Hall, adjoined McCoy Hall on the
west, facing on Eutaw Street. A gymnasium and a "cage" for
indoor lacrosse and football practice lay to the east, across narrow Garden Street, with their backs on Howard Street. We had
no green lawns and no playing fields. The only available outdoor
sport was pitching nickels on the Garden Street sidewalk. The
athletic teams had to go out to the suburbs for practice games.
This was a place for study, not for campus life. We undergraduates numbered about 150 among 300 graduate students and
(across town) about 300 students of medicine.

The college curriculum was sensibly arranged in five groups
centered, respectively, on classical languages, modern languages, history and economics, mathematics and physics, and
chemistry and biology. Every freshman had to take English, a
modern foreign language, a science, and a historical subject.
Other courses came later, according to the group and the individual student's option as approved by his advisers (this system
anticipated what was later called the "core curriculum"). My
memory as to my own original choice of a group is now, after
more than seventy years, somewhat confused. Having been well
grounded in Latin by Edward Lucas White, I thought at first to
enroll in Group 1, but the university catalogue for 1906, I find,
listed me in Group 2. At any rate my adviser was Kirby Flower
Smith, professor of Latin, who kindly approved my transfer to
Group 5 the next year, when I suddenly discovered that I was
born to be a biologist.

Constrained as the Johns Hopkins undergraduates were by
the studious atmosphere of a primarily graduate university,
they still felt the occasional need for fun. On one fine spring
morning by some sort of thought transference it occurred to a
lot of us all at once that the day was much too fair to be spent
indoors. So two dozen of us slipped out of college, took the

Howard Street trolley car to its terminus at Lake Roland, and set off on an all-day ramble over the countryside, merry as colts kicking up their heels in a pasture. Dean Griffin expressed his concern over our irregular conduct; contagious spring fever was simply not in his book.

We students whose pranks sometimes vexed the dean once saw him the victim of a presidential prank. Mr. Remsen (he was always so addressed) had occasion to talk to the undergraduates on some matters of college policy. Dean Griffin opened the meeting, yielded the rostrum to the president, and took a seat on the front row. During a somewhat tedious passage of the president's discourse, he began to doze, and the president saw him nodding. With a wicked gleam in his eye, Mr. Remsen stopped speaking for a moment and then said, "On this point I should like to hear the dean's opinion," to which Dr. Griffin, waking, could only stammer his vague assent.

Mr. Remsen, one of the great organic chemists of his time, was a man of the laboratory, not inured to academic ceremonial. At a commencement in my student days he was awarding degrees to the senior college class, forty strong. The graduates came on the stage in groups of five, standing before the president to receive their diplomas and hear him pronounce them bachelors of arts. When the eighth and last group came along, Remsen's mind wandered a bit; he declared them to be doctors of philosophy, "with all the honors, rights, and privileges to that degree appertaining." A titter from the audience alerted him to his slip. The five mistitled youths were leaving the platform. Turning in their direction, the president shouted, "Hold on, boys, I made a mistake. You're not doctors of philosophy, you're only bachelors of arts."

All freshmen had to take English 1, Rhetoric. To its teacher, John C. French, I owe thanks for careful if not brilliant instruction in English composition. Dr. French gave me good grades, especially after an upperclassman advised me to strike a pathetic note in my themes. The second year of English, devoted to literature, was taught by elderly Herbert Eveleth Greene. The boys made fun of his gentle ways and called him "Ma Greene," but he taught me to enjoy Chaucer, God bless him.

Except in English my grades were mediocre until I found my niche in biology. For my poor record in political economy I blame my lack of interest more than any fault of the professor, "Tubby" Barnett, who had a sense of humor and ample enthusiasm for his subject, but neither he nor the assigned textbook convinced me that there was anything interesting in economics. For an even worse performance in advanced algebra, I partly blame a sour, unhappy professor, who need not be named here. I had enjoyed geometry and algebra and had handled them well at the Boys' Latin School, but I really had no head for more subtle branches. Physics was also difficult for me, even though we had the honor of being lectured to by Joseph S. Ames, who was to become president of the university. He was impressive and likable. At one of his lecture-table demonstrations the apparatus refused to behave properly. Dr. Ames, who had a bad stutter, was flustered and exclaimed "all this experiment d-d-demonstrates, gentlemen, is the p-p-perversity of inanimate objects."

The end of the freshman year, in June 1904, found me suddenly without occupation. I had been working hard and was too tired to pick up at once the leisurely ways of summer vacation. Home was uninteresting, books were dull; the weather was hot, and the outdoors had no charm. In short, I was in the grip of a depression, the first of three that have overtaken me at widely spaced periods of my life. I moped about the house and wished that I were anywhere else. I talked of wanting to go to sea. My parents, more concerned, I think, than they let me know, dealt admirably with this crisis. They bought me a round-trip ticket to Boston on a ship of the Merchants and Miners line that then regularly ran between Baltimore and New England; they put some money in my purse, gave me as a precaution a letter of introduction to a business friend of my father's on Beacon Hill, and packed me off on the first long journey I had ever made alone. I was seasick on the three-day voyage and homesick at Boston, but I pulled myself together, went to the YMCA for advice about a lodging house, and settled down for a fortnight. I systematically visited the city's historic buildings, was impressed by the murals in the public library, rowed a boat on the pond in the public gardens, and took the trolley car to Lexington and Concord. When I presented my letter of introduction to father's friend he welcomed me like a long-lost nephew and took me to dinner at the Marblehead Yacht Club. Before my stay was over gloom had given way to cheerfulness. At home during the rest of the summer I found plenty of things to keep me contented until college reopened.

In my second (junior) year, I signed up for American history under Charles M. Andrews, who had distinguished himself at Johns Hopkins and was to continue a notable career at Yale. He taught us as if we were graduate students, by learned lectures accompanied by references for outside reading. Although I had an incipient liking for history and in later years have written much on the history of my profession, I was too immature to learn at the graduate student level and was relieved when I was permitted to drop the course.

Languages went better. Latin with W. P. Mustard was a delight; who could fail to enjoy Horace? I even translated one of his little poems, *Persicos odi, puer, apparatus,* for the college paper. German composition was taught by formidable Henry Wood. Although he was American-born, he was steeped in the German university culture, had married a baroness, and looked like a Hofgeheimrat. But he could unbend, as I discovered when I decorated the margin of an exercise in composition with a sketch of a railway train and a signpost marked "Zu Berlin." The paper came back duly corrected even to my signpost, which now read "Nach Berlin." French literature went well under the guidance of competent, good-natured Murray P. Brush, who impressed me as a man of affairs rather than an academic. (In fact he succeeded E. H. Griffin as dean and later became president of the Carnegie Institute of Technology at Pittsburgh.) I was admitted to a small special class in advanced French composition led by Brush's colleague Edward C. Armstrong, who paid us the compliment of trying out on us a textbook he was writing, on the French verb.

One idle day at Glencoe in the summer vacation of 1907 I found on Dr. Gorsuch's bookshelf an old volume of reports of the U.S. Department of Agriculture containing an article by the eminent bacteriologist Theobald Smith on his discovery that Texas cattle fever is transmitted by ticks. Fascinated by the story I decided then and there that I wanted to study biology. When college opened in the fall, with the consent of my adviser I transferred to curricular group 5, dropped Latin, and enrolled in Biology 1. Working at the microscope or listening to the clear lectures of Prof. Ethan Allen Andrews I felt, for the first time in my life, in easy command of what I was studying. This was where I belonged. The next year I took comparative anatomy under R. P. Cowles with equal satisfaction. In the six trimesters of biology I never made a grade lower than 95 percent. At my request Dr. Cowles kindly gave me and an equally enthusiastic classmate, Martillus Todd, informal instruction in sectioning and staining animal tissues for microscopical study.

During the senior year my interest in biology was reinforced by a brief look at another life science. Dean Griffin had for many years conducted a sort of finishing course, compulsory for all seniors, entitled Logic, Ethics, and Psychology. In 1909 he turned the spring trimester over to an extraordinary newcomer to the faculty. John Broadus Watson, who was already stirring up American psychologists with his behaviorist concepts, was not happy at having to take time from his research and his graduate students to teach lowly undergraduates, but he nevertheless gave a series of brilliant lectures based largely upon his own work on the behavior of animals and human infants. From several of the collegiate professors, men whose primary duty was to teach the undergraduates, I gained much —H. E. Greene, W. P. Mustard, W. J. A. Bliss (physics), and Edward Renouf (chemistry). But the university also wisely expected some of its foremost scholars and scientists to teach an undergraduate course.

Such outstanding men, whether or not they were good pedagogues, could not fail to inspire especially susceptible students. That is what J. B. Watson did for me. His enthusiasm and interest stimulated me greatly. Into a term paper I wrote for him I put a lot of hard thinking and some simple but original observations, and I was rewarded by a special message of commendation scribbled on the margin of my paper over the initials J.B.W.

So far I have said little about college friends. Because we undergraduates were mostly day students, we were thrown together less intimately than if we had been living in dormitories. Sam Chew, as I have said, was my closest friend. The son of a scholarly physician, he was deeply read in English literature and liked to let people know it. For this I am grateful; Sam taught me a lot, but some people thought him a bit precious.

Sam became chief editor of the *News-Letter*, the students'

fortnightly paper, and gave it a literary flavor by publishing his own poems or essays in almost every number. I was news editor under him and in our senior year succeeded him as chief editor when he tired of the job. Toward the end of the year I was too busy to carry on, and another of my 1909 friends, Hamilton Owens, took over. To get the copy together, edit it, and see it through the press later proved to have been useful practice for our life's work. Sam became professor of English at Bryn Mawr, Owens became the brilliant chief editor of the Baltimore *Sun* newspapers, and I have been editing scientific and scholarly journals during much of the past half-century and am still at it.

Another college friend who influenced me by the example of his scholarship, more lightly borne than Sam's, was Arthur Bloomfield, son of Maurice Bloomfield, the professor of Sanskrit. He was a year ahead of me at the Boys' Latin School, in college, and in medical school, and went on to be resident physician of the Johns Hopkins Hospital and finally professor of medicine at Stanford University.

During all my seven years in college and medical school Johns Hopkins held the national collegiate lacrosse championship. Almost every able-bodied undergraduate played the game. Too light, slow, and awkward for the varsity, I tried out for the class team and got to play in a couple of interclass games as a substitute defenseman. In my senior year, when the university was just beginning to develop the Homewood site, we played on the brand-new athletic field on University Parkway—the only time in the university's history when sports took precedence over scholarship.

In the spring of my senior year I was elected class poet and perpetrated for our graduation volume a merry encomium on the Class of Nought-nine that was just above the level of doggerel. I was, however, never to be more than an occasional poetaster. Not long after, on a fine hot June day, we seniors, thirty-seven strong, presented ourselves for graduation. Nine members of the class received their diplomas with honors, having won high grades in all courses taken. Five of these were elected to Phi Beta Kappa. I was not among them. An odd circumstance comes to mind, which I can mention now without offense. All these star students, so far as I recall, led useful lives and several of them, I know, were prominent in their communities, but not one of them was known widely enough to be listed in *Who's Who in America,* whereas three members of the class who were chief editors of the *News-Letter* made *Who's Who.* I can think of several possible explanations of this fact, not necessarily disparaging of the honors men, but the statistical sample is too small for useful conclusions.

Twice a year, on commemoration day and at commencement, all the university's members, young and old, joined in a pageant worthy of alma mater's worldwide fame. Whenever I recall my college days, the first picture memory brings back is that of the academic processions on such occasions, we undergraduates marshaled first into the hall, then the graduate students, the faculty, the distinguished guests, the trustees, the president, sometimes the governor of Maryland; often the archbishop of Baltimore, James Cardinal Gibbons, came to show the ancient respect of his church for academic learning. I hear the orchestra playing the triumphal march from *Aida.* I see the colorful robes of a hundred universities; I see myself, among the least in that great company, but one of the proudest to be there.

On the eve of my graduation in 1909, Professors Andrews and Cowles urged me to stay on for a Ph.D. in zoology and arranged for me to spend the summer at the U.S. Bureau of Fisheries laboratory at Beaufort, North Carolina. So it was that one afternoon in late June, with a suitcase in one hand, a microscope box in the other, and my camera slung around my neck, I boarded at Light Street wharf in Baltimore the southbound Chesapeake Line steamer *City of Norfolk.* That evening after dinner, as I sat on deck enjoying the cool breeze off the water, the stars in the clear night sky, and the lighthouses as we passed them one by one, I wondered how I should use the ten weeks before me; my teachers had left me completely on my own, with only meager suggestions for the summer's work.

Beaufort is a pleasant town on Bogue Sound, a southwestern extension of Pamlico Sound, the wide internal waterway protected from the ocean by a hundred miles of sandy barrier reef. Eighteen miles northeastward along the reef, Cape Hatteras faces the alternating calm and fury of the Atlantic. At the laboratory, a neat frame building on a small island just off Beaufort's waterfront, I was welcomed by the superintendent and assigned to a plainly furnished bedroom for which, with meals, I was to pay a moderate charge. The Johns Hopkins biology department, having cooperated scientifically for years with the U.S. Bureau of Fisheries, had the use of a work table in the big laboratory room, which I was now to have, together with an aquarium tank supplied with running seawater, the use of a rowboat whenever I needed it, and trips whenever I liked on the station's collecting boat, a small motor trawler of fifty or sixty tons' displacement.

Best of all, I was to have the daily companionship at work, at meals, and in hours of relaxation, of seven or eight experienced biologists, scientists and teachers who proved to be always willing to counsel a nineteen-year-old novice. The senior of these, Henry Van Peters Wilson, a veteran summer worker at the station, was professor of zoology at the University of North Carolina and a specialist on the structure and phylogeny of marine sponges. George H. Parker, professor of zoology at Harvard, was studying nerve transmission in invertebrate animals. E. P. Lyon, then at St. Louis University, later dean of the University of Minnesota's medical school, was at work on the respiration of sea-urchin eggs. A quiet, serious young Quaker professor at Earlham College in Indiana named Binford was making studies of the local stone crab for the Bureau of Fisheries. There were a couple of other biologists whom I have forgotten and a friendly student of about my age, from Professor Wilson's department, who was assisting the superintendent of the station in experimental hatching of sea turtles.

R. P. Cowles, whom I had asked for advice in planning my work at Beaufort, had suggested that I follow up a study he had published in his doctoral dissertation, of a large marine worm of uncertain affinities called *Phoronis*. I dug one out of the sandy bottom of the Sound, but on reflection I felt that such an undertaking would require more experience than I possessed. I looked through my microscope at some of the marine protozoa and the fascinating larvae of echinoderms and crabs to be found in any sample of Bogue Sound water and the beautiful eggs of the southern sea urchin *Toxopneustes*, so transparent that in recently fertilized ova I could see the sperm head approaching the egg nucleus and the formation of the first mitotic spindle with its chromosomes. These preliminary explorations of the vast panorama of aquatic life spread out before me suggested that the best use I could make of this precious opportunity was to give myself a systematic course in the comparative anatomy of marine invertebrates to supplement my college course in vertebrate anatomy.

Taking down from the laboratory bookshelf a textbook of invertebrate biology and checking the laboratory's list of locally available species, I made up a selection representative of each of the more important phyla, a protozoan, a flatworm, a roundworm, an annelid worm, a crustacean, a mollusc, an echinoderm. The warm waters of the harbor, the sound, and the ocean provided me with all the specimens I needed. Picking my animals out of the sand, from the wharf piles, or from the daily catch of the trawler, I examined the smallest specimens under the microscope, dissected the larger ones, photographed those that I could pose before my camera, and carefully sketched the others. At that time of year many of these creatures were spawning; I could observe their embryonic development as well as their adult structure. Books and journals were at hand for comparison of authentic descriptions with what I saw. Able consultants were also at hand; Wilson, Parker, Lyon, and Binford were always willing to advise me. Few universities could have provided better consultants.

The protozoan that I chose to study intensively was *Cothurnia,* a charming creature living in millions on the wharf piles and seaweeds and any other relatively firm underwater structure. The tiny pear-shaped single cell of an individual animal, too small to be seen without a microscope, lives in a transparent goblet-shaped "test" to the bottom of which it is attached by a short stem. The longer stem of the goblet is attached to whatever firm base the individual has settled upon. The cell body is capable of extending itself into a long trumpetlike form, so that its oral end can be protruded through the open end of the test to catch, with the aid of its beating cilia, whatever particles of nutrient material may drift by it. From time to time the cell divides into two; one of these daughter cells remains in the cup, while the other goes into contortions that change its shape into that of a slipper with cilia along the sole and finally breaks loose from the bottom of the cup. Its sister cell (or mother, whichever you choose to call it) accommodatingly draws down from the opening of the test, the free cell escapes into the outer world, swims away, and soon attaches itself to some firm surface, develops its own new test, and repeats the cycle of life. Sometimes, however, the stay-at-home cell blocks the way out and prevents its sister from leaving. Unable to escape, the free cell struggles wildly for a few hours and, when it has used up its stored energy suddenly swells into a ball and goes into pieces.

Watching this little drama (it may take, under the microscope, six or seven hours) I thus witnessed several times a rarely observed phenomenon, the death of a protozoan. Ordinarily these one-celled creatures do not terminate their lives by death but by division into daughter cells. This was my first piece of original research, unless we count the simple tests of personal imagery I made for J. B. Watson's term paper in the previous spring. When I returned to Baltimore in early fall of 1909 I wrote up my observations on *Cothurnia*, illustrated them with a page of pen-and-ink drawings, and offered them to Professor Andrews for publication in "Notes from the Biological Laboratory," which occasionally appeared as a number of the *Johns Hopkins University Circulars*. This three-page work heads the list of my 240 or more journal articles.

While at Beaufort I also made a modest beginning in experimental biology by repeating Jacques Loeb's experiments, published ten years before, in which he caused unfertilized sea-urchin eggs to undergo development by treating them with dilute solutions of inorganic salts. He used the ova of a northern genus, *Arbacia;* I had ova of *Toxopneustes* in plenty. The laboratory shelf provided magnesium chloride, which I carefully diluted with seawater to the exact concentration prescribed by Loeb. My experiments worked. I had the thrill of seeing the unfertilized eggs divide, and was able to keep them alive until the embryos began to metamorphose into the adult stage. Jacques Loeb, far more experienced than I in nursing the fatherless embryos, had succeeded in carrying them through metamorphosis.

We lived in almost monastic seclusion at the laboratory. Beaufort offered little in the way of diversion. The town, in fact, was rather oblivious of us. Some pious citizens, I believe, worried about the presence of a pack of evolutionists. To less sophisticated people our doings were obscurely mysterious. E. P. Lyon returned one day from a visit to shore and at lunch reported that someone had addressed him as "Dr. Gudger," the name of a Carolina ichthyologist who had often spent his summers at the station. Said Parker, "That's just the local term for a biologist; we are all gudgers here."

For me to row my boat on the sound or have a long summer evening's chat with my elder fellow scientists was entertainment enough. There was plenty of good conversation at the dinner table, and lighthearted banter. G. H. Parker was a notable wit and Lyon could be almost equally humorous. At lunch one day the subject was a floating cage that Parker had built to keep sea urchins alive for experimental use. Lyon said it wasn't sufficiently buoyant and wouldn't hold enough sea urchins. Parker, in mock indignation, said, "That float would hold everybody at this table!" "Bet you five dollars it won't," said Lyon. Parker took him up, and the showdown was set for that evening after dinner.

At the appointed hour the eight of us, having taken the precaution to appear in our bathing trunks, assembled at the station dock, where Parker had moored his float. One by one he ushered us aboard. Standing shoulder to shoulder we had barely room left for Parker himself. Jeering at Lyon because the craft was still afloat, he stepped aboard. The float promptly sank and dumped us all in the harbor to the accompaniment of Lyon's taunts.

I was sorry to leave Beaufort station at the end of this, to me, wonderful summer. An inexperienced youth, uncertain of my talents and capabilities, I had been admitted to the companionship of experienced men of science and had found the intellectual strength to study complex natural phenomena on my own initiative. Watching with fascination the life and death of a microscopic organism, I had begun a career of scientific research.

Back in Baltimore in September I was faced with what seemed to me a momentous decision, whether to enroll as a graduate student in zoology or to begin the study of medicine. I could be sure of a welcome from Andrews and Cowles, but Professor Jennings was the unknown quantity. I had never had a word from him; still, the distinguished man was known to have little interest in undergraduates. His leadership would be essential if I aimed at a Ph.D., but this was not fully guaranteed by the kindly encouragement of his colleagues. Moreover at Beaufort I had read some recent articles on protozoa as carriers of disease and had vaguely thought of a career in medical protozoology. My parents, I felt, would prefer me to study medicine, but forebore to counsel me directly.

The only family advice I received came from a cousin, Dr. William S. Baer, head of the orthopedic clinic at the Johns Hopkins Hospital. Instigated (as I must suppose) by my father, Billy Baer invited me to dinner at the University Club and in a long tête-à-tête conversation urgently recommended that I study medicine. "Not everyone can become a professor of biology," he said. "That takes brains; but anybody can make a living in the practice of medicine. Better get your M.D., and then, if you have the brains, you can try research. If not, you will have a profession to rely upon."

I believe (though with only our general family background to support the conjecture) that my parents had a deeper reason for their gentle concern about my choice of a profession than a wish for my practical welfare. In the minds of evangelical Christians distrust of Darwinism still lingered. My father's Wesleyan faith was deep and untroubled; my mother's was perhaps more reflective—she once said to me that she wished she knew more about evolution—but I think that both of them feared that a career in biology might lead me away from the altars of home and church.

Be that as it may, toward the end of September 1909 I went over to the Johns Hopkins Medical School and applied for admission. In those days there were no hordes of candidates to be screened months in advance; I was immediately accepted—my college grades in biology saw to that—and a few days later I joined my seventy new classmates in the study of human anatomy.

My decision, I now see, was not as momentous as I thought in 1909. My temperament and my talents, such as they were, would inevitably have made me a scientist and professor, whichever discipline I chose to follow, but I am glad that I chose medicine.

MEDICAL
STUDENT

3

THE PRECLINICAL YEARS

The medical school of the Johns Hopkins University, when I entered it in October 1909, was foremost in the United States. Other schools, notably Harvard, the University of Michigan, and the University of Chicago had eminent faculties and good students, but only Johns Hopkins possessed the full complement of a distinguished senior faculty; a strong array of associate and assistant professors; students all of whom were fully college-trained; a first-class hospital under its own control; ample laboratories and libraries. A critical historian, Donald Fleming, has said, "The Johns Hopkins Medical School had made out as early as 1900 some claims to be the best system of medical education in the world." Years later when I was informally advising the premedical students at the University of Rochester, I gave them my formula for rating a medical school: multiply the distinction of the faculty by the quality of the students and divide by the number of students. Cunningly devised to give the then small Rochester school a high standing, my formula would nevertheless have awarded first place in 1909 to the Johns Hopkins Medical School with its seventy or eighty students to a class.

Certainly the department of anatomy, in whose dissecting rooms and laboratories of histology and neurology I was to spend my first two trimesters, had a distinguished staff whose teaching and example, though I did not know it at the time, were to determine my career for the next half-century. I think it was the strongest anatomical department in the English-speaking world. Its chief, Franklin Paine Mall, then forty-seven years of age, had reoriented the teaching of anatomy in America by combining in one discipline gross and microscopic anatomy, anatomical neurology, cytology, and embryology. Warren H. Lewis had charge of the dissecting rooms, assisted by Eliot R. Clark. Florence R. Sabin and Herbert M. Evans taught histology and neurology. Four of these five professors and instructors, all M.D.'s, were, or would some day be, members of the National Academy of Sciences. Four of them and two students working in the laboratory that year, Lewis Weed and I, would be presidents of the American Association of Anatomists.

Franklin Mall was a quiet, diffident man looking younger than his age and physically unimpressive. The students' nickname for him was a diminutive, "Johnny" Mall, but his shyness and reserve concealed a searching mind. He had radical ideas about teaching. Unlike all other professors of the subject since Galen, he thought that systematic lectures on gross human anatomy were unnecessary. We were to learn by dissection and by informal discussion with our teachers. We might use a textbook, choosing one from among the four or five then put out by various publishers, but we were never assigned passages to study. How we used the textbook was our own affair. The medical students invented a story that when Mall's first child was born, his wife asked him how to bathe the baby. "Just put her in the tub," he said, "and let her work out her own technique."

Dr. Mall occasionally visited the dissecting rooms where we worked every morning, and he made a round of the two histology laboratories almost every afternoon when the histology class was in session. Sometimes he merely looked over our shoulders and said nothing. Now and then he answered a question directly and clearly; more often he made a remark obscurely related to the work in hand. Watching a student painstakingly tracing the course of a long nerve, *N. peronealis*, for example, he might suddenly ask, "Where does the Monument Street trolley car go after it passes our building?" This sort of pedagogy he explained to me four years later, when I was a teaching assistant in his department; he wanted the student, as he freed the nerve from surrounding tissues, to think where it began in the spinal cord, where it would end in the foot, and what kind of impulses it carried.

Some of the students, accustomed to didactic college teaching, did not appreciate such cryptic pedagogy nor the freedom Mall gave them to learn by doing rather than by listening to lectures or memorizing a textbook. One of these in an earlier class, Bertram Bernheim, was so deeply disappointed by what he considered neglect by Mall and his staff that he illicitly obtained part of a cadaver from the anatomy laboratory, took it in the summer vacation to his home on a Kentucky horse farm, and repeated the dissection. In 1948, when he had become a widely known surgeon, he published a book about his education at Johns Hopkins, in which he sharply criticized Mall's method of teaching anatomy. In a review of the book, I pointed out that he had done just what Mall wanted us to do, learn for ourselves, and thus he owed to Mall the intellectual independence that had made him a pioneer in the new field of blood-vessel surgery.

I have spoken of "dissecting rooms" in the plural. At Johns Hopkins, thanks to another of Mall's innovations, the study of gross human anatomy by dissection was conducted, not as in most other schools, in a large, often noisy, and sometimes unkempt dissecting hall, but in a series of small, quiet, impeccably clean laboratory rooms. One day during the year I spent as teaching assistant in Mall's department after taking my M.D., I found myself alone with him in a small laboratory room where the staff met for lunch. He had just come from morning rounds in the dissecting rooms and was at the sink, washing his hands clean of the carbolic smell of the cadavers whose tissues he had been handling. Mall suddenly said, "I'd hate to be an archaeologist; it's such dirty work." I hadn't the slightest idea what he meant, but the remark stuck in my mind, and twenty years later, when I read Florence Sabin's biography of Mall, I understood at last. "You must know, my young friend," he was thinking to himself, "that the teaching of anatomy used to be dirty work, done in large noisy halls, with little respect for the dead, on decaying cadavers, for purely practical ends. But you are privileged to do your teaching in these small, quiet, clean laboratory rooms that I designed. You work in an atmosphere of scientific inquiry. For you and your students, anatomy is clean work. Your teachers have made it so." He did not think it necessary to tell me this in so many words; he expected me to feel it.

Each of the dissecting rooms accommodated eight to twelve

students, four to a table. Warren Lewis, Eliot Clark, Charles Essick, and an assistant each presided over two rooms, exchanging their sections each half-trimester, so that each section was taught in turn by one of the four. I began with the enthusiastic but somewhat finicky Eliot Clark, who insisted on perfect dissections, scorning a cut nerve or ragged muscle.

Warren Lewis, on his daily visits to the dissecting rooms, was a formidable quizzer, insistent on accurate detail. At the time, I believe, he was unhappy over the breakup of his first marriage. He was frightening; when he stepped into our room the chatter of young people at work gave way to silence as we waited to hear who would get the first question. On one such occasion one of the students was so startled by Lewis's sudden appearance that he flung his right hand, holding a scalpel, across his left wrist, cut a superficial vein, fainted and, when he regained his wits, found Dr. Lewis carefully bandaging the wound. If this picture of our professor of gross anatomy in 1909 misrepresents him, I have made up for it in the affectionate obituary article I published in *Biographical Memoirs* of the National Academy of Sciences (1967), in which I tell of his notable career and that of his second wife, Margaret Reed Lewis, herself a very productive scientist.

Florence Sabin, then thirty-eight years old, was a friendly, plainly dressed woman whose face was lighted by the glow of intelligence and humanity. Her concern for her pupils prevented her from leaving us to study for ourselves as much as Mall and Lewis did. She lectured weekly on histology and neurology, interpretatively rather than didactically, highlighting recent research. She told me later, when I became her teaching assistant, that she discarded her notes after each lecture, to force herself to keep her facts up to date. I felt at home in her well-organized laboratory course in microscopic anatomy and enjoyed it more than any formal study I had ever undertaken. Thanks to my summer at Beaufort, I had more experience with the microscope than most of my classmates. To fully appreciate the marvelous structure of the body's tissues one needs not only the optical instrument but also eyes trained to perceive what the lenses bring to sight.

My growing interest in anatomy led me, late in the first year of medical studies, to ask Dr. Sabin to preside over an informal "journal club" of like-minded students interested in keeping up with current publications in anatomy and related fields. She kindly agreed and met us weekly to hear one of us report on some recent article, after which she would lead the discussion of the work. She was the very pattern of a stable and self-controlled scientist. Her research demanded great manual dexterity. It was amusing, therefore, to hear her tell a story of extreme absent-mindedness on her part. A member of the journal club reported on a French study of abnormal behavior resulting from local damage to the brain. One patient, a chef, had done various absurd things with his pots and pans. Dr. Sabin, opening the discussion, said with a smile that she hoped she was not developing a similar case of apraxia; that very morning, cooking an egg for breakfast while thinking of a research problem, she had forgotten the frying pan and dropped the egg directly into the gas burner.

Eliot Clark I remember as an attentive teacher, overintent on detail, less inspiring than Sabin, more direct than Mall. He became professor of anatomy at the University of Georgia, later at the University of Pennsylvania. About Herbert Evans, most vivid of these five eminent anatomists, I shall have much to say in subsequent chapters, for I was to join him at Berkeley six years later.

I was the youngest member but two of our class of seventy-odd men and women, high-standing graduates of colleges all over the nation, of such quality that any one of us might wonder how he could hold his place in competition with men from Yale who had studied biochemistry under Russell Chittenden, the Princetonians who had been pupils of the inspiring zoologist Edwin G. Conklin, or such a fellow student as John Morton, trained as a naturalist at Amherst and Woods Hole; or those whose personal heritage presaged high talents—Frederick L. Gates, son of John D. Rockefeller's principal philanthropic adviser; Francis Trudeau, whose father was the famous specialist on tuberculosis; Aristine Pixley Munn, daughter of a wealthy insurance magnate; or Gilbert Horrax and Edgar Erskine Hume, whose polished manners and social charm promised smooth careers; or scions of southern gentry like the Kentuckian Henry Cave or Linton Gerdine from Athens, Georgia. Among these outstanding people there were four in particular, of widely different backgrounds, with whom I found special compatibility that led to strong friendships—Fred Gates; Daniel Davis, son and grandson of distinguished admirals; Edgar Hume, youngest member of the class; and Grover Francis Powers. These friends were welcome guests at my home in Roland Park, and all won my family's high regard. From each of them I learned much in various ways. Edgar Hume took me to my first opera when after my twenty-first birthday I felt free to disregard the Methodist ban on theatergoing. Daniel Davis and I took a walking tour together in the Virginia mountains in the spring of 1910. I long cherished Fred Gates's friendship and mourned his death in mid-career.

Grover Powers became the closest friend of my lifetime. I shall have much to record of our daily association in medical studies, our two long summer journeys together, a break in our friendship that still puzzles me, the happy resumption of brotherly regard in later years, and his devoted career as professor of pediatrics at Yale. Grover was two years older than I and more mature. He came from West Lafayette, Indiana, and had attended college at nearby Purdue University. His elderly parents were members of a small sect called Advent Baptists. He had therefore been brought up, like me (though in a narrower environment), under the social restraints of evangelical puritanism. Like me also, but with greater internal stress, he was growing away from the intense faith and strict rules of his family's religion. The strain of this transition, I think, accounted in part for an air of quiet melancholy that he sometimes wore. He loved his parents and respected mine.

My father was, as I have mentioned, superintendent of the Sunday school at Broadway Methodist Church, a few blocks from the Johns Hopkins Hospital. For some years he had managed to recruit as teachers some of the medical students with Methodist backgrounds who from a sense of duty were willing to devote their Sunday afternoons to expounding the Bible story and Christian morals to East Baltimore boys. Among those who had helped in this way, before my time, were Guy Hunner, a leading Baltimore gynecologist; Benjamin T. Terry, future editor of the *Journal of Experimental Medicine*, and Charles Bunting, professor of pathology at the University of Wisconsin—quite a strong Sunday school faculty! Filial affection drew me into this service, which I could still perform without a sense of hypocrisy, and Grover accepted my father's invitation to join us.

On the first Sunday that he took a class, I pointed him out to my fourteen-year-olds, mentioning that he came from the West. "Oh," said one lad, "is he a cowboy?"—a query all the more ridiculous because Grover at twenty-two was the gentlest, most sensitive man I have ever known, of almost feminine refinement. He was a bit overweight, slightly balding, slow of gait, totally unathletic. But in our student days and travels together he was a friend and brother, an intellectual companion, a generous sharer of pleasures and hardships alike.

There were seven or eight women in the class. This was my first intimate experience with the other sex as fellow students. I was, I think, a little scared of these capable, serious women in their mid-twenties, a couple of them near thirty, who were bent only on a professional career; they wanted no masculine gallantry nor even social deference. One of them, however—handsome, rosy-cheeked, friendly Dorothy Clark—could not avoid admiring glances and was popular with all the men. One of our classmates, in fact, was conspicuously smitten by her charms throughout the four years of medical school. He was heartbroken, and the rest of us were jealous, when Dorothy got engaged to a resident psychiatrist who was not even a Johns Hopkins man. After I went to California in 1915 I never chanced to meet any of these feminine classmates again and lost track of them all, except that I have heard that sensible, sturdy Augusta Scott became a competent psychiatrist in New York and hardheaded Pearlie Mae Stetler, whose parents when they named her must have expected her to grow up a sweet young thing, acquired a busy practice as a general surgeon in Chicago.

In a large room next to Professor Mall's office and communicating with it, places were set aside at a bench under the windows for a few students and occasional guests of the department who were carrying on original research. I remember seeing at work there Walter Dandy, the future neurological surgeon, and Lewis Weed, destined to inherit Mall's chair. The example of these older students led me, toward the end of the second semester, in the early spring of 1910, to knock at the professor's door and ask for the privilege of undertaking research under his guidance. If he accepted me I expected Dr. Mall to assign me a problem, some bit perhaps of his own research program, but the first question he asked me was what I proposed to investigate. I had not thought about that; I simply wanted to work with him.

I asked for a few days to prepare a project and began a systematic search for some topic that might impress him favorably. I knew that for several years he had been developing the idea that compound organs are composed of structural units— small models, so to speak, of the whole organ, each with its own blood supply and drainage, repeated many times to make up the organ. He had developed this concept by a masterly monograph on the liver, published in 1906, and another on the spleen. One of his students had similarly analyzed a salivary gland; the nephron (glomerulus and tubule of the kidney) is obviously such a unit. Nobody, I found, had as yet looked at the pancreas in the light of Mall's ideas, so I told him that I wanted to look for a structural unit of that organ. This argumentum ad hominem was effective. I was accepted, providing that Warren Lewis would certify that I knew enough gross anatomy to be exempted from a customary second-year review course, to allow me time in addition to the two free afternoons a week set aside as encouragement to students to choose elective work. I passed Lewis's easy informal quiz and was given the run of the students' research laboratory.

My project called for following the duct system of the pancreas in embryos and fetuses by injecting the main duct with an opaque fluid (India ink) and then making the gland tissues transparent by a well-known process that I need not describe here. Pig embryos were readily available at Hohman's slaughterhouse, three blocks from the medical school. Herbert Evans, an expert at fine injections, taught me how to make the glass cannulas, with tips one-hundredth of an inch in diameter, through which I was to inject the ink under a dissecting microscope. This project was not to be completed in a few months. I worked at it whenever I could find time, throughout my four years of medical school, until I had assembled a full series of injected embryonic and fetal specimens and established a structural unit. I do not recall that Dr. Mall ever gave me direct guidance, although he followed my progress and was encouraging. As I began to write up my findings, he called for successive drafts, pointing out needed additions or revisions. When he declared the seventh draft acceptable, he assigned a professional illustrator to prepare figures from my specimens and sketches. In December 1913, six months after I received my medical degree, I presented a brief account of my findings and demonstrated my best specimens at a meeting of the American Association of Anatomists held in Philadelphia and was gratified by favorable comments from several experienced anatomists, including Prof. George H. Piersol of the University of Pennsylvania. My complete article, "The Structural Unit and Growth of the Pancreas of the Pig," appeared in the *American Journal of Anatomy* for May 1914.

The third trimester of the first year was devoted to physiology and physiological chemistry (nowadays called biochemistry). William Henry Howell, professor of physiology and dean of the medical school, was Mall's opposite as a teacher. In appearance a dignified, thoughtful academic, as Cecilia Beaux painted him in a brilliant portrait now at the school, Howell was direct in discourse and in action. He gave us a long course of systematic lectures spoken without notes in English so perfect that they could have been taken down and used for printer's copy. The lectures were, in fact, abstracts of Howell's textbook, then in use in many American medical schools. In the class laboratory Howell was assisted by Donald R. Hooker and Charles D. Snyder, both kindly teachers and good scientists but sadly dull lecturers. In the laboratory we worked on assigned experiments as carefully planned for us as were the professor's lectures. Howell was actively engaged in research, chiefly on the clotting of blood; Hooker had pioneered in the clinical measurement of blood pressure; Snyder was investigating the physiology of muscle; but for me the course lacked the thrill that anatomical studies had given me.

Walter Jones, who led the teaching of biochemistry, had neither Mall's subtlety nor Howell's polish. Lean and dour, with features now scowling, now derisive or humorous, he prowled about the laboratory looking at our steaming flasks and bubbling retorts, loudly commending the more skillful students and bawling out those he thought clumsy or stupid. His vividly personal lectures made biochemistry seem a battle of wits between the scientist and the contents of his flasks.

One of these discourses, repeated annually, was so notorious in the school that upperclassmen used to return to hear it again, filling the back of the hall and waiting for the cues for noisy applause at the climactic moments. I believe that Jones himself looked forward to this annual occasion. In his lecture he dealt with the purine bases, a fighting topic for him because some of his own research in that field had been sharply contradicted by an equally intense German chemist. When in our year Jones reached the purine bases, the audience again overflowed the lecture room. Jones waited outside until we all were seated and silent, then came in dramatically at the front, strode to the blackboard, seized a piece of chalk, and without a word wrote in large letters the name of his opponent, Alfred Schittenhelm, then turned to the audience and snarled, "The gentleman whose name I have written here—I cannot bring myself to pronounce it—has erroneously declared . . ." and was off on a fascinating fifty-minute polemic on the molecular structure of adenine, guanidine, theobromine, and caffeine. After the final burst of applause, he smiled sardonically and left the hall.

I enjoyed Jones's dramatics but was not a very apt pupil. Because of my late decision to study medicine, I had not studied organic chemistry in college and therefore had to wrestle with the more complex organic compounds without much knowledge of the simpler ones. But I must have scraped through the final examination.

One of the great strengths of the Johns Hopkins Medical School has always been a pervading interest in the history and literature of our profession. The Medical History Club at Johns Hopkins is, I believe, the oldest medicohistorical society now active in the United States. It met, in my day, in the medical amphitheater, where at almost every meeting the great man of the school, Dr. William H. Welch, and a group of senior professors sat in the front seats. I began to attend its sessions at once, and missed hardly a meeting in the six years 1909–1915 and again when I was back in Baltimore, 1919–1923. Another stimulus to my latent interest in the history of medicine was a collection of medical classics in the school's library, then in the physiology building. These books, once at the Warrington Dispensary in Lancashire, England, were installed in a locked bookcase just inside the library door, where they were visible to all comers through the glass doors. Among the fine old volumes bound in leather or parchment were good early editions of Harvey on the circulation of the blood, the *Fabrica corporis humani* of Vesalius, and the Giunta edition of Galen. In my leisure hours—few they were—I used to get the key from the librarian and leaf over the pages of these records of the earlier days of our profession. Many of the Warrington books of course were in Latin. Though I was not fluent in that language I could read it well enough to get the flavor of their contents. When I had gotten well into my research on the pancreas, I wanted to learn about the men who in past centuries had laid the foundations of our current knowledge of that organ—Regner de Graaf, who in 1664 first noticed the pancreatic secretion; Wirsüng and Santorini, who first described the pancreatic ducts, whose embryonic development I was now tracing; Langerhans, the medical student who discovered the pancreatic islets in 1869.

De Graaf's *De succo pancreatico* led me to his teacher at Delft, Isbrand van Diemerbroeck, whose magnum opus, a textbook of anatomy, is among the Warrington Dispensary books, in an English translation of 1689 by William Salmon—the most amusing book on human anatomy I have ever looked into, full of facts, gossip, philosophy, and pseudophilosophy, even a chapter on the location of the soul in the body. Diemerbroeck's *Anatomy* led me to his *De peste* (1646), a book on bubonic plague narrating his own experience during heroic service in an epidemic in Holland. Among the remedies he listed was the ancient and honored cure-all theriac (Venice treacle), made up of as many as 150 ingredients. Theriac and mithridatium had a long and fascinating history. Chaucer, for example, mentions theriac in the *Canterbury Tales,* when the host of the Tabard Inn cries: "By corpus bones, but I have triacle. . . . myn herte is lost for pity of this mayde." Fascinated by this masterpiece of therapeutic credulity, I began to collect references to it in earlier medical literature, a task facilitated by that marvelous work, the *Index Catalogue of the Library of the U.S. Surgeon-General's Office.* By the time I was graduated from medical school I was ready to complete an essay, "Mithridatium and Theriac, the Most Famous Remedies of old Medicine," which I presented while an intern, at a meeting of the Johns Hopkins Medical History Club on January 11, 1915.

The end of my first year in medical school left me in a happy mood, more confident of myself than ever before and sure that I was on the right track, although I could not see as yet whither it would lead me. In that summer of 1910, my parents went to Europe for six weeks, leaving my brother and sister and me to visit with various relatives. I stayed with a young married couple, cousins of mine, John Baer and his wife, who lived near us in Roland Park. In need of rest after that exciting year, I enjoyed an idle vacation—occasional tennis with my brother, quiet walks in the country, a day at the Baltimore County Fair at Timonium, where my kinsman Dr. Dickinson Gorsuch was showing his prize-winning Ayrshire cattle. The Baers had a good library, and I devoured, among other books, their complete set of Rudyard Kipling's novels and short stories. This and an equally large set of works by the polymath John Fiske kept me in reading matter for the six weeks' stay.

In the first year of medical school we had studied the fundamentals of normal human structure and function—anatomy, gross and microscopic, physiology and biochemistry. In the second year we turned to the study of diseases as seen by the pathologist and the bacteriologist, and to the curative agents of the pharmacologist. Dr. William H. Welch, the professor of pathology, was sixty years of age in 1910, with white hair, a trim pointed white beard, kindly features and the rather prominent abdomen of a connoisseur of good Maryland food. His combination of personal dignity with easy courtesy to students had won for him the affectionate nickname of "Popsy." The first time I ever talked with him revealed this affability and also gave me a hint of his prodigious memory. He knew by name practically every member of the faculty and every student he had taught. I was waiting for a streetcar across from the pathology building, my seven-pound textbook of anatomy under my arm, when Dr. Welch joined me with a friendly nod and said, "Your book tells me that you are one of our students, but since I didn't recognize you, you must be a first-year man." "Yes," I said, "I'm George Corner." This placed me for him; he had known my grandfather of the same name, who was one of the founding trustees of the Johns Hopkins Hospital. From that meeting through the rest of his life Popsy never failed to recognize me at sight.

In 1910 Dr. Welch had already attained the distinction later awarded him by President Herbert Hoover, who called him "our greatest statesman in the field of public health"—and the president might well have added, "in medical education." In the year when he taught my class he was elected president of the American Medical Association; since the foundation of the Rockefeller Institute for Medical Research (now Rockefeller University) in 1901 he had been chairman of its board of scientific advisers; in 1906 he was president of the American Association for the Advancement of Science; and in 1913 he was to become president of the National Academy of Sciences. These important posts and endless demands for his advice had left him no time for research and were beginning to limit his teaching. He met our class once a week, with occasional absences when one of his staff had to take over, sometimes on short notice. His lectures were quite informal; it is reliably reported that he seldom prepared them in advance and sometimes had to be reminded before class what his topic was for that day. He sat at ease in a chair at the front of the classroom and spoke impromptu in clear, polished English. Whatever the topic, be it inflammation or arteriosclerosis, cholera or pneumonia, he stated the relevant facts, never failing to include something about the history of the subject, perhaps an allusion to Hippocrates or Galen or an insight he had gained in his postgraduate days in Germany, from Carl Ludwig or Robert Koch—making the windows of his classroom seem to open not upon the drab roofs of East Baltimore but upon the world of scientific medicine.

During our attendance at Dr. Welch's course of lectures in the fall of 1910, when airplanes were still a novelty, an aviation meet was held at Halethorpe, a southwestern suburb of Baltimore. Among the pilots who took part was the young Frenchman Hubert Latham, who had won a reputation for daring by several flights over European cities. A wealthy Baltimorean confined by chronic illness to his bedroom in his St. Paul Street residence offered Latham a bonus of one thousand dollars if he would fly over Baltimore so that the invalid could see him. Latham agreed and planned to fly a wide loop over south and east Baltimore up to Mt. Royal Avenue and Charles Street, then southwestward, in sight of his sponsor's house, and back to Halethorpe. This route would take him over the Johns Hopkins Hospital—great news for the medical students. Unfortunately my class was scheduled to attend, at the exact hour of Latham's flight, Dr. Welch's weekly lecture. Such was our respect for Popsy and his superb lectures that all seventy of us gave up seeing Latham and went to class in the pathology building.

Latham flew precisely on schedule. In the middle of Dr. Welch's discourse we heard the distant rumble of the airplane's engine, growing to a roar as it passed almost overhead. We heard shouting in the streets, and then the noise faded as the plane went on to the north and west. We had heard, but not seen, the first flight of an airplane over Baltimore. Next week at the same hour Popsy began his lecture with a complaint against us all. "I wanted to see that airplane. Why didn't you tell me? That was a historic event, and you all sat there listening to me!"

Unlike Franklin Mall, Dr. Welch did not teach in the student laboratory where we studied sections of diseased tissues under the microscope. He left the teaching there to a junior staff of four or five men, of whom the principals were George H. Whipple, resident pathologist of the hospital, and Milton C. Winternitz, assistant resident pathologist. Whipple was then thirty-two years of age. If I had known that I was to be closely associated with him in the latter part of his distinguished career and was to be his biographer, I would have studied him more closely in 1910–1911. All I knew of him then was the quiet courtesy, concise speech, and professional assurance with which he explained things that puzzled me as I looked through my microscope.

Winternitz was Whipple's opposite. Only twenty-five years of age (he had taken his M.D. at twenty-three, as I was to do) he bubbled with enthusiasm, talked long and loudly, and enjoyed bantering with the students. One day when four or five of us were sitting around a table intently studying a tray full of viscera from a recent autopsy, Winter came up behind me and said, "Study hard, boy, study until your head aches!" To which some devil made me reply—the first and only time I ever tried to insult a superior—"Hard study may give you a headache, Doctor Winternitz, but I can take it." "That's the way to talk," said he, giving me a genial slap on the back, and grinning, he went on to the next table.

When Dr. Welch was out of town on his lecture day, one of these two instructors had to give the lecture. George Whipple told me years later that he and Winter divided the session's topics between them, and each prepared himself in advance to substitute for the chief. They did very well. I recall Whipple's thoughtful, well-organized talks and Winter's sparkling chats; but Whipple said that when Dr. Welch did appear, the two of them sat in the back row and heard Popsy do with elegant spontaneity what one or the other of them had laboriously prepared himself to do. This was a great trio that we students were privileged to hear. Whipple went on to be dean of the University of California's school of medicine, then was called to organize the new medical school at Rochester, New York. He shared the Nobel Prize in 1934 for his researches that led to a curative treatment for pernicious anemia. Winternitz became dean of Yale Medical School and led it brilliantly toward its present distinction.

There is an excellent photograph of the three of them sitting side by side, which I used in my book *George Hoyt Whipple and His Friends*. Seen thus together, they typify for me three aspects of medical science—Welch, bearded and portly, standing for the hieratic tradition in medicine, its long history, its Hippocratic image of the father-physician, its intellectual dignity; Winternitz representing the ever-youthful curiosity of science, its prying search, its excitement in discovery; Whipple, the steady, solid accumulation of observed facts and the deductions and analysis by which they are put to use.

The instruction in pathology was followed by a course in bacteriology led, under Welch's remote supervision, by W. W. Ford, a pleasant man who had done some good work on mushroom poisons. The course did not greatly interest me, because, as I now perceive, the great era of major discovery in bacteriology was over and the study of viruses had not yet begun to revitalize the field of microbiology. It puzzles me now to recall that another related field, that of immunology, was scarcely given a place in either Welch's or Ford's teaching, although Welch was certainly familiar with it, as with everything done by pathologists in the remote and recent past. I suppose the explanation is that immune reactions were as yet largely empirical phenomena, for example, the production of diphtheria antitoxin, not yet theoretically explainable and therefore hardly teachable. The old side-chain hypothesis, which Dr. Welch barely mentioned to us, was inadequate. Within a few years the development of a chemical theory of immunity was well under way, led by Karl Landsteiner at the Rockefeller Institute.

The course in pharmacology in the spring of 1911 was taught by John J. Abel, who a few years before had achieved the isolation and chemical characterization of adrenalin. Dr. Abel made pharmacology a fascinating as well as a useful subject. He was fifty-three years of age but seemed older. In his informal, rambling lectures he brought us close to the great pioneer days of modern physiology and pharmacology in Germany, where he had studied seven years with Ludwig and Schmiedeberg. Tall, slender, with scanty iron-gray hair and a goatee, he came to the student laboratory at every session, sharing with an assistant or two our guidance in a well-planned series of experiments on drug action. In one experiment that I remember vividly, we practiced the treatment of acute morphine poisoning. We first overdosed our rabbit, then saved him from death—"Don't let him rest, keep him moving, and fill him up with caffeine." A year later, in Labrador, Grover Powers and I put the lesson into practice.

We loved John Abel's combination of absent-minded discourse with great scientific knowledge. At the time he was working on a heart-regulating substance extracted from the poison glands of a tropical toad. A member of our class, Daniel Davis, found in a bookseller's catalogue the offer of a good copy of William Withering's classical work of 1785 on his discovery of the potency of the foxglove plant, *Digitalis purpurea,* in relieving cardiac dropsy. The bookseller's price of fifteen dollars was too large for Davis, but he collected twenty-five cents from each of his classmates, and we presented the book to Dr. Abel at the last session of the course, to his great delight. Years later, at Rochester, I bought another copy of *Account of the Foxglove* for the school library. The price had risen to $150. I suppose that if Dr. Abel's copy should come on the market now, it might bring $1,500.

Up to World War I a tradition lingered on from the days when Mall, Welch, and Abel were young men, that a trip to Germany was part of the education of ambitious young American medical men and students. My father had heard me speak of this, and toward the end of the school year in the spring of 1911 he generously offered to finance for me a summer at a

German university center. I opted for Freiburg-im-Breisgau, in southern Germany, where several of my younger teachers had recently worked, and proposed to Grover Powers that he join me. Shortly after classes ended we sailed from Baltimore on the North German Lloyd ship *Main.* Landing at Bremen after a smooth eleven-day crossing, we spent a day visiting Bremen Cathedral and other sights, then traveled by train to Cologne and a day later took the Rhine steamboat to Mainz. We lingered a couple of days at Heidelberg, where we saw a "Feierabend" with illumination of the castle, and then went on to Freiburg by train.

Freiburg was (and I hope still is, after being bombed in two world wars) a handsome little city set against dark green hills where the river Dreisam comes tumbling out of the high Black Forest onto the valley of the Rhine. It has a noble cathedral and a charming park, many old houses, a tall gate tower surviving from the medieval town's defenses. We looked at once for lodging and first interviewed a genial landlady who had a couple of pink-cheeked daughters about eighteen and twenty years old, very curious about us two American students. The rooms were pleasant. I thought it a great opportunity to improve our conversational German, but Grover was adamantly opposed to the eager landlady and her nubile daughters. We finally settled at the obviously safe Pension Villa Hoven on Wimpfelingstrasse, where the other roomers were university students, some of them Russians, a polite but not charming lot, rather boisterous at table. I do not like people who at mealtime compare the food to pathological tissues. One of the medical students created a big laugh when a dubious-looking pudding was brought in, by exclaiming, "Aha, ein Carcinom!"

At the university offices we obtained for a few marks *Hörerkarten* enabling us to attend lectures and demonstrations. We also found notices of a vacation course in German for foreigners, to begin in mid-July after the university courses ended, and we both signed up for that. Early in our stay we met a friendly Englishman named Kettle, a London medical graduate who had been spending a year in the laboratory of Ludwig Aschoff, Freiburg's celebrated professor of pathology. He took us to call on Aschoff, who politely welcomed us to his lectures. A man evidently of intense energy, he had a military haircut and two deep scars from one corner of his mouth to the ear, relics of his student days in one of the aristocratic fraternities *(Korps)* that maintained the custom of dueling with swords.

Aschoff was a lecturer of declamatory vigor, very positive and emphatic. At a session we attended, he demonstrated the long bones of a man who had died of a degenerative bone disease, emphasizing every point of his discourse by driving his autopsy knife into the softened bones until he almost cut them to shreds. We attended also some operations by the professor of surgery, Kraske, and medical lectures by De la Camp, professor of medicine. Sitting in De la Camp's lecture room one hot morning, after an overheavy dinner the night before, I suddenly felt dizzy, put my head down, and awoke to find myself on a wheeled stretcher in the corridor outside the amphitheater, attended by the head nurse of the medical clinic and De la Camp's chief of staff, who was holding my legs in the air. Somebody told me later that when the professor learned what had happened, he told the audience that he had tried in vain to persuade the Ministry of Education to improve the ventilation of the amphitheater, "and now that young American faints in the bad air." Grover took me home in a cab to the pension, where I stayed in bed for a day, attended by a kind local doctor who called me *Herr Kollege* and would not accept a fee.

One day De la Camp demonstrated a case of typhoid fever, a great rarity in Germany because of superior public hygiene but no novelty to us, for in Baltimore we had seen several autopsies on people dead of typhoid. Every July the Johns Hopkins Hospital cleared two wards to receive the summer inflow of typhoid patients, and the surgical service was on alert for emergency operations on perforated intestines. We second-year students could have given De la Camp pointers on the pathology of typhoid fever.

By pinning up a notice in the university registration office, Grover and I each found a student to take walks with us every few days, conversing in German one day and English the next. Grover's companion was the son of an elderly pharmacist who joined us now and then for a stroll in the Stadtgarten. One afternoon he gave me a long story of his hatred for the Prussians, who had conquered Baden in the wars of 1849 and 1866.

South Germans being very friendly people, we easily made

acquaintances. They were surprised by our teetotalism but put it down to American eccentricity. The summer course for foreigners was excellently taught by junior university professors and teachers from secondary schools. Two of the latter, whose names I forget, invited us to join them on a weekend walking tour in the Vosges Mountains, across the Rhine valley from Freiburg. The goal of our tour was the grand restored castle Hoh-Königsburg in southern Alsace, where there were several hundred Sunday visitors in the castle grounds merrily drinking beer served by black-robed nuns from a nearby convent.

Our companions were very agreeable, and we alternated conversation in German and English, greatly to the benefit of Grover and me and, I hope, also of our companions, whose English was better than our German. But our language has its pitfalls. In a crowded restaurant at the end of luncheon on the second day out, one of the teachers rose suddenly, as if to leave the table, and in response to my inquiring glance showed me his purse to indicate that he intended to settle the bill, saying in English loudly and clearly enough to be heard throughout the room, "I want to pee!"

That summer a great event occurred in Freiburg. The university's enrollment for the first time reached 3,000 students. A festival was declared by the rector, at which there was a procession of faculty and students and brass bands through the main streets of the city. The fraternities *(Körper)* marched in uniform with banners, followed by the less aristocratic *Burschenschaften* and all sorts of lesser student societies, from the chess club to a small antialcohol society. In the middle of the procession, alone in an open barouche over which a floral canopy had been erected, rode the hero of the day, a pudgy little *Fuchs* (freshman) whose belated arrival had sent the enrollment up to the magic 3,000. After the procession there was a dinner outdoors in the Stadtgarten for faculty and students and anyone else who had the necessary marks to pay for the meal. Beer and oratory were unlimited, but I saw nobody drunk or disorderly. I often sadly wonder how many of those merrymakers were to fall before French, British, and American guns in World War I, only three years off. Our English friend Dr. Kettle, who left for home before we did, told me an almost incredible thing. When he went to pay his farewell respects to Professor Aschoff, he expressed the hope that they might meet again, before long, in England. "Yes," said Aschoff, "I shall go there some day with our army."

During the last two weeks of our stay in Germany, Grover and I went on a long walking tour in the mountains of the Black Forest with knapsacks on our backs and bergstocke in our hands. We started northward along mountain trails as far as Hornberg, an old town on the Breigach, a lovely little stream that is one of the sources of the Danube. This is the finest country I know for a casual tour on foot—a land of high wooded hills, picturesque old villages, and ruined castles. The footpaths are mostly easy, they are well marked and kept clear by the Schwartzwaldverein, and there are good inns on every mountain and at every valley crossroads. The people were everywhere friendly. Many of the other young wanderers we passed on the trails carried guitars and swung along singing folksongs. Passers-by always gave us a friendly "Guten Tag" or "Grüss Gott." We had superb maps. One need never get lost in the Schwartzwald, and there was nothing to fear except rain. Once we got thoroughly soaked and at the end of the day had to wait for dinner in our room, in our pajamas, while the housemaid dried our jackets, trousers, underwear, and boots at the kitchen fire.

From Hornberg we walked southward along the riverside highway to Triberg, another ancient town on the Breigach, dominated by its castle; then by Villingen to Donaueschingen and southwestward to climb the Feldberg, about 4,000 feet high, from which in clear weather one can see the snow-clad Bernese Alps far to the south. From the Feldberg we descended to the Höllenthal—which for its green beauty should be called the vale of heaven, not of hell—and down to Freiburg, coming at last over the Kanonenplatz to see the sun setting across the wide Rhine valley, with Freiburg Cathedral silhouetted against the evening sky.

When in early September we had to leave for home, we had a few days left for Switzerland and Paris. Our first stop was at Basel, of which I now remember nothing except the paintings of Arnold von Boecklin at the art museum, especially the dreamlike *Die Toteninsel*. These deeply poetic works touched a romantic chord in my youthful spirit (not entirely stilled at eighty-nine, after a lifetime in science), as did also the poetry of Boecklin's contemporaries Alfred Tennyson and Edgar Allan Poe. From Basel we traveled to Lucerne, and again, of that place I have only a general memory of lake and mountains and a handsome town, but I retain a vivid mental picture of another masterwork of the romantic period, Thorwaldsen's *Lion of Lucerne,* carved out of the solid rock. Grover and I felt that it would be quite unenterprising for two young men in Switzerland not to climb a mountain, so from Lucerne we took an afternoon train to the foot of Mt. Rigi (5,900 feet) and with our Schwartzwald rucksacks once more upon our backs walked up to the summit over an easy trail, stayed over night at the mountaintop hotel, and with a few other sturdy tourists rose at dawn to watch the sun rise magnificently over the high mountains.

Interlaken was our base for an ascent of the Jungfrau by the cogwheel railway to the Jungfraujoch at 11,000 feet, where we had an awesome view of the peak towering 2,600 feet above us, with the whole massif of the Bernese Alps for a backdrop. Finally, on our way to Paris we stopped at Lake Geneva for a couple of days and on a beautiful afternoon crossed the lake by steamboat to Evian. We must have visited the city of Geneva, but if so I do not remember it. I wonder why the Swiss cities, Basel, Lausanne, and perhaps Geneva, left such slight marks on my memory. I suppose that the mountains overwhelmed their image. We spent three or four days in Paris seeing the usual sights recommended by the guidebooks, gazing at Napoleon's tomb, climbing the steep streets of Montmartre, and riding the ascenseur to the top of the Eiffel Tower.

In mid-September we sailed for New York on a small ship of the French line—I forget her name. We were on our way home and ready to begin the clinical years of the medical curriculum.

4

THE THIRD YEAR

In October 1911 my classmates and I began the second half of the medical school's curriculum. Upperclassmen had told us that the third year, in which we were now to be introduced to the study and treatment of patients, was the hardest of the four years. To me it was a long, dogged effort to grasp the overwhelming mass of facts and theories of internal medicine, pediatrics, surgery, obstetrics, and gynecology that was placed before us. I think that I was rather dazed by it all; my memories of the year 1911–1912 are blurred, as if I had been walking through a maze.

At that time the work of the third year was centered on the outpatient department of the hospital, where we took the histories of the patients' illnesses, examined them under supervision, observed the diagnostic procedures and treatment of our teachers, and wrote out their prescriptions. The Johns Hopkins Hospital dispensary (to use the old-fashioned term) did not then match the high standards of the rest of the institution; its waiting room was a dismal place where ailing people sat on benches awaiting their turns to see the doctor. The examining rooms were equally dismal. A general movement to improve the management and equipment of outpatient services in teaching hospitals, begun by Dr. Richard Cabot at the Massachusetts General Hospital, had not yet reached Johns Hopkins. The quality of instruction varied with the instructors, from that of experienced practitioners like Louis Hamburger (internist) and T. Caspar Gilcrist (dermatologist) to that of a young opthalmologist whose teaching was so inadequate that some of us were moved to complain to the dean. The instruction was excellent in the major branches of internal medicine and surgery, which were well established in the hospital on a university level. The weakness was in specialties that were still headed by local practitioners who could not devote sufficient time to their teaching. There were notable deficiencies, for example, in ophthalmology, laryngology, and psychiatry, all three of which were shortly to be reorganized and properly manned.

One or two amusing minor items about the dispensary work bob up in my memory. Caspar Gilcrist had a diet list that he declaimed to patients with acne, "no cakes, no pie, no candies, no pickles, nor anything else you like!" And I once had a call for help from a young woman clerk at the drug counter. According to custom, I had put my initials on a couple of prescriptions ordered by the physicians in charge: a gargle for a sore throat and an ointment for a skin eruption. The first patient came back next day to complain that she couldn't gargle with the ointment. The clerk, fearful of losing her job if the doctors learned of her carelessness, begged me to write new prescriptions and an explanatory letter to the other patient, who had begun to treat her eczema with the gargle. I could see no reason not to settle the matter as requested.

We spent six mornings a week in one or another division of the dispensary. From noon to one o'clock daily there was a lecture by a senior professor or his chief aide. The afternoons were given over to various ancillary courses—clinical microscopy, surgical pathology, pharmacy, practical therapeutics, and bandaging. Two afternoons each week were left free so that students might take elective courses or work independently. By neglecting the electives offered on those afternoons I could get over to the anatomical laboratory to put in a few hours on my research on the pancreas. One elective course, however, I could not put aside. In the third trimester Harvey Cushing, W. S. Halsted's most brilliant colleague, conducted a course in experimental surgery once weekly—a course so popular that students had to draw lots for admission. I was successful in the draw and so had my first introduction to Cushing, then well on his way to recognition as one of the world's greatest neurosurgeons. The next year he was called to a senior chair at Harvard. I was to be honored in later years by his friendship and generous interest in my studies in the history of medicine.

Professor Halsted, surgeon-in-chief, gave a clinical lecture every Friday noon. He was fifty-nine years of age, dignified, taciturn, elegantly dressed. We students knew nothing then about his now well-known addiction to cocaine, which he conquered, and (it is now said) to morphine, which he at least controlled. Those experiences made him very shy and reserved. Lecturing in the old surgical amphitheater he spoke in tones so low that he could scarcely be heard in the upper seats, and even down front he seemed at times to be mumbling to himself. His lectures were over the heads of third-year students but must have been inspiring to his resident staff; he dealt with important but obscure problems such as the necessity of avoiding "dead spaces" in surgical wounds or whether or not, when ligating a large artery, to tie off also the accompanying veins. At the operating table Halsted was painstaking, precise, very slow, and unspectacular, always striving to cause the least possible trauma to body tissues and to produce minimal bleeding.

His senior colleague, John M. T. Finney, was outgoing, practical, efficient at the operating table, and a very clear expositor of the diagnostic and operative procedures that we might expect to see in practice. Dr. Finney had made a place for himself in Baltimore's philanthropic and educational affairs and in the spring of 1911 had been offered the presidency of Princeton University in succession to Woodrow Wilson. His declination of this offer was followed in December, to the great satisfaction of his students, by promotion to a full professorship.

The professor of internal medicine was Canadian-born Lewellys F. Barker, tall, blond, and handsome, the very model of an upper-class Nordic. After some years of postgraduate experience in anatomy and pathology at Johns Hopkins, he went to the University of Chicago as professor of anatomy. When in 1905 William (later Sir William) Osler resigned the Johns Hopkins chair of internal medicine to become Regius Professor at Oxford, Barker was surprisingly called to succeed him. Barker made up for his limited experience in the practice of medicine by keen intelligence, industrious reading, a good memory, and a distinguished personal presence, but his Saturday noon clinical lectures, staged with almost theatrical polish, were redolent of the monographs and textbooks from which he had largely gleaned his information. Barker's senior associate, William Sydney Thayer, gave the Thursday lecture in internal medicine. A cultivated New Englander always wearing a flower in his buttonhole and a gracious smile on his lips, he was a thoroughly experienced practitioner of internal medicine and had done excellent research on malaria. As we found out the next year, Thayer was a superb exponent of medicine at the bedside. Any member of our class who might fall ill, given the choice of a physician, would have asked for Thayer if his ailment was medical and for Finney if it was surgical.

We had also, in the third year, a weekly lecture on obstetrics by another of the senior professors, J. Whitridge Williams, a tall, broad-shouldered man nicknamed "Bull" Williams because of his strong features and forceful manner. A humorous teacher, he embellished his chatty, informal talks with quotations from two books—the Bible and *Tristram Shandy*—telling our class, "I never quote any other books, but you students are such damned heathen you don't know which I am quoting."

One morning he was demonstrating the use of obstetrical forceps of the formidable axis-traction type. An obstetrical manikin was placed in front of the class, a dummy made of metal and rubber in the shape and size of a pregnant woman's lower abdomen and pelvis, with a dummy leather baby in its simulated uterus. Dr. Williams inserted the forceps, got its curved blunt blades on the fetal head and began to deliver the leather baby with a firm pull. The handles of the forceps suddenly came off, the professor was thrown off balance and fell headlong backward. His shoulders struck the floor with a thud. Undaunted but muttering a curse, he got up and repeated the performance, only to have the handles again give way. Over he went once more but scrambled to his feet and exclaimed, "Obstetrics is a dangerous specialty!" Dr. Williams had earlier that year been appointed dean of the school as successor to William H. Howell. In later years I had occasion more than once to be grateful for his consideration and sound advice.

Our crowded schedule left little time for diversion. Evenings were for study, Sunday for church with my family and my Sunday school class. Occasionally, however, I took an evening off, at a symphony concert or to hear some well-known speaker.

Grover Powers and I went one evening to hear Sen. Robert M. La Follette, an incomparable political orator. During my student days I heard several of the country's best known public men— Edward Everett Hale (during my visit to Boston in 1907); William Jennings Bryan repeating his famous "Prince of Peace" religious oration; Theodore Roosevelt, shortly after his African safari, addressing a Methodist convention; Billy Sunday, the evangelist, campaigning for souls.

Edward Everett Hale was very old, an impressive relic of bygone days. Roosevelt, not the grinning Teddy of the cartoonists, was serious, thoughtful, with a naturalist's interest in the animals and people he had met in Africa. He spoke with respect of the Methodist missions he had visited, recalling to the delight of his audience the names of their missionaries. Billy Sunday was a tasteless showman, expert in stirring the emotions of his huge audiences of unthinking people. Bryan, when I heard him at a large meeting of the Baltimore YMCA, was no more than a fluent Chautauqua lecturer, though he had the platform presence that had made him famous as a political orator. La Follette excelled them all, I thought, in ability to touch the heartstrings of an audience. Crusading for the Progressive party's proposed reforms, he spoke for two hours without a break and left me wishing for more. I was convinced of his sincerity and almost dazed by his oratory, but I cannot remember now any words of his address.

In the spring of 1912 Grover and I heard another crusader whose simple appeal was to affect both our lives. Wilfred Thomason Grenfell, on tour through the eastern states to win support for his medical mission in Newfoundland and Labrador, speaking in a Baltimore church told about his chain of hospitals, nursing stations, and schools, his summer cruises in the little hospital ship *Strathcona*, and winter visits of mercy to families isolated by snow and ice. He appealed not only for financial support but also for volunteer doctors, nurses, and medical students to serve in the summer, when his stations were busiest. His charming English informality, his quiet eloquence, and the prospect he offered of an adventurous summer in the north gripped us both. A few days later we each wrote to the Boston headquarters of the Grenfell Association, volunteering our services for the approaching summer.

We were accepted and about the middle of June took the Federal Express overnight to Boston for a day's briefing and thence traveled by railway through Maine and Nova Scotia to North Sydney on Cape Breton Island, where we boarded the ferry for the night crossing of Cabot Strait to Port aux Basques, Newfoundland. From there the narrow-gauge Newfoundland Railway took us on a long loop across the island to Lewisporte on the east coast, where we had to stay overnight in the home of a local family, waiting for the coastal steamer *Prospero* to carry us northward. Two days later, after several stops at little fishing ports, *Prospero* docked for several hours at St. Anthony, the site of Grenfell's largest hospital, his orphanage, and the mission's principal school. Here we learned that we were to go on to Battle Harbor, about sixty-five miles farther north across the Strait of Belle Isle, at the southeast angle of the Labrador coast.

The next morning we saw our first sea ice as *Prospero* pushed slowly toward land through a loose floating pack and finally dropped anchor off the entrance to Battle Harbor. The town of fifty or sixty white-painted one-story frame houses stood on the landward shore of a little rocky and treeless island separated from the mainland by a narrow channel locally called "the tickle," in which three or four small icebergs were stranded among floating ice pans. Looking into the tickle, we could see that the low foreshore of the island, just beyond a rickety wharf, was covered by a fish flake—a crude wooden platform a half-acre in extent on which a recent catch of codfish, split and salted, was drying in the sun. At the head of the wharf was the town's general store, an outpost of a trading firm in St. John's, Newfoundland. North of the store and a little above it stood the two-story mission hospital, the town's most conspicuous building. Near it was a one-room schoolhouse and the cottage of the mission doctor, John Grieve, and his family. There were a couple of churches, but I do not recall a resident clergyman. Across the tickle were a few more fishermen's houses. Behind the town the island rose seaward to a rocky summit perhaps two hundred feet above sea level, on which stood the mast and shack of a government radio station. Around the summit lay patches of last winter's snow, and beyond it in the open Atlantic many large icebergs glistened in the morning sunshine. Neither on the is-

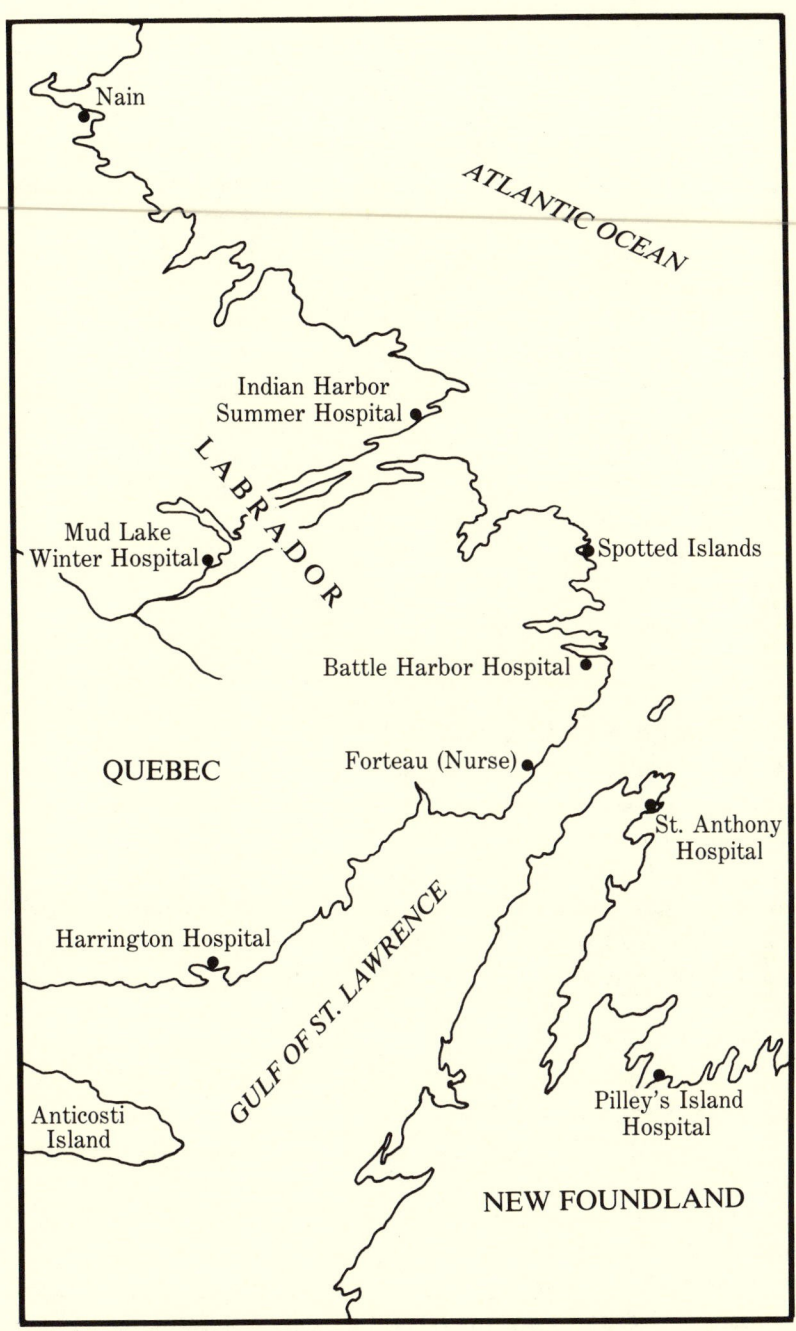

Map illustrating stations of the Grenfell Mission (Royal National Mission to Deep Sea Fishermen) in Newfoundland and Labrador in 1915.

land nor on the mainland were any trees or tall shrubbery to be seen. A grim place, you will say—nothing but rocks and ice and the pounding sea, but I was happy there, and (I think) useful, for two summers.

Prospero was too big to enter the tickle. We were taken ashore in the mission's six-oared boat, skippered by Louis Fallon, a University of Pennsylvania undergraduate who had been with the mission a couple of seasons. Ashore at the hospital, Dr. Grieve heartily bade us welcome.

The hospital, we found, had beds for twenty patients in the men's and women's wards, two verandas for open-air patients, a small operating room, and a room used variously as pharmacy, dispensary, and clinical laboratory. The building also had a small hall for Sunday religious services, used in time of need as a dormitory for unexpected patients or visitors. The staff made the best of a few small bedrooms, a dining room, and a sitting room with a view over the tickle. The mission fleet included a small schooner, a launch, a skiff for harbor use, and the large rowboat for meeting ships offshore.

John Grieve, our chief, was a hardy Scot about thirty-eight years of age, a medical graduate of Edinburgh University. He and his wife lived the year round at Battle Harbor. During the winter, when the Labrador ice pack made the hospital inaccessible by boat, Grieve made medical calls in the neighborhood by dog sledge and annually made a long trip to distant villages along the Labrador shore of the Gulf of St. Lawrence and the Atlantic coast. Thanks to his Scottish pluck and endurance and the skill of his loyal dog drivers (the Murphys of Battle Harbor, father and sons), he had become one of the most extensive sledge travelers in the country. Some of his trips included practically every house from Forteau to Nain, a round trip of fifteen hundred miles.

His staff in the summer of 1912 consisted of a salaried head nurse from the Sick Children's Hospital of Toronto, three volunteer nurses from first-class U.S. hospitals, and a housekeeper. There were six college students, three of them from the University of Pennsylvania (Fallon, Morton McCutcheon, who became a professor of pathology there, and William D. Stroud, who became professor of cardiology); two jolly Californians; and a very likable freshman named Stephen Woodbridge from one of the New England colleges. These collegians helped about the boats and in the general work of the station. Our housekeeper was a lively, talkative woman of thirty-five years from western Canada, accustomed to roughing it on the prairies, she told us, with her pinto pony. All these people proved to be competent for their various duties. In the living room in leisure hours there was merry conversation, or McCutcheon, a talented guitarist, would entertain us, sometimes with his own compositions. Dr. Grieve told us that he was expecting an addition to our company, a young volunteer named Betsy Copping, who was going to open the Battle Harbor schoolhouse for a couple of months to give the village children a summer's schooling.

From time to time we had interesting visitors. Early in July 1912, a party of three on their way to the mission's northernmost station at Indian Harbor, at the entrance to Hamilton Inlet, stayed with us for a few days. Their leader was Dr. Harry Paddon, a quiet young man just out from England; his companions were Miss Mina Gilcrist, a trained nurse, and Frank Babbott, just graduated from college, who had volunteered for the summer in order, he said, to find out whether he wanted to study medicine. Soon after they reached Indian Harbor, Paddon developed a deep palmar abscess that had to be drained under general anesthesia, an operation requiring a surgeon with a steady hand and some knowledge of anatomy. Obviously Miss Gilcrist had to be the anesthetist and Babbott the surgeon, although he had never held a surgical knife in his hand. Paddon showed Babbott how to proceed and described the anatomy of the bones, muscles, blood-vessels, and nerves of the palm of the hand. The three joined in prayer for heavenly guidance; Paddon lay down on the operating table, Miss Gilcrist put him to sleep with ether, and Babbott cut down on the abscess. All went well; the incision healed promptly. Before long Paddon and Miss Gilcrist were married, and in the autumn Frank Babbott went to medical school. He became president of the Long Island Medical College.

In August a middle-aged English visitor of the tweedy sort dressed in elegant sports clothes named Layard came ashore from *Prospero* and received the hospitality of the mission. He said he was related to Henry Austen Layard, the famous excavator of Nineveh, but he was traveling for fishing, not for archaeology. With a local guide he went into the mainland forest and brought back some beautiful salmon, a welcome change from the codfish and tinned meat of our daily diet.

The housekeeper had a staff of five or six Labrador girls for housework in the wards and staff quarters and in the kitchen. They were there partly to get the work done and partly to gain experience in household management, hygiene, and cookery that they could take back to their villages.

The housekeeper had to feed thirty-five people, the sick and the well, on a diet every article of which, except fresh fish and berries, had to come, in tin cans or barrels, by vessel. She must concoct a milk and egg diet, when ordered, from tinned milk and egg powder; and she had to feed invalids who were deeply suspicious of custards, broths, and such unfamiliar things, and complained that they were not given salt pork and "sinkers."

The people of southern Labrador were mostly of British ancestry, descendants of Devonshire and Somerset men who settled in the harbors to avoid the long voyages from England to the fishing grounds off Newfoundland and Labrador. The permanent population, the "live-yeres," was very small. I heard it estimated at twenty-five hundred. But as June sunshine and west wind cleared the bays of ice, there came a sea caravan of a thousand schooners from Newfoundland, Nova Scotia, and even New England, and hundreds of fishermen and their families by steamer—in all, twenty or thirty thousand people. Of these summer colonists, the schoonermen moved from place to place seeking a catch; the remainder had their regular homes with shacks in which to live, keep the fishing gear and boats, and salt the fish. Battle Harbor was strategically placed to serve these migrants as well as the live-yeres. Every fishing vessel passing to Labrador for the summer or southbound for Newfoundland in the fall must course within sight of Battle Island. I have seen thirty-five sail becalmed off the island at one time.

Our medical work did not differ greatly from that of a small village hospital and dispensary in the United States, and yet there were special conditions which added immensely to the burdens and, one might add, to the interest of the situation. I am describing what I saw in 1912 and 1913. First, there were the widespread occurrence and disastrous results of tuberculosis. In the absence of statistics it was estimated that one death in three in Newfoundland and Labrador was caused by this disease, besides those in which an intercurrent infection carried off a tuberculous patient. The blame for this could fortunately be traced with certainty. Spitting was the national sport of the fishermen, both indoors and out; when it was practiced by an infected man in a tight, overheated one-room shack, among a family of underfed children, the result may be imagined. A lad was admitted to Battle, and died the next day, whose sputum showed at least five hundred tubercle bacilli in every field of the sample taken for study. He had been lying for seven months in a room also occupied by six brothers and sisters and had never in his life been told that it is wrong to spit on the floor.

Strangely enough, another serious disease of this northern country was one that everyone thought of then as peculiar to the Far East, namely, beriberi, or endemic peripheral neuritis. About 12 percent of admissions at Battle Harbor were cases of this disease. In etiology the northern cases agreed with the experience of physicians who attributed the disease to a diet formed chiefly of polished rice, the husks of which are discarded in the process of polishing, thus removing a substance necessary to prevent neuritic degeneration. In the north the winter diet consisted largely, sometimes entirely, of tea and bleached white flour. This diet lacked the same substance which is wanting in polished rice but is present in the husks of rice and wheat and in fresh meat, i.e., vitamin B-1 (although in 1912 we did not know what it was). A fairly well-off family in the Strait of Belle Isle failed to get their winter supplies because of an early freezeup and had to subsist through the dead of winter on a few barrels of flour and a little tea; they had absolutely nothing else, not even sugar. At the end of February four of them were attacked by the paralysis of beriberi. In March they got some fresh game and immediately began to improve, but one of the boys could never walk again.

In the spring of 1913 an epidemic of pneumonia invaded many harbors, with an unusual number of fatalities. The other common respiratory ailments were frequent, notably enlarged tonsils and adenoids. Scurvy, of course, and all the forms of disease due to malnutrition were prevalent. In most cases the faulty diet was due not to starvation but to the people's ignorance of how to lay out their resources for proper food. Accidental injuries and wound infections sent many of the fishermen to the mission dispensaries; violent pyogenic infections of cuts caused by fishing tackle were frequently seen.

Skin diseases, especially eczema, caused much suffering among the fishermen aboard schooners, where it was next to impossible to keep clean. Scabies was prevalent, and pediculosis was the bane of the nursing staff—it was found in every ward patient. The mission doctors did no obstetrical work except when called in complicated cases—not from unwillingness, but because of the slowness of travel and because the patients favored lay help. Cardio-renal arteriosclerotic disease was common, a fact to be blamed on the constant exposure and dreadfully hard work of the fishermen. A man told me that the nets belonging to his crew were set in a place three miles from his schooner. He and his mates had pulled their heavy boat the six miles three times a day, in gale and calm, all summer long. Let the reader try a few minutes at a fifteen-foot sweep in a heavy sea and he will appreciate what hard labor really is.

In the hospital Grover Powers and I kept neat histories of every case, recording complete blood counts, analyses of stomach contents, and in a few cases pathological reports based on freehand razor-blade sections. We found time for such work and the routine physical examination in spite of numerous other duties, being, as the mission magazine said, "house surgeons, house painters, and stevedores."

That summer Dr. Grieve put all the male volunteers at hard labor as a pick-and-shovel gang, with himself as working foreman, excavating and blasting out a new reservoir on top of the island to collect melted snow and rainwater to augment the hospital's water supply. The gang of diggers represented eight universities from Edinburgh to Pasadena. Another more risky task in mid-July was to dynamite a small iceberg that had stranded in the tickle, threatening to block the hospital boat *Strathcona* from mooring there. A more routine assignment in which we all took turns, medicos as well as collegians, was to pull an oar in the big rowboat bringing passengers and freight from coastal steamers anchored outside the tickle.

But Powers and I were in Labrador primarily for medical work, and we had some interesting experiences. We diagnosed what must have been the northernmost case of malaria ever seen. The patient, a schoonerman, said that he had never been south of Boston, where he had visited during the past summer. Where he could have been bitten by a mosquito carrying the parasites I found in his red blood cells remains a mystery. Another remarkable case was that of a man who came in with a large irreducible inguinal hernia, with four inches of small intestine in the scrotal sac, which was badly inflamed. When Dr. Grieve operated on the man, on opening the sac he found a fish bone about an inch and a quarter long, which had perforated the intestine and passed into the hernia sac, setting up the inflammation that brought the man into the hospital. The question was what to do with the infected loop of intestine with its ragged, inflamed surface. If replaced in the abdominal cavity it might cause a general peritonitis. To excise it and rejoin the cut ends of the intestine would necessitate a tedious operative procedure in an infected field. Grieve simply put the herniated loop back in the abdomen, after which step he closed the inguinal ring. We had no antibiotics in those days; the next week was an anxious one, but the man recovered smoothly.

On an outpatient call I had one of the most embarrassing experiences of my brief clinical career. One night I had gone to bed after a rather indigestible late supper of tinned sardines and potato salad. The call came just as I had settled down to sound sleep. Men had rowed across the harbor in the black night to fetch a doctor for a boy they said was desperately ill. Thick-headed from interrupted sleep and a bit dizzy, I dressed hastily and went back with the men. As our boat touched the shore below a fisherman's home, someone came out of the house with a lantern shouting, "Tell the doctor to hurry, Jack's mighty bad." We finished the trip with a breathless scramble up the rocky shore. I could feel the potato salad bobbing up and down in my stomach.

My patient, a boy of seventeen, was in bed surrounded by nine or ten alarmed relatives in the stifling hot and fetid air of the sickroom. Pale and sweating, he was groaning with acute abdominal cramps. The clinical history was brief but helpful. He had been gorging himself all afternoon on the little red berries that grow among the rocks of that rugged coast. It was a simple case of gastric distention. I called for a basin, put it under his chin, and stuck a couple of fingers into the back of his throat. It worked. Up with a rush came the half-digested berries. The sight and smell were nauseating. My head was splitting and my stomach went out of control. I leaned over the basin and splashed the remains of my salad and sardines over the patient's berries. We both felt better at once. Somebody brought towels and while the women were mopping him up, I wiped my face, muttered my excuses, and went outdoors. The cold night air cleared my head. I went inside once more to make sure my patient was comfortable and then left him to his greatly relieved family. The men rowed me back to the mission. I spent the next day in bed, suffering as much from humiliation as from a lingering sick headache. But when Grover Powers returned from a follow-up visit to my patient, he told me that Jack's parents regarded me as a hero. "The poor little doctor, he was so sick himself, but he cured our boy."

A schooner bound north to fish for cod came into the tickle to put ashore one of her crew, Steven Collins by name, who had been seized by a convulsion and had fallen over the galley stove. He had lain in his bunk, semiconscious and filthy, for three days on the way to Battle Harbor. It was my turn for an outpatient call. I went out to the schooner to see the man and get him ashore. His shipmates were dumbly helpful, but they were no more experienced than I in getting a helpless man off a ship. At Johns Hopkins that spring I had heard a brilliant series of lectures on uremia by Professor Barker, but he had not taught us how to carry a heavy, stuporous sailor out of the schooner's cramped forecastle, up the companionway steps, aft along he deck, and over the side into a skiff banging against the schooner; still, I had to take command of the operation. Fortunately we did not spill him into the harbor.

On the ward, when we got Steve undressed and cleaned up, we found his chest badly scorched and blistered. His legs were swollen, and his urine was loaded with albumin. Dr. Grieve came to see him and prescribed the usual treatment of the time for uremia—a diuretic, hot packs to sweat off fluids, plus a stiff dose of morphine for the pain of his burns. Three or four hours later Grieve returned and, finding Steve quiet, ordered another injection of morphine and left for an urgent sick call across the tickle. Saying that he might be gone for hours, he left me in charge. "If he convulses, hold him down the best you can." In an hour Steve went into a severe convulsion. He was too big and muscular for me to handle alone. I sent for Grover, and the two of us managed to keep Steve from falling out of bed. As the convulsion ceased, I noticed that Steve was breathing only eight times a minute, then six, then four. I looked at his eyes; his pupils were contracted to pinpoints. He had been given too much morphine.

Looking back, I suppose that he was not actually dying of morphine poisoning on top of his renal block and his burns, but a respiratory rate of four per minute alarmed me. Remembering the rabbit we had treated in the pharmacology course the previous year, we began to apply what we had learned. We had been trying to reduce the fluid in his body; now we poured strong coffee down his sluggish throat. We had been trying to keep him quiet; now we eased him out of bed, and each of us taking an arm, we walked him, stumbling, up and down the ward for an hour. He had no more convulsions, and his breathing gradually returned to the normal rate. Dr. Grieve had not yet returned. When we felt it safe to leave Steve to the night nurse it was well past midnight. We went to bed to get a little rest before the next day's work began. For me, and I think for Grover, too, this was a heartening experience. We had borne for the first time complete responsibility for a human life and had met the emergency with professional competence.

The fisher folk of northern Newfoundland and of Labrador, viewed as hospital patients, were admirable in some ways, annoying in others. The deeply pious nature of the people took outward effect in a spirit of listless dependence on Providence, so that necessary treatment was postponed, or operations were declined, in spite of every argument. A man brought in with a fractured hip proved to have had chronic gastritis for eight years, with vomiting after each meal for the past two years. The patient said that he had never bothered to see a doctor and, moreover, that as he had stood his ailment so long, he would rather continue vomiting than be put on a milk diet. A woman sixty-two years of age appeared at the dispensary bulging with an ovarian cyst which after removal weighed twenty-eight pounds. She and her family greatly feared operation but finally gave permission. During her convalescence her husband came to visit her and on leaving said, "Well, Doctor, so ye've come through with this terrible thing. Who'd 'a thought it? But then, all things is possible with the Lord. And now, Doctor, since ye've done so well by me wife, I just think I'll let ye test me eyes."

Tradition and superstition were held with tenacity, oftentimes blocking the efforts which were being made to teach the prevention of common ailments. A prejudice against dark flour seems to have arisen in days when darkness meant dirt, but it caused useless expense for bleached flour and led to the occurrence of beriberi. The people were invariably surprised if they were told that medicines were not necessary or were inadvisable for their complaints, and left unsatisfied if they were not given pills and potions. Large doses of bitter drugs were preferred and were faithfully taken with much satisfaction on the part of the patient.

It was always amusing to see with what naive surprise they regarded certain things which were very familiar to us—the clinical thermometer, for instance, which was thought by many to be a kind of medicine. The bathtub was the greatest novelty. "Doctor," said one of the patients, "has I got to strip off me clo'es and git into that thing? You folks be shockin' hard on us pore sailors." The art of bathing had to be taught and its performance supervised. How often would you bathe if in winter you had to melt every drop of water from snow and in summer the water about your schooner was only six or eight degrees above freezing?

Navigation along the Atlantic coast of Labrador was a precarious business. North of Belle Isle there were no aids to seamen such as lighthouses or channel buoys. Steersmen found their way by landmarks on shore or by the spray from waves breaking over a hidden rock. In foggy weather they stayed in harbor. One beautiful clear moonlit night in August we were awakened about midnight by long whistle blasts from a steamer in distress about a half-mile off the north entrance to the tickle. Everybody turned out, and the men, including Grover and me, took the mission rowboats out to the ship, a small freighter. Coming into Battle Harbor from the north, the pilot had failed to see a partly submerged rock because the sea was so quiet that there were no waves to break over it. The ship was taking water and was already down by the stern. We took a couple of passengers ashore and returned to help the ship's crew load their boats and ours with some valuable freight—bales of fox and arctic hare pelts. The passengers, patients for the hospital, were admitted and the crew was put on mattresses in the meeting hall. After a few hours sleep, in the morning I walked out to the end of the island to see what had happened to the ship. The wind had risen and a strong sea was running. She was breaking up; only the bow was still visible. On a rock by the sea sat her old skipper. He had been sitting there all night, bowed with grief as he watched her slip into the sea.

A fortnight after Powers and I first arrived at Battle Harbor, *Prospero* again appeared off the south end of the tickle. We were by that time regular members of the boat crew when we were not required on the wards or in the operating room. As we pulled under the lee of the ship, I saw a bright-eyed girl with light brown hair smiling down at us, evidently pleased that she was to be rowed ashore by six nice-looking young men. This was the expected schoolmarm, Betsy Copping. She looked so young that I would have thought her about nineteen years old, but I learned later that she was twenty-three. She became at once a happy member of our hospital family, and I found her very good company—alert, well read, and interested in everything that went on around her. When I exhibited the photographs I was always taking of people and scenes on the island, Betsy, I thought, showed the most intelligent appreciation of my pictures. In turn, I was touched by her womanly interest in the dozen children in her little school.

Busy as we all were, Betsy and I had little opportunity for private conversation, but one afternoon we climbed, or rather scrambled, to the summit of the island and sat there a couple of hours looking at the rough sea and glistening icebergs, and talking mostly about ourselves. She came, she told me, from Massachusetts (her clear, precise New England speech had already told me that). Her father was an English-born Congregational minister, pastor in a New Hampshire mill town, Salmon Falls; her mother was a native of Maine. When she was a child, the family had lived in Acton, Massachusetts, near Concord. Later, when her father had a church in Stratham, New Hampshire, she was a star pupil at nearby Exeter's Robinson Seminary. At graduation from that excellent high school, she was valedictorian of her class. She had had one year at Simmons College, Boston, training for librarianship, but a temporary illness and the chronically tight budget of a minister's family took her out of college and into school teaching—the first grade in a public school—a work for which she had a marked natural talent. Like me, but a year earlier, Betsy had heard Wilfred Grenfell talk about his mission; she had volunteered for service there and had spent the winter of 1911–1912 happily and healthily, in charge of the mission's school at St. Anthony. She had postponed her return to New England because Dr. Grenfell asked her to carry on at Battle Harbor during the summer of 1912. She showed me with pride a little golden badge, a gift that Dr. Grenfell gave to especially helpful volunteers.

In turn I told her about my family, my medical studies, and my research on the embryonic pancreas and spoke of my plans for a medical career, to all of which she listened with gratifying attention. That was our only tête-à-tête, but when she left for home, early in September, we parted with a promise to continue our friendship by mail. A half-century later, reminiscing about our summer on the lonely island, so far away and so long ago, we both recalled that bright afternoon of youthful confidences, when each of us had separately felt a warm sense of companionship and attraction, one to the other, too new and surprising to be at once confessed.

In mid-September Grover Powers and I went home to resume our studies, traveling aboard *Prospero* to St. John's and thence by a larger ship of the same line to New York. We had a distinguished fellow traveler on the trip to St. John's. Sir Edward Morris, prime minister of Newfoundland, was campaigning along the coast for reelection to the provincial parliament. At each port of call, St. Anthony, Little Harbor, Fogo, Twillingate, and other smaller places, Sir Edward with his two or three companions went ashore to make a stump speech, Grover and I trailing along to hear him. A man of impressive physique and a friendly shipmate, he seemed to us at first to be little more than a small-town politician. His speeches consisted almost entirely of promises to do something for the community —better roads, a telephone line, a new dock. Two years later, when World War I began, his great abilities took him into the highest war councils of the Empire and won him in 1918 the unusual honor, for a colonial statesman, of elevation to the peerage as Lord Morris. While Grover and I were in St. John's awaiting the steamship to New York, Sir Edward and Lady Morris invited us two young travelers to dinner and an informal evening chat at their official residence.

From New York, Grover went to Indiana to visit his parents, and I to Baltimore. Joining our family in welcoming me at home, our black cook, Emma Grant, said to my mother: "The trip done him good. Last spring he could scarce lift a chair. Now he carries his trunk upstairs hisself!"—and to me, "Mr. George, I hope you didn't fall in love with none of them heathen Norwegian girls when you was way up north."

5

THE FOURTH YEAR

I enjoyed my fourth year as a medical student more than the third. There was more time to think for myself, a little more opportunity to develop personal interests. There were fewer facts to cram and more to learn by doing, and quite often there came a friendly and beautifully expressed letter from Betsy Copping, who was teaching school in Methuen, Massachusetts, twenty-five miles outside Boston.

Our work was centered on the hospital wards, two trimesters on the medical service and one on the surgical. On the ward each student had his own patients, assigned to him in turn when admitted to the hospital. We wrote a preliminary statement of the illness and the patient's previous medical history, made a physical examination, recorded the blood pressure and pulse, made blood-cell counts, and tested the urine for albumin and sugar. In case of respiratory disease, we examined the sputum under the microscope for tubercle bacilli and pneumococci. Comparing notes with the intern, we prepared ourselves to discuss the case, if called upon, with the senior professor on ward rounds. Sir William Osler, the first professor of internal medicine at Johns Hopkins, claimed as his special merit that he taught medical students on the wards. Osler had moved to Oxford eight years before my time, but he had left behind him associates and pupils well trained in the art. I recall with admiration the clear, wise, humane Oslerian discourse of teachers like William Sydney Thayer, Louis Hamman, Thomas R. Boggs, and Charles R. Austrian and their courteous handling of the patients, who if not too ill to care seemed to enjoy them, or at least to appreciate being at the center of a ring of concerned people —the professor, the intern, the head nurse of the ward, a junior nurse or two, and the six or seven students attached to the ward.

One episode on Ward O comes vividly to mind. Professor Barker was discussing the illness of a young woman from the slums, half-witted and badly spastic from a chronic degenerative disease of the nervous system. Wishing us to observe her peculiar gait, he helped the patient out of bed and walked with her along the ward. It was a picture for Rembrandt or Goya—the ill-formed, stumbling black girl in her wrinkled hospital gown, the tall, handsome, elegantly dressed professor at her side, guiding her with grave courtesy; the riveted attention of the students.

Sometimes a bit of comedy broke through the professional dignity of a ward round. The patients in a teaching hospital are not merely specimens of disease, to be observed by the students and lectured over by the professors. They are people, and if they have not been muted by overwhelming illness, they may let you know it. The urbane Dr. William Sydney Thayer stood at the bedside of an elderly black man suffering from severe cardiac insufficiency. Thayer was trying to get one of my classmates, not the brightest in the group, to suggest a suitable diet for the patient. The student having produced no ideas on the subject, Dr. Thayer said, "For instance, would you recommend a dinner of ham and cabbage?" The student said "Yes, that would be good," whereupon the patient entered the discussion. "Gawd, no, Doctor: done et some ham and cabbage last week. That's what brung me here."

The previous summer in Germany, I had heard another patient intervene in a discussion between teacher and student. Bernhard Krönig, professor of gynecology at Freiburg-im-Breisgau, had examined a woman under light anesthesia in an anteroom prior to operating. He gave one of the senior students the privilege of palpating the uterus. When the young man finished, Krönig asked whether he thought that the ailment was curable by operation. "Ja, Herr Professor," the student said. "Ich glaube dass es sich ausheilen kann." The anesthetist must have been letting up on the ether; the patient, dimly reawakening to a world of pain and fear, began to wail: "Nein, nein, ich sage nein! Es kann sich nicht ausheilen!" "Weg mit der Kritik," said Krönig, and the orderly wheeled her into the operating room, where, I trust, the professor's ministrations proved her gloomy prognosis incorrect.

Ward work, watching surgical and gynecological operations, and attending the noonday clinical lectures kept us busy until lunchtime six days a week. Numerous elective courses were available in the afternoons. One such opportunity I did not want to miss. Max Broedel, the school's celebrated medical artist, offered a weekly course in medical illustration. His pupils in 1910 included two or three junior members of the faculty and seven or eight students. Max's skilled hand and bantering tongue kept us admiring and amused. He used to tease me by comparing my art work with that of my cousin Thomas Cromwell Corner, Baltimore's leading portrait painter. To start me off he had me draw in charcoal the toothless skull of an old man. As my drawing neared completion Max could not resist adding a highlight here and there or deepening a shadow, until I feared that as a work of art the picture was becoming as much his as mine. When he was satisfied with it he said, "Take it uptown to Bendann's (an art dealer); he'll put it in his window as a genuine Corner."

On April 12, 1913, while I was at work in the students' research room of the anatomy laboratory preparing my paper on the embryonic development of the pancreatic ducts, I had a glimpse of the celebrated William Osler. He had come over from Oxford to give the principal address at the dedication of the Phipps Psychiatric Clinic and was in the laboratory for a chat with his friend Mall. Instead of leaving the professor's office by the door into the corridor, Osler came through the adjoining research room, and just as he entered it, Max Broedel came in from the corridor and saw Osler. With joyful cries of "Max!" and "William!" the two men rushed together and flung their arms around each other in happy reunion. I began to see what people meant when they spoke of Osler's charm. Next day at the dedication ceremony I saw it even more. Telling the crowded audience of Baltimore people how happy he was to be back with old friends, he named some of them whom he saw in the front rows. "There's Hal Thomas, whose grandfather was a trustee of the hospital; over there I see my old friends Brent Keyser and

Blanchard Randall," and he named two or three others. He had won his audience in the first three minutes.

During the school year 1912–1913 Battle Harbor was much on my mind. I intended to return there for another summer and spent a good deal of time on activities in one way or another related to that aim. Wishing to do what I could for the Grenfell Mission, I had lantern slides made from about thirty of the best of the negatives I had made of scenes and people on the island, and I let it be known in Methodist circles that I was prepared to give talks about Labrador. My father, pleased by this under-taking, financed the making of the slides. Since many of the older churches and Sunday schools in Baltimore were not yet wired for electricity, I had to project my pictures with an old-fashioned limelight lantern with its oxyhydrogen burner sup-plied by two heavy cylinders of gas, a forty-pound load to get to the meeting places by cab. My classmate Daniel Davis enjoyed serving the cause as my projectionist, which he did expertly. During the winter I gave about a dozen of these illustrated talks, with small financial gain for the mission but excellent experience for me in public speaking.

I spent almost every Friday evening during the academic year at Broadway Methodist Church with a little club for boys fourteen to sixteen years of age that had started with my Sun-day school class. The region of East Baltimore around the church was deteriorating and offered few decent diversions for the children of the lower-middle-income class then living there. Motion pictures were not yet being shown everywhere, and there was no television. My boys suggested a club, and the church provided a room. The Boy Scout movement had not yet reached the United States. Many Protestant congregations at that time maintained units of the Boys' Brigade, a military-style organization, uniformed and armed with dummy rifles, but I had no taste for mock-soldiering and ran the club along the lines of another, more imaginative boys' club movement called Knights of King Arthur. We opened our meetings with a sword on an improvised altar, in words of knightly import. How to occupy the boys during the rest of our two-hour sessions was my problem. I solved it that winter by telling them about my summer on Battle Island. I happened to mention that Dr. Grenfell had adorned his hospital and school at St. Anthony with appropriate scriptural verses cut out of wood. When I told them that these wooden letters had been made by people interested in the mission, the boys volunteered to make an inscription for Battle Harbor Hospital. At my request Dr. Grenfell suggested words from the Gospel of St. Matthew 25:40, "Inasmuch as ye have done it unto one of the least of these my brethren, ye have done it unto Me." We spent our Friday evenings (even on the night before my final examination in internal medicine) cutting out the foot-high letters from half-inch pine boards. We sandpapered them, had a couple of messy evenings painting them white, then shipped them to Battle Harbor.

I had another, quite different, construction project of my own for Battle Harbor. In 1912 Dr. Grieve had operated on several children for enlarged tonsils. As his anesthetist I had noticed how inconvenient was the administration of chloroform (which Grieve, as a Briton, preferred to ether) by the standard method of pouring it on a cloth mask placed over the patient's face. I would put the child to sleep, then remove the mask so that Grieve could work on the throat; the anesthesia would begin to wear off; he would wait while I plied the chloroform again; and so on two or three times. At the Johns Hopkins Hospital I had seen a new method, by which ether was vaporized by an electric heater and delivered into the pharynx through a tube attached to the oral speculum, leaving the surgeon a clear approach to the tonsils while maintaining a constant state of anesthesia. For Battle Harbor, where there was no electricity, I developed a similar apparatus using a vaporizing tank (a quart-sized can from an ice-cream freezer surrounded by hot water), into which ether dripped from an engineer's oil cup controlled by an adjustable needle valve. The tank was immersed in a basin of hot water to vaporize the ether. The anesthetic vapor was propelled through the pharyngeal tube by air pressure from a rubber bulb held by the anesthetist. A metal worker constructed my apparatus for a few dollars from parts I bought at a hardware shop. To test its safety and effectiveness I applied to the experimental surgery laboratory, where Dr. Roy D. McClure kindly permitted me to act as his anesthetist in ten operations on the thyroid gland that he was doing on large dogs. It worked well, and at Battle

Harbor next summer I used it in several operations without mishap, to the great satisfaction of Grieve's successor, Arthur Wakefield.

For greater usefulness at Battle Harbor in 1913 I needed more intimate experience in the routine of the operating room than I would get in medical school as one of a class of seventy-seven students. A cousin of mine, Firmadge Nichols, a recent medical graduate of Johns Hopkins, was resident surgeon at St. Agnes Hospital, a suburban institution operated by nuns of a Catholic nursing sisterhood. He willingly accepted me as a volunteer on his wards and in the operating room one day a week. I needed, of course, official permission to absent myself from the school for this purpose. One of the signs of greatness in men and institutions is judicious flexibility. Both the dean, Dr. J. Whitridge Williams, and Dr. J. M. T. Finney, who had charge of student affairs under the austere surgeon-in-chief, W. S. Halsted, granted my unusual petition, and every Thursday of the last trimester I went to St. Agnes to serve as a weekly visiting member, so to speak, of the resident's surgical team, usually as "instrument man." Thus I got the feel of operating room procedures.

The patients I saw and the operations in which I took part were the usual run of general surgery, with one unforgettable exception. A young woman, pregnant at full term, was brought in bleeding to death internally from premature separation of the placenta. Preparations were immediately begun for a caesarean section, at which I was again to be instrument man, but it was too late. While the nurses were readying a blood transfusion, increasing pallor and a failing pulse told us the woman was dying. Dr. Nichols, though not a Catholic, was in duty bound to assure the unborn infant the hope of heaven through the rite of baptism. The operating room became the scene of a religious ceremony, all the celebrants—the head surgical sister, the doctors, and I masked and capped and clad in operating gowns instead of clerical vestments. The sister opened a flask of physiological salt solution, by emergent necessity mystically transformed into holy water. I handed Nichols a large scalpel. An assistant resident had his fingers on the patient's wrist feeling the pulsebeat. A few minutes passed in deep silence. Then the pulse watcher dropped the woman's arm, with a signal to Nichols. With rapid strokes he widely incised the abdominal wall, exposed and opened the uterus and lifted the baby into the world it would never see. Before there was time even to learn whether or not it was breathing, the sister poured a few drops from her flask upon the infant's head, intoning with measured solemnity the ordained words, "I baptize thee in the name of the Father and of the Son and of the Holy Ghost." But we had lost our fight for the child's eternal bliss; it, too, had ceased to breathe and was doomed to languish forever outside the gates of Paradise, a wistful shade among the multitude of other infants who died in the womb, unbaptized, forbidden ever to look upon the Father in his glory.

My readers may ask why I have not mentioned Grover Powers in connection with these activities and projects so closely related to our service in Labrador. We had been close friends for three years; we had made two journeys together in foreign lands; we had roomed together on shipboard, in the Black Forest, and at Battle Harbor without even a passing disagreement except once, when at Freiburg he would not agree to take rooms in the house of the too-friendly landlady and her potentially alluring daughters. I was therefore puzzled and distressed when in the autumn of 1912 Grover suddenly began to avoid me and when in the course of our studies we chanced to meet was mournfully uncommunicative.

After some weeks of perplexity I wrote him a note expressing my sorrow and asking what I had done to distress him. To this he replied by a letter of six pages vaguely telling me of his unhappiness about my attitude toward him, without citing any specific instances of discourtesy or neglect on my part. After more than sixty years I still do not fully understand what had troubled him, but in retrospect I see that in the makeup of this gentle, sensitive man, there was a streak of almost womanly sensibility that had its role in our intimate friendship. In our Black Forest tour it was I who plotted the daily stages of our travel on foot, it was I who had first thought of volunteering for the Labrador mission. On the other hand he was protective of me; I remember once hurting his feelings by testily refusing to take his advice to wear my overcoat on a windy day. One night at Battle Harbor in the room we shared, after we had put out the lights and gone to bed, I was dropping off to sleep when

Grover rose from his cot, crossed the room, and touched my shoulder. When I sleepily asked him, "Grover, what's up?" he said, "I just wanted to feel that you were there." Whatever affection he felt for me was never expressed more explicitly than in the episode just mentioned. Grover's sudden change of manner may have resulted from something approaching jealousy. Had I wounded him by letting Daniel Davis share in my lectures instead of himself? Had he divined my deepening affection for Betsy Copping? In these or some other ways had I denied his need for my exclusive regard?

The rift persisted during the two years I remained in Baltimore after our graduation, when Grover was on the pediatrics house staff of the Johns Hopkins Hospital. In fact our friendship was broken for twenty years. In the mid-1930s when he was professor of pediatrics at Yale, I resolved to bring this sorry situation to an end. I wrote to Grover saying that I was going to attend a scientific meeting in New Haven and hoped to see something of him when I was in town. He met me at the railway station with a beaming smile and drove me on a sight-seeing tour around the city. We were brothers again. Stopping his car on the high point of the East Rock Drive to enjoy the view over the city and the university, Grover said simply that he had been wrong in his attitude to me in 1912 and 1913. I forbore asking what had disturbed him. During the remaining decades of his nobly useful life, I saw him several times with unmarred affection. At his funeral in 1968 I sat in a pew behind his wife and son and grandchildren, silently sharing their grief.

In the spring of our fourth year in medical school the dean's office posted a list of the twenty-five men and women who stood highest in the class, of whom twenty would be appointed resident house officers (the Johns Hopkins term for interns) on the respective clinical services. Those standing highest had the choice of services; medicine, surgery, gynecology, obstetrics, pediatrics. I stood tenth in the class and therefore was reasonably sure to get an appointment to gynecology, which I wanted. Grover Powers was eleventh and chose pediatrics.

My peace of mind about the next stage in my progress was, however, soon dispelled when I received a note from Professor Mall asking me to call at his office. He offered me an assistantship for teaching and research in his department. I replied that

I had planned to take an internship in gynecology, hoping to make a career as practioner and teacher and, if I was capable, to do research in that field. In that case, said Mall, I would be wise to spend ten years in a preclinical science such as anatomy before becoming a clinician. Gynecology, he said, was not keeping up with the advance of medical science; the field needed a new stimulus from the laboratory side. When I pointed out that a temporary stay in an anatomical or physiological laboratory (his was really both) would deprive me of experience in diagnosis and treatment, he reminded me that Lewellys Barker had been called from the anatomical laboratory of the University of Chicago to be professor of internal medicine at Johns Hopkins. I could not be so optimistic as to assume that a similar thing would happen to me, and moreover I did not want to lose the experience of internship and therefore asked Dr. Kelly whether he would postpone my appointment to his house staff for one year so that I could have a year with Mall to explore the possibilities of research on the ovarian cycle. As it happened, the time was opportune for such a request. The advisory board of the medical faculty had only that year yielded to the individual heads of clinical departments authority to choose their interns. Dr. Kelly was thus free to do as he pleased. With Tom Cullen's advice and perhaps a word from Dr. Mall, he agreed to put off my internship until 1914. Since the appointment to an assistantship in anatomy would not take effect until September 1913, I was free to return to Labrador for the summer. On commencement day, June 10, 1913, at the Academy of Music on Howard Street, we of the graduating class received our diplomas from the hand of President Ira Remsen. Before I could leave Baltimore, however, came the ordeal of the state board examination for the license to practice medicine, three days at the medical and chirurgical faculty on Cathedral Street in ninety-degree weather.

On the day after the examination I took the Federal Express once more on my way north. Betsy Copping, forewarned that I would stop over in Boston for a day or two, had written to say that fortunately she would be staying in town that weekend. She must have let her family know about the young Baltimorean she had met at Battle Harbor, for at the Parker House Hotel I found a note from her cousin Robert Gordon, a fellow in English at Harvard, inviting me to join him, his wife, and Betsy at a Saturday evening "pop concert" of the Boston Symphony Orchestra. The next evening she and I decorously attended the evening service at Park Street Church and after the final amen bade each other a reluctant farewell for the summer. Next morning at the office of the Grenfell Association I was shocked to learn that Steven Woodbridge, the likable college boy at Battle Harbor the previous year, had developed tuberculous meningitis and was lying mortally ill at his home in a Boston suburb. I went out to see him and stood at the bedside with his bravely composed mother. Steve recognized me but could speak only a few words. I too could say little; I had not been a physician long enough to know what to say to a mother whose only son was dying. A farewell grasp of her hand and a look of sympathy had to suffice as I left to start the next stage of my journey.

Next morning as the train chugged through New Brunswick and Nova Scotia, I was surprised to find myself deeply depressed, let down after the excitement of graduation and the stress of the state board examination, sorrowed by two partings from cherished friends, one for a long summer, one forever, and grieved by the contemplation of disease that my profession was powerless to cure. I had accepted with my diploma a lifetime burden of responsibility for other people, whether as physician or teacher; how could I be sure that I would measure up to the unforeseen tasks I faced? I don't know how long this melancholy state might have lasted, but the dining car served a good lunch, and in the late afternoon the train stopped for a while on a siding in green country beside one of the Bras d'Or lakes, as the sun was going down in a fair sky. I stepped off the train and stood gazing at the lovely scene. Suddenly it occurred to me that I was young and healthy, that I had been trained at a great school and admitted to a great profession. What other young doctors had done I, too, could do. The memory of that moment of insight— a sort of private epiphany—has lasted all my life, bidding me take courage to go forward when fatigue and indecision threatened to overwhelm me.

At Battle Harbor I found that I was to have a new chief; John Grieve had been promoted to Harrington Harbor Hospital on the St. Lawrence coast of Labrador. Dr. Arthur Wakefield, who had taken over, was quite different from the steady-going Scot, his predecessor. An Englishman of what I call the fox-terrier type, Wakefield was sandy-haired and blue-eyed, sharp-nosed, slightly exophthalmic, a man of quick movements and rapid speech. He had played Rugby football, the roughest of English college sports, and had been the doctor on one of the British Mt. Everest expeditions. At least once while I was with him he proved his physical toughness by taking a swim in the icy sea. When he and I went on a sick call together on foot over the hills across the tickle, although he was fifteen years older than I, he had me breathless trying to keep up with him. He had studied medicine at the London Hospital. I believe that he came out to Labrador from love of adventure more than from missionary zeal—but so, come to think of it, had I.

My duties that summer were much like last year's but with less pick-and-shovel work or house painting and more responsibility for medical service. Dr. Wakefield recognized my possession of a medical degree and a license to practice by having me do some surgery, including a tonsillectomy or two and excision of a subcutaneous cyst in a man's scalp, under local anesthesia. With my homemade ether machine I was the anesthetist in several major operations.

One task assigned to me by Dr. Wakefield awoke my scientific interest, though to no avail. On a recent visit to his English home, Wakefield had talked about the problem of beriberi in Labrador with a biochemist in one of the London medical schools who was working with rice hulls, trying to extract the unknown substance whose lack in a diet of polished rice somehow caused the peripheral neuritis. He gave Wakefield a recipe for an extract of wheat bran. We had in the hospital a couple of partially paralyzed beriberi patients. I made up the extract as directed, by soaking bran in a weak solution of acetic acid. A muddy-looking, vinegar-flavored mess, it had no appeal to the patients to whom I laboriously administered a cup of it twice daily. After a couple of weeks we abandoned the experiment by mutual consent. We were only a little ahead of the age of vitamins.

I took my share of the outpatient calls, which often meant cold, damp travel in small boats or tramping over soggy turf among the rocks. Only once was I in real danger. One windy afternoon a boat came into the harbor manned by six young oarsmen and an old skipper. They came from a village eight miles away—I forget its name—across the mouth of St. Louis

Bay, which juts into the mainland immediately north of Battle Island. The men had come to get medical help for Henry Fequet, the principal man in their village, who, they said, was painfully ill with stomach cramps. After the men had a rest and a cup of tea, I put on my oilskins and boots and took my seat in the stern of the boat beside the skipper. After we got out of the tickle into the bay, the wind from the north became much stronger, with a heavy sea running before it. A half-mile out, the waves were about eight feet high. Pulling as hard as they could, the men made very little headway. After a quarter of an hour of no progress at all, the skipper decided not to gamble eight lives against Henry Fequet's one, but to return to harbor was now also a gamble. To turn the boat in the heavy seas meant a serious risk of swamping it. None of us could have made it to shore in the icy water. The skipper was closely watching the oncoming waves. I held my breath when he ordered the turn. Instantly and in perfect unison the men on the port side backed water while those on the starboard side pulled ahead; the skipper leaned heavily on his steering oar, and the boat swiftly came about in the slack water between two waves—perfect timing and as smart a piece of oarsmanship as one could ever hope to see. For the next few minutes the going was tricky, with following waves threatening to poop the boat, but soon we were in the sheltered water of the tickle. The men stayed all night at the hospital. In the morning we set off again on a calm sea.

Henry Fequet and his family lived high up on a rocky shore —"a wonderful upright and clifty place," said the skipper. I found my patient in bed surrounded by solicitous relatives, but he said he had taken a turn for the better. I found no fever, no abdominal masses or tenderness, no irregularity of the heart, nothing wrong with his lungs. There were no symptoms of gallstones or intestinal obstruction. At the Johns Hopkins Hospital he would be x-rayed and would have his gastric juice analyzed and his heart tested by that recent invention the electrocardiograph. All I could give him was verbal reassurance and soda mints. Since he did not call us again during the rest of the summer, I concluded that I had not missed anything serious.

They brought me another patient, a girl three years old, emaciated and coughing. I wished that I could call a consultation with my pediatrician friend Powers. Feeling helpless I prescribed a diet of milk and eggs. No eggs were to be had in the village, but somebody said that an old woman at Pity Harbor, three miles away, had some hens. One of the Fequet boys guided me along the cliff tops to see if the old woman had any eggs to spare. She gave me half of her stock—two eggs. On the way back to Fequet's place I walked very cautiously, for a stumble would ruin my entire therapeutic resources. The child's mother gratefully took the eggs and said, "Doctor, I'll fry one good right away." I hastened to recommend soft-boiling it and added an urgent plea to bring the child to the hospital if she did not do better.

Returning to Battle Harbor late that afternoon I was dozing in the stern of the boat when a chilly feeling awoke me and I found that we had run into a fog so thick that the sight of shore was completely blanked out—a situation as dangerous in its way as yesterday's wind and waves. We were right in the wide mouth of St. Louis Bay; if we went only a few degrees off course, we might find ourselves in the open Atlantic with night coming on. The skipper, I could see, was worried. He ordered the men to ship their oars, then took a pocket compass from a locker under his seat, put it on a thwart amidships, and took a vote of all hands as to the direction we were headed when we lost our landmarks in the fog. Averaging the vote he set a course by compass. The men rowed in silence for an hour until we heard dogs barking and found that we had come straight into the tickle at Battle Harbor.

The only part of the outpatient work that I disliked was hauling teeth, as our patients called the operation, but I could not decline their appeals. Our outpatient bag contained one pair of dental forceps that had to be used on incisors and molars alike, regardless of their shape. Fortunately (for me) in that land of scantily nourished people and neglected oral hygiene, decaying teeth were not too tightly set in their sockets. I managed to get them out and never broke anybody's jaw.

In mid-June we had unexpected visitors. A small fishing vessel came into the tickle and there disembarked the Arctic explorer Donald B. McMillan and his six companions of the Crocker Land expedition, bound for the farthest north to find the island Peary thought he had seen northwest of Axel Heiberg Land. Their ship, loaded with supplies for a stay in the Arctic that was to last two years but actually lasted twice that long, had struck a rock in the Gulf of St. Lawrence in the vicinity of Forteau. They were forced to wait at Battle Harbor until another ship could be obtained from St. John's. I enjoyed talking with the young scientists of the party, the geologist Elmer Ebklaw; Maurice Tanquary, the zoologist (both from the University of Illinois); and Ensign Fitzhugh Green, U.S.N., physicist and engineer. McMillan himself, a very agreeable man, chatted with me one day, explaining the complexities of the Eskimo language, which he was industriously studying. The doctor of the party, Harrison Hunt, is described by Everett S. Allen in his biography of McMillan, *Arctic Odyssey*, as "an outdoorsman in splendid physical shape," and so he looked when I met him. Actually he was taking the risk of a long stay in the far north with only one kidney, the other one having been removed some years before. He told me this himself, in words that showed that he recognized the gamble, but he kept in good health during the whole stay of four years. The party was with us for a few days until the old sealing steamer *Eric* arrived to carry them on to their base on Ellesmere Island.

I have a hazy memory of meeting at Battle Harbor Clarence Birdseye, the founder of the quick-frozen food industry. According to his entry in *Who Was Who in America*, Birdseye was at that time working as a trapper on the Labrador and Newfoundland coasts. He must have visited our mission; or have I confused him with Ebklaw and Tanquary? He conceived the quick-frozen process by observing that fish taken out of the water and into the air at temperatures far below zero Fahrenheit froze so rapidly that their tissues were not altered by crystallization of water contained in their microscopic cells; and when thawed after storage they retained a naturally fresh flavor.

I have said little thus far about Dr. Grenfell. He made his headquarters at St. Anthony and visited the outlying stations only occasionally. In Baltimore I had heard him speak once; he came to Battle Harbor three or four times. These brief contacts, and his books, all of which I read, were sufficient to win my total admiration. Among all the good and able men I have known in a long life, there were two, either of whom I would have most eagerly chosen as my companion if I were to be cast away on a desert island. One of these was Stanhope Bayne-Jones, of whom

I shall have more to say in a subsequent chapter; the other was Grenfell. Both had qualities most essential for such a role—physical vigor, intelligence, resourcefulness, unselfish companionship.

Part of Grenfell's charm was an almost boyish impetuosity. Once in a leisure hour at Battle Harbor one of the nurses said that she would like to climb an iceberg. "Let's go," said Dr. Grenfell. With five or six of us he rowed out into the tickle, where a small berg was stranded, its above-water portion sloping gradually enough to make a climb possible. Holding the end of a long rope, which we all grasped firmly, Grenfell scrambled to the top of the berg, followed by the rest of us. Snapshots of this jolly little adventure made good conversation pieces at home next winter.

I asked Dr. Grenfell whether there was any truth in a story I had heard about a far greater piece of impetuosity on his part. Crossing from Southampton to Montreal on a Canadian Pacific liner, he was greatly attracted by a young woman from Chicago, who found him interesting enough to be granted a full share of her time during the voyage. On the last day before docking in Montreal he asked her to marry him. "But you don't even know my name," she exclaimed. "What difference does that make?" said he. "It's going to be Grenfell." This story, he assured me, was true and had led to an enduring marriage.

Love of adventure, I think, was responsible for his choice of a career as much as his unostentatious but deep, almost fundamentalist Christian piety. To bear hardship while seeking to do good was a lifelong duty. In the wheelhouse of his ship *Strathcona* he tacked up a motto from Virgil, *Forsitan et haec olim meminisse juvabit*—"Someday even this will be a happy memory." He spoke in public with easy informality and wrote well. His *Adrift on an Icepan* is a classic of suspenseful adventure; *Labrador, The Land and the People* is learned enough to be assigned reading for graduate students in geography. But his best gifts were the sincerity and charm that drew people to work with him.

In September 1913, Dr. Grenfell asked me to join the mission staff and spend the next winter in charge of his small station at Pilley's Island in Notre Dame Bay, Newfoundland. This was a great surprise. He had seen me at work only once, and that occasion was marred by a minor calamity. He made an unannounced stop at Battle Harbor and came to the hospital while I was in the operating room doing a tonsillectomy with the now obsolete wire snare. I was seated at the head end of the operating table, with the needed instruments lying in a sterile towel pinned to the sterile sheet covering the operating table and to my operating gown, forming a kind of hammock over my knees. The door of the room opened, and in came Dr. Grenfell. In my surprise, forgetting that I was a surgeon at work, I did what any mannerly young man would do under more usual circumstances —I rose respectfully to my feet. Down went the instruments clattering to the floor. I had an embarrassing ten minutes while the nurse picked them up and resterilized them. I suppose, however, that Grieve and Wakefield had given Dr. Grenfell a generally good report on my work.

At Pilley's Island I would have had a house, a trained nurse to help me, and a dog team with a driver for winter travel. The offer appealed mightily to my love of adventure and novelty, but I knew in my heart that a winter with the mission, not to mention the whole career that was implied in the offer, in solitary medical and surgical practice before I had even an internship, in an isolated village without educated companions and without a library, was not for me. Furthermore I had accepted Dr. Mall's appointment for the next academic year. After I reached home I was again surprised to receive a letter from the pastor of a small town on Prince Edward Island, Canada, saying that the community had lost its only physician and inviting me to take his place. I was offered a house and a ready-made practice. How the pastor got my name he did not say; he probably had applied to the Grenfell Association in Boston for assistance in finding a doctor. These two unsought calls to practice medicine were reassuring. Billy Baer's dictum of four years earlier was evidently true; if I did not make good at teaching and research I could still go into general practice.

In September I returned to my home by ship to Lewisporte, then by the Newfoundland Railway to Port aux Basques, the night ferry to North Sydney and rail to Baltimore, with a stopover, of course, at Boston. When on the first leg of this journey *Prospero* stopped at St. Anthony, I was given a valuable parcel to carry to Boston with me. The mission had started a home industry for fishermen's wives, the weaving of homespun woolen cloth. My parcel was a sample bolt of this material for the Grenfell Association. Arriving at North Station, Boston, at 11:00 P.M. on the fifth day of my journey, I decided to walk to the Parker House Hotel. I did not know the local streetcar routes well and did not want to spend my scanty cash on a taxi. So I set out on foot with the cloth under my arm. I must have looked shabby and in need of a good wash. There were no air-conditioned railroad cars in those days. Through the open windows, in the summertime, came a swarm of cinders from the locomotive. They got in the passenger's hair and down his neck and smudged his face. My suit was wrinkled, and the paper around my bolt of cloth was beginning to frazzle.

A block or two from the railway station a policeman stopped me and demanded an explanation of the bundle I was carrying through the streets at that hour. My story of a five-day journey from a place he had never heard of did not impress him. "You're a common thief," he said. "I saw you in Scollay Square a week ago. You're coming to the station house with me." He refused to accompany me to the Parker House, where I had registered on the trip north in June and where somebody could verify my signature even if my face and clothes were not recognizable. So we walked in glum silence three or four blocks to the police station. There I was stood up in front of a high bench behind which a sergeant on night duty glared at me. He, too, did not believe my tale of traveling from Labrador, though I should think that not even a Boston thief would be able to invent so exotic a story. The sergeant asked whom I knew in Boston who would identify me. This was getting serious; it looked as if I might be in for a night in a cell until somebody from the Grenfell Association could be summoned in the morning to identify me. But I had the whole next day planned; a good rest at the hotel all morning, a visit to the Grenfell office to deliver the bolt of cloth, the afternoon with my friend the Yankee school teacher, and at night, departure from South Station for Baltimore, where I had an important engagement the following evening—the wedding reception of my cousin John King.

In despair I told the sergeant that Dr. Harvey Cushing, professor of surgery at the Peter Bent Brigham Hospital, knew me, but my heart quaked with the thought of what the sometimes irascible Cushing might say if he was called at midnight. Next I mentioned a medical classmate, Gilbert Horrax, then an intern at the Lahey Clinic. The sergeant seemed reluctant to disturb even an intern's slumber. The breakthrough came when I produced a membership card of the Johns Hopkins University YMCA. The sergeant, evidently impressed at last, said, "If you're telling the truth, you've had a good education, I'll say that." After a bit more palaver he told me that I could go—no apology, no sociable words of farewell from either the policeman or me.

So I got my bath, some sleep, and a good morning's rest. Betsy Copping was glad to see me and proposed an afternoon trip on the excursion boat to Nantasket—a great idea. There is something specially romantic about the combination of a pretty girl and a boat. When my train pulled out of South Station that night I was ready to forgive the Old Bay State for its officious policemen, considering that it had also produced my delightful friend.

FINDING
A CAREER

6

ASSISTANT AND INTERN

Even before I received my diploma and license to practice medicine, doors had been opened for me to three widely different careers by way of a leading American gynecological clinic, the foremost department of anatomy, and the most famous medical mission. I had put aside Grenfell's call to Newfoundland; this coming year, though I did not know it, would decide between the other two careers.

I was, of course, no stranger to the Johns Hopkins anatomical laboratory when in the fall of 1913 I took up my appointment as assistant in anatomy; I had worked there in the student's research room on my study of the development of the pancreatic ducts. Now I had a room to myself on the third floor, with a microscope and a microtome, glassware and trays, and the lesser equipment of a microscopist's laboratory. I was the youngest member of Professor Mall's staff of eight people. My teachers of four years before—Mall, Warren Lewis, Florence R. Sabin, Herbert M. Evans, Eliot R. Clark, and Charles Essick—were all still there. That fall there were also three new members, each of whom had taken his doctoral degree only a few months before. Edmond Vincent Cowdry, a Canadian trained at the University of Chicago under R. R. Bensley, was six years older than I. Having been an assistant and instructor in college biology classes while a graduate student, he ranked as associate, equivalent to assistant professor elsewhere. He was destined for a long and varied career as cytologist, pathologist, and gerontologist; he became professor of anatomy at Peking Union Medical College and later for many years was at Washington University, St. Louis. While at Johns Hopkins he continued pioneer research begun at Chicago, on mitochondria, tiny granules found in all cells of animals and plants. Cowdry was, I believe, the first Ph.D. in the Johns Hopkins anatomy department. As such, and because of his seniority and teaching experience, he was (I thought) in a kindly way rather patronizing toward me and the other new assistant, Paul G. Shipley, but he and I remained casual friends throughout his career, which ended in 1975. Shipley, a Yale M.D., was a competent anatomist but not highly original. He remained with Mall for a few years and then became a pediatrician. He died comparatively young. Essick, who left after a few years to take charge of his family's optical factory, was the only one of the group who did not continue in a research career.

Cowdry, Shipley, and I were assigned to assist Dr. Sabin in teaching the first-year course in histology. This was held three afternoons a week, in two large rooms where the students sat at their microscopes studying the tissues of the body and the cells of which they are composed. Dr. Sabin, with womanly concern for the young men working with her, would not let us do any of the chores that go with running a laboratory class. She saw to the preparation of materials used in the course, including the upkeep of the collections of sections of the various tissues and organs issued to the students for reference during the course. She also arranged for fresh tissues from the nearby slaughterhouse and from small laboratory animals that were studied in class. We assistants had only to appear in the laboratory at 2:00 P.M. on class days, ready to spend the afternoon answering the students' questions, teaching them how to stain and mount sections or to tease out bits of fresh tissue for examination under the microscope, and pointing out significant details in the sections—the give and take that make up the teaching of mature students. All of them had studied biology, some of them with America's foremost college teachers. They all knew how to use their microscopes and textbooks; some of them were older than I. I had expected that at first I might be nervous or hesitant, working with these superior young people, but such was not the case. To be well informed, accurate, clear, and concise for three hours at a stretch can be fatiguing, but I greatly enjoyed teaching and soon felt that I could succeed at it.

The histology course went on through the fall trimester and was followed in the winter trimester by the course in anatomical neurology, a study of the internal structure of the brain and spinal cord. For this course Dr. Sabin, aided by a technician, had with immense labor prepared a continuous series of cross sections of the brain stem and spinal cord, specially stained to show the nerve-cell groupings (nuclei) and fiber tracts. Each student had a set of these sections mounted on glass slides. Their study with the microscope, aided by models and charts and elucidated by Dr. Sabin's carefully prepared lectures, constituted the work of the course. I took part in teaching this subject also, having taken the course four years before, but I found the complexity of the brain more baffling than the structure of the other organs and tissues. I never gained a sense of full competence in teaching anatomical neurology like that which I had in general histology, either at Johns Hopkins or later at Berkeley and Rochester, where circumstances compelled me to take part in the instruction in neurology.

Dr. Mall expected each member of his staff to offer an elective course for a few students on some topic related to the staff member's special interests. Warren Lewis offered, for example, advanced instruction in the anatomy of the muscular system; Dr. Sabin led a group interested in the blood cells; Eliot Clark taught osteology. When Dr. Mall asked me what topic he might put me down for—these electives were listed in the school's catalogue —I said that I would like to offer a dozen weekly sessions on the history of anatomy. Obviously surprised, he said dubiously that I would not have many applicants. His manner suggested that this was a kind way of expressing doubt as to my qualifications for such a program. He did not know how many hours I had stolen from other reading to examine the medical classics in the Warrington Dispensary collection and to burrow in Fielding Garrison's newly published *History of Medicine*, but he listed my course in the catalogue, and ten students signed up. I assigned to each the life and work of a great anatomist of the past— Galen, Vesalius, Leonardo da Vinci, William and John Hunter, Karl Ernst von Baer, and so forth. At each session the student of the day presented a half-hour sketch of his particular anatomist, and I provided continuity by discussing other workers and other discoveries in the same period. My pupils, or I might more correctly say "my fellow students," worked quite seriously on their essays. Their work and mine also was of course amateurish, but I gained a broad foundation for subsequent writing and teaching of the history of medicine. At the last session the class presented me with a copy of Sir William Osler's *Man and Medicine*, signed on the flyleaf by each member of the group.

The strength of Professor Mall's anatomy department was immediately apparent. Where else could be found under one roof nine anatomists, all competent teachers, all engaged in research, seven of whom were or would become full professors in leading universities, recognized as productive scientists by fellow anatomists around the globe? Mall himself was at that time investigating the spiral structure of the muscular walls of the heart that enables the ventricles to wring themselves empty at each beat. I used to see him in his laboratory over a steaming stewpot, boiling a heart from the dissecting room in an alkaline solution so that he could separate the layers of cardiac muscle. Warren Lewis and his talented wife, Margaret Reed Lewis, had well under way their fundamental experiments on tissue culture. Florence Sabin was studying by novel methods the embryonic development of blood cells. Herbert Evans had brought home from Freiburg Carl Goldman's spectacular method of staining the tissues of living animals with acid azo dyes and was using his bright blue rats to understand the activities of macrophage cells. Eliot Clark was studying the growth of lymphatic vessels into embryonic and regenerating tissues. Essick was working on brain structure, Cowdry was finding and describing mitochondria in various organs and tissues. Shipley was beginning to study the poison glands of a tropical toad, from which our professor of pharmacology, Dr. John J. Abel, had recently isolated a cardiac stimulant.

Four years before Dr. Mall had made me choose my own topic for research. Now, having found that I was able to find my own way, he set me a specific problem, one close to his own interests. He proposed that I should study the development of the corpus luteum of the mammalian ovary. What he had in mind can be explained quite simply even to readers with little

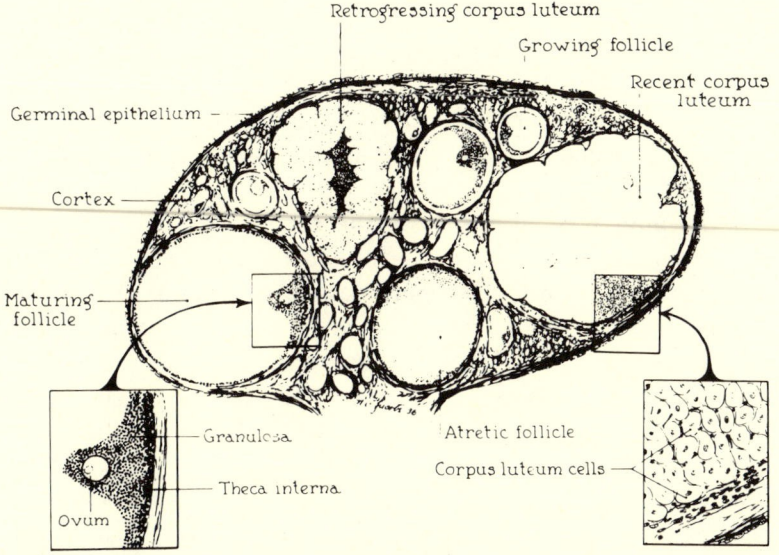

Figure 1. Diagram showing structural elements of the mammalian ovary. From G. W. Corner, "The Sites of Formation of Estrogenic Substances in the Animal Body," Physiological Reviews 18 (1938): 154.

knowledge of biology, although it called for long study and led me into thirty years of investigation of the female reproductive cycle.

The ovaries of all animals from coelenterates to our own species contain ova (egg cells) which when released and fertilized by sperm cells of the male develop into embryos. In the ovaries of mammals each ovum is enclosed by protective cells, which as the egg matures form a fluid-filled sac around it, known as a follicle (figure 1). From time to time, and in most mammals at regular cyclic intervals, the follicles (usually one at a time in women, ten or more in the sow) rapidly enlarge, rupture, and discharge the ovum into the oviduct (Fallopian tube), through which they proceed to the cavity of the uterus. If fertilized by timely mating with a male of the species, they divide into mulberry-like masses, which become hollow, attach themselves to the lining of the uterus, and develop into embryos. Meanwhile the emptied follicles do not disappear. The cells that line them greatly enlarge and fill or nearly fill the cavity, forming the corpus luteum (so-called because in some species, including the human, its cells are filled with yellow pigment). Blood capillaries spread from the follicle wall into the corpus luteum, organizing it to produce, as we now know, a potent hormone (progesterone) that prepares the lining of the uterus to receive the embryos. In pregnancy the corpora lutea persist, at least until the embryos are well developed, and in many species throughout the whole period of gestation.

Dr. Mall was interested in the corpus luteum because it seemed to offer a possible means of determining the age of early human embryos. For his embryological collection, one of the foremost in the world, he was almost daily receiving human embryos and fetuses from miscarriages, gynecological operations, and autopsies. When normal, these specimens could be ranked in order of size, but many were malformed. There was no way to date all of them precisely from the time of ovulation. It was known that domestic animals (i.e., the cow, sheep, sow, and dog) ovulate at a time closely related to estrus ("heat"), but women do not exhibit any such cyclic sexual urge. The time relation of the human cyclic phenomenon of menstruation to ovulation was not known. Since the corpus luteum begins to form immediately after ovulation, precise knowledge of the stages of its formation and development might provide a key to the age of the embryo.

So Dr. Mall gave me, to begin my study, sections of corpora lutea from a dozen cases of early pregnancy in his collection, but these told me little or nothing. The specimens had been fixed and stained with various fluids and dyes; some had been mangled by surgical procedures. At best, human material was going to be very scarce. I must build a foundation for such research by turning to some more favorable source. At Hohman's slaughterhouse two or three blocks away from our laboratory, sows, many of them pregnant, were being butchered six days a week. Their uteri and ovaries had no commercial use and could be had for the asking. I could get them warm from the carcass and prepare the corpora lutea for microscopic study by uniform fixation and staining.

In the course of the year, from October 1913 to May 1914, I collected 128 pairs of ovaries from pregnant sows, observing and measuring the embryos and fetuses in each case. By careful study of the constituent cells of the corpus luteum I could divide my specimens into seven stages of pregnancy with sufficient reliability that I could recognize the stage from the microscopic evidence alone. This survey of the development, maturity, and ultimate degeneration at the end of 160 days (the term of gestation in the sow) was very instructive to me but did not promise much help with Mall's problem. He was especially interested in very early pregnancy. The youngest embryos of swine that I could recognize were at the stage of five somites (embryologists will understand), i.e., about twenty days after ovulation, as we now know. This limit was set by the fact that I did not know how to recognize earlier embryos. Very early embryos of ungulates (swine, sheep, cows, deer, etc.) are not spherical blastocysts like those of many other animals; they are spun out into long stringy tubes looking like threads of mucus. I did not know this, but I was in good company. The great Dr. William Harvey, discoverer of the circulation of the blood, wishing to show King Charles I how life begins in the uterus, killed several of the royal deer in the first few days after mating. When he found in their uteri only what he thought was stringy mucus, he was forced to suppose that the uterus secretes the embryos just as (he says) thoughts are secreted by the brain. Early pig embryos are similar to those of deer; I, too, did not recognize them, so I could not seriate my earliest corpora lutea by comparison with corresponding embryos. This had to wait for a later stage of my own development.

Dr. Mall thought my monograph "The Corpus Luteum of Pregnancy As It Is in Swine" worth publishing and allowed me again the services of the skilled illustrator Alice Haswell. Mall, having very recently been enabled by the Carnegie Institution of Washington to organize alongside his Johns Hopkins department a Carnegie department of embryology, had begun a handsome series of monographs entitled *Contributions to Embryology*. My article was printed as number 5 of the first volume, in which number 1 was written by Dr. Mall himself— high company, I thought, for a mere assistant in anatomy.

I sent a longhand preliminary draft of the article to my friend Betsy Copping, with some trepidation because in those still prudish days she might regard ovaries, uteri, and pregnancy as topics unfit for the eyes of a modest young woman. In fact she wrote without any sign of embarrassment that she had read the draft—the first formal scientific report she had ever seen—with admiration of what she was pleased to call my accomplishment in research.

In spite, however, of the approval of the two people whose opinion meant most to me—the professor and the schoolmistress—this monograph, of all my 240 papers in scientific and scholarly journals, is the one I would now most willingly see blotted out. It added little to knowledge of the sow's reproductive cycle; it did not support Mall's notion about dating early human embryos, which indeed I had come to consider impractical. Although my description of the lutein cells at the various stages of pregnancy had been based on current methods of European investigators, the cytology of the day was soon to be superseded by new concepts. While making the study, however, I had learned much. I had chanced to begin my study of the mammalian female reproductive cycle with a species whose cycle turned out to be so comprehensible as to constitute a model against which to compare the more complex cycles of other species on which I was later to work. The familiarity I had gained with the gross appearance and structural details of the sow's ovary was of immense value to me six or seven years later when I studied prenatal mortality in swine and when I worked out the entire reproductive cycle of the sow, and later still, when I began a successful effort to isolate the hormone of the corpus luteum. The year with Mall and his distinguished colleagues had enhanced my self-confidence; it had shown me that I was capable of using the techniques of anatomical research and that I could teach medical students with some measure of success and much personal satisfaction.

In the Christmas week of 1913, the American Association of Anatomists held its annual meeting in Philadelphia at the University of Pennsylvania. I qualified as a researcher when I reported the results of my research of the past four years on the structural unit of the pancreas and the development of the duct system, and I was elected a member of the association. I was to be for eight years its secretary-treasurer and for two years its president. At that time its membership was undergoing a change. The proportion of M.D.'s, who were mostly interested in practical anatomy, was diminishing, and Ph.D.'s especially trained for research were coming in. These young newcomers tended to rate themselves, as a class, superior to the M.D.'s. Four or five of them were elected members at the Philadelphia meeting, among them Davenport Hooker and Stacy Guild. A decade later, when Guild and I were both associate professors at Johns Hopkins, Stacy told me that in 1913 Hooker and he, discussing the new members, agreed that Corner was a promising young chap, even though he was only an M.D.

In the spring of 1914 my thoughts were much on Betsy Copping, whose letters continued to arrive every few days. I realized that I had quite fallen in love with the image they presented of a charming and intelligent young woman, reinforcing my memories of her as I had seen her at Battle Harbor and in those brief meetings in Boston on my trips to and from Labrador. How she felt about me I could not be sure. Her letters and mine had remained on the level of warm friendship; for all I knew, that might be all she had in mind. I might even have New England rivals for her affection. As for me, pen and paper could no longer suffice. I must go to see her and find out and, if the signs were propitious, offer myself as a formal suitor. For this campaign I had the summer before me; my internship would not begin until September. All I needed was a plausible excuse to be somewhere near her parents' home in southern New Hampshire, to which she would return when school was over, and a little cash for travel. I got a list of summer camps in southern Maine and was soon signed up as camp physician by Camp Kineo on Long Lake, near Harrison, Maine, about sixty miles from the parsonage at the mill town of Salmon Falls. Betsy had chosen another setting, however. When I wrote she said that she would be happy to have me visit her, but she had made plans for a quiet vacation at rural Tamworth, New Hampshire, where an old friend, a Mrs. Hoag, took boarders. If I cared to come there on my way to Camp Kineo, Mrs. Hoag would be glad to have me stay at her house.

I arrived at Tamworth on a Friday afternoon in early June. It was indeed a romantic place, a village of white clapboard houses on a little stream in a valley between the Sandwich range and the Ossipee Mountains. Betsy and I were Mrs. Hoag's only guests so early in the season.

On Saturday, as Betsy had planned, we took a long walk part way up Mt. Chocorua and had lunch at a little place on the mountainside. It was a fine day, the mountain views were lovely, the lunch good, my companion altogether charming. We were so happy together that I could not risk prematurely voicing my heart's desire; if she said me nay, how dismal would be the rest of my visit! Returning to Tamworth later in the afternoon, we found the valley road along the brook very dusty; we were thirsty but, having no cups, must perforce dip the cool water with our hands. Kneeling together by the brook, side by side and almost cheek by cheek, to satisfy mutual need, I felt as if we were joining in a primal rite of spring. I might have spoken then; I could have put an arm around her and like a lover in some romantic novel have uttered passionate words of undying affection. But the words failed me—and again, what if she said no? Betsy, I think, had been sharing my romantic mood and was disappointed when I let the precious moment slip, for after we rose and resumed our route to the village, her gay chatter gave way to wistfulness; we talked of only trivial things. But before we parted in the evening she asked me to go to church with her the next morning.

The church was all a meetinghouse should be, bright in the summer air. June flowers brought from village gardens adorned the chancel. The people were reverent, the hymns well sung, the preacher eloquent. He spoke of our hopes of Paradise; to sit beside Betsy in the pew and hear her sweet voice mingling with the village choir was heaven enough for me. When our hands touched as we two shared the hymnal, I saw a sudden blush on her cheek and heard a quaver in her voice that told me her thoughts were less on heaven than on me.

When the last amen had died to silence and all the church-door greetings had been said, a cloud had hidden the sun and a light rain was falling. But when I suggested that we should walk for a while along the valley road, Betsy was willing. "I have my umbrella," she said, "and you shall be my rain-beau." When we had passed beyond the village and were alone on the road, walking close together beneath her umbrella, all my reticence forgotten, all rhetoric foregone, I told her in plain words that I loved her deeply and asked if I had a chance to win her for my own. She scarcely waited for my words to end. "Of course you have," she said, and said no more. I, too, said no more; what more to say? The words we each had longed for had been spoken, our hearts were filled with thoughts too deep for words. We walked on together in silence until it was time to return to Mrs. Hoag's for midday dinner. Those few words had sealed our betrothal and pledged us to a marriage that was to come sooner than we thought and lasted for more than sixty years.

The next day was rainy, and we spent most of it in Mrs. Hoag's sitting room, getting reacquainted with each other in our new relationship. I had brought along my cherished volume of poems by the English physician-poet Robert Bridges and read to my fiancée some of his beautiful love lyrics. We talked bravely of a long engagement; I would work hard during my internship, hoping to be chosen for the residency, which meant a wait of five years before we could marry; house staff appointments at Johns Hopkins Hospital were for single men only. Betsy would continue teaching school. She had been asked to be principal of the small public school at Salmon Falls, but she did not wish to live at home and preferred to continue teaching the first grade at Methuen. On Tuesday, coming down from the clouds of romance, I reluctantly left her to join the Kineo campers on their way to Long Lake.

On the whole the summer was pleasant enough and a good preparation for the arduous year ahead of me, but I did not see Betsy as often as I had hoped. She came once to the nearest railway station to meet me, and we dined happily together at a nearby restaurant. When camp broke up in mid-August, I was invited to stay at the Salmon Falls parsonage for a few days, where I at last met my reverend father-in-law to be, a gentle spirit and a liberal, thoughtful preacher—and his wife, not as contented as he with life in a village parish, but a devoted housewife skilled at making both ends meet. Seemingly satisfied with Betsy's choice of a future husband, they both gave me a kindly welcome.

The department of gynecology of the Johns Hopkins Medical School and Hospital, when I joined it in September 1914, as one of three incoming interns, was staffed by highly competent men. Howard Atwood Kelly, its chief, and Thomas S. Cullen, his senior colleague, were not only expert surgeons—Dr. Kelly was the most dexterous operator I have ever seen—but also accomplished pathologists and diagnosticians with wide-ranging experience in female urology and abdominal, as well as pelvic, surgery. Their textbooks and monographs were known around the world. Both of these eminent men had active practices in the city, Dr. Kelly at his private sanitarium on Eutaw Place and Dr. Cullen at the Church Home, a few blocks down Broadway from the Johns Hopkins Hospital. We saw little of them except in the operating room. Other visiting surgeons on Kelly's staff were Guy L. Hunner and W. W. Russell, also practitioners in the city. The resident gynecologist that year was James Craig Neel, four years out of medical school and already a masterly surgeon; his assistant residents were, in descending order of seniority, Veeder N. Leonard, William Dunn, and my classmate Walter Holmes. The two other interns were Hugh M. N. Wynne and Leslie Redelings. Both these immediate colleagues of mine went on to long careers in practice and part-time teaching of gynecology in medical schools, Redelings at San Diego and Wynne at Minneapolis.

The intern's duties were numerous and varied, lasting from before breakfast to late evening. He had immediate charge of the medical work on a public ward, with responsibility for the general care of the patients, although his head nurse had much to teach him and could be a wise adviser in times of perplexity. The patients saw more of the intern than of his superiors on the staff, and thus he was their principal source of information, the recipient of their confidences and complaints and often of their gratitude. A woman leaving my ward after recovering from a major operation at which I had been the third assistant said: "Goodbye, Doctor. Next to God and Dr. Kelly, I owe my life to you." "Yes," I said modestly, "we were a good team."

We interns were in the operating room every morning, five or six days a week, from eight o'clock until noon and at any hour when an emergency case took precedence over all other duties. The rest of the day we were occupied on our respective wards. During the greater part of my intern year I had charge of Ward H, for white women. Before breakfast I made a quick round of the ward with a nurse and after lunch began the day's routine. I greeted each new patient on arrival and questioned her about her general medical history and present illness, writing the story down on the official forms as part of the patient's permanent record. We had of course been trained in history taking as students on the medical and surgical wards, but gynecological histories present special problems. In the first place they call urgently for tact. One has to ask very intimate questions. One of my first patients exclaimed, "Doctor, you look so young, but you know all about women."

Then there was the matter of foreign languages. My German was good enough for the purpose; my college Latin helped a little to decipher broken English interspersed with Italian or Spanish; but I was completely stumped by a woman who spoke only Lithuanian. No bilingual visitors turned up to help me. Finally I found on one of the medical wards a woman patient who spoke German and Lithuanian but no English. Since she was not confined to bed, I took her to the bedside of my patient, where I framed my questions in German; the interpreter translated the German into Lithuanian, in which tongue the patient replied; the story came back through the reverse stages, and I wrote it down in English. Fortunately the patient's ailment was diagnosable by the physical signs, which supported what I had learned by the trilingual interview. When she was convalescing from her operation I reviewed the history with a niece who came to visit her and found we had elicited the relevant facts.

After taking a new patient's history, with stethoscope at hand I made a careful physical examination, including the pelvic region, in the presence of a nurse. I made the necessary blood-cell counts and tested the urine for albumin and blood. With all this information in hand and duly recorded, I then made my provisional diagnosis, to be checked by my immediate supervisor, an assistant resident, and by either the resident or one of the senior visiting men.

Since nearly all our patients required surgical operations, and because in those days we did not send them home as soon as is now the practice, the intern got to know and understand them. Late one evening the night nurse called me in great alarm, saying that one of our patients had suddenly become paralyzed. Hastily dressing and going to the ward, I found the young woman lying stiffly in bed, unable to move her legs and badly frightened. I could find no physical reason for her inability to move her legs. The knee jerks were active and so was the Babinski sign (toe reflex) in both feet. The nerve pathways from skin to spinal cord and back to the muscles were therefore intact, and so evidently were the muscles of the limbs. This was a clear case of psychogenic paralysis, something I had read about but never seen. In this case I could well understand the situation. The patient had come to the hospital ten days before, suffering with a very extensive and painful ulceration of her urinary bladder, for which she had undergone, elsewhere, lengthy and unskillful treatment. Craig Neel had taken special interest in the case, but improvement was initially slow. She was discouraged and worn out by long suffering. That night, waking from sound sleep she felt her legs tingling and her knee joints stiff and concluded that she had been paralyzed. All she needed was sympathy, positive assurance that the paralysis would wear off, and a dose of phenobarbital to quiet her alarm.

Another unhappy patient gave me a bad half-hour. This was a mountaineer woman from a remote valley in West Virginia who had been brought to the hospital and left there alone. Advised that she needed an operation for a pelvic disorder that had caused her severe backache but did not threaten life, she broke down in fear of the knife, decided to go home, and insisted on having her street clothes brought. The head nurse's arguments were unavailing. There was no legal way to restrain her, but while she was dressing I was summoned. Rejecting my advice she left the ward, descended the stairs to the long corridor with me holding onto her sleeve, still trying to persuade her to return to the ward. At the front entrance on Broadway, as a last resort, I left her beside the doorman and hurried back to the office of Dr. Ralph B. Seem, assistant superintendent of the hospital. To my breathless appeal for help, he said with a derisive grin, "She's your patient, Doctor." By the time I got back to the front door she had disappeared. We never heard from her again. I suppose the police picked her up and sent her home.

I happened to notice one day that among the twenty patients on my ward there were natives of ten different European and American countries. A whim seized me that on my nightly round I would bid each good night in her native tongue. So, beginning with those whose languages I had studied in school, I got the others—the Italian, the Pole, the Czech, and the rest—to teach me the words for "good night" in their respective tongues. Thereafter I recited the appropriate phrase at each bedside as I made, with the night nurse, my last round of the day. There was at first nothing more to this routine than a bit of boyish showing-off and the hope of getting some of the patients to sleep with a laugh instead of groans or the tears of loneliness. I soon found that the salutation was something more than a jest. These women, lying in two rows of identical beds along the ward, were touched by the individual greeting, and each was set apart, if only a little, as a person in her own right. In the case of one who was difficult to handle, the simple formula of "Buena noche, señora" helped to break down fear and let us ultimately bring some comfort to the hurt spirit as well as the body.

In the operating room we had a continuous sequence of patients mostly with the familiar gynecological conditions—pelvic inflammatory disease, fibroid tumors of the uterus, carcinomata, ovarian tumors, tubal pregnancies, relaxed pelvic outlets. The work would have been monotonous except that people's ailments, like other aspects of their personalities, are never quite the same in any two people. It was always instructive, of course, as we assisted master surgeons, to watch them at work. Dr. Kelly's well-known evangelical religious views gave rise to apocryphal stories about him, for instance, that he prayed for each patient before an operation. If so, he did it inaudibly and invisibly; I once heard him ask an assistant resident to close an operative incision so that he (Dr. Kelly) could have a little time before the next operation to go over his notes for his Bible class meeting that evening, but I never saw him pray in the operating room. I think the story arose from the sight of us all before an operation, each man bowed over a rectangular basin of mercuric chloride solution with folded arms in the fluid. Incidentally, this practice and the previous hard scrubbing of our hands with green soap and brush caused a rash on my sensitive skin, so that for some weeks I could not scrub up for operations and served as anesthetist instead, administering nitrous oxide gas for brief operations, ether for long ones. Nowadays interns have been relieved of that duty, which has been taken over by specialists. I fortunately had no ill success or alarms in the series of two or three hundred patients I anesthetized. The only really worrisome case was that of a doctor's wife whose husband was permitted to witness the operation but, knowing that Dr. Kelly's experience with the knife could be trusted, chose to stand by me, watching my every movement.

For my worst embarrassment in the operating room, I take

some credit to myself even though at the critical moment it involved what looked like flagrant disrespect for my distinguished chief. He was operating before a group of students and visiting M.D.'s, on a woman who had an immense unilocular ovarian cyst holding about a gallon of fluid. I was the lowest member of the team, standing opposite Dr. Kelly to pass instruments and thread needles. At his side stood an assistant resident, Walter Holmes. The tumor was flabby and heavy, like a rubber hot water bag, but with much thinner walls, in places paper thin, and was densely adherent to the surrounding pelvis and lower abdomen. Dr. Kelly with consummate skill had freed the top and sides and was working his way between the tumor and the underlying ureters and great vessels. To get better visibility and more working space, he told Holmes and me to put our outstretched gloved hands under the tumor and lift it a little. As he was finally cutting it away, I saw to my horror a tiny rip at the top of the sac, through which a few drops of fluid were exuding. We had been taught that ovarian cyst fluid sometimes contains malignant cells. It must not be allowed to drip into the patient's body. A moment later Dr. Kelly cut the tumor free. There was a surge of fluid in the flabby sac and the rip widened. A trickle of fluid started down the side of the tumor. I had to act instantly. There was no time to ask Dr. Kelly for instructions or arrange a procedure with Walter Holmes. I pushed my hands farther under the slithery cyst, taking full control of its weight, and with a sudden heave flung it out of the field of operation, over the edge of the table, and squarely onto the slightly prominent abdomen of Howard Atwood Kelly, world-famous professor of gynecology in the Johns Hopkins University. The tepid muddy fluid drenched him from the waist down.

For a tense moment, I saw over the professor's mask a pair of wrathful eyes, but quickly realizing why I had done it, he turned toward the watchers in the stand and mildly said, "The doctor thinks I didn't have my shower bath this morning."

One morning in the spring of 1915, Dr. Kelly had finished his own operations and had gone elsewhere in the hospital to visit the convalescents while the resident's team operated on a woman from a public ward. In spite of his skill, Neel found himself in trouble. The patient's internal condition was much worse than expected; Neel had a large task of excision and repair. Two hours went by, and the patient began to weaken. The anesthetist—that was my part in the team—found it necessary to warn Dr. Neel to hurry, but Neel could not hurry. The pulse became so weak and rapid that I could not count it. The usual precautions against shock, such as we had then, were instituted, and we all worked on in grim silence broken only by Neel's worried inquiries to me about the patient's condition and my doubtful replies. The students were getting restless in the stands. In short, we were almost dangerously rattled, when the door opened and in came Dr. Kelly. "How are you getting on?" he asked. "Badly," said Neel. "I'm afraid we're going to lose her; wouldn't you like to scrub up and help me?"—a suggestion that would have cost a precious ten minutes at least. By this time Dr. Kelly was behind Neel looking over his shoulder. "Oh, no," he said. "You are doing an excellent piece of work. I can't add anything. You have a hard job there, Doctor, but that's the way I'd do it myself."

He came to the head of the table and asked me about the pulse. "One hundred and eighty," I said, "the last time I could count it." "Yes," said Dr. Kelly, taking the pulse himself, "I can barely feel it. I see you're doing all the right things," and then to the students, "The doctor is giving a very nice anesthesia; you'd do well to study the chart afterward." I don't remember that he said anything more. He remained a quarter of an hour calmly watching us work and then paid Neel the best compliment of all: he went out of the operating room and disappeared, leaving behind him five young men who felt as if they had been knighted on the field of battle. If we were to lose our patient on the table, the chief was witness that we had made a valiant fight. But we did not lose her, and a month later she was well.

Another day, Dr. Kelly had finished the removal of a fibroid tumor of the uterus, having passed all but the last stage of closing gaps in the pelvic peritoneum and suturing the abdominal incision. Wishing to leave to keep an appointment, he asked his first assistant, William Dunn, one of the assistant residents, to finish the operation. Dunn was a good surgeon, but he had a slight mishap; with his suture needle he accidentally punctured a vein under the peritoneum. The escaping blood made a pool that began to spread widely, raising the peritoneum over it like a large blood blister. Dunn, taking alarm, tried to clamp the bleb, but it continued to spread. Without warning he suddenly fainted, falling forward over the patient's body. The operating room orderly coolly stepped forward and dragged Dunn out of the room. Walter Holmes, the third assistant resident, in his second year out of medical school, who had been assisting Dunn, was now for the first time in his life in responsible charge of an operation. He took the operator's place, punctured the swelling hematoma with the point of a knife, mopped up its contents, found the bleeding point, tied it off, and calmly proceeded to close the incision. As anesthetist I watched with admiration this superbly competent action of my former classmate. Holmes after his residency became the leading gynecologist in Atlanta, Georgia.

Our work tied us closely to the hospital. Every Sunday one of the three interns had the afternoon off. I, of course, went to Roland Park to dine with my family. Occasionally when the wards were quiet one of us would take care of two wards, allowing a fellow intern to have a free evening. My greatest pleasure was given me by Betsy Copping's letters, arriving every day or two, more delightful than ever, now that she could freely express her love for me and her hope for our future together.

One evening when I was sitting in my room writing to Betsy, there was a knock on my door and in came Dr. Frank R. Smith, a middle-aged physician of English birth who was acting editor of the *Bulletin of the Johns Hopkins Hospital,* a monthly journal of considerable distinction (now called the *Johns Hopkins Medical Journal*). He was an experienced editor; Sir William Osler had trusted him for editorial advice on the original draft of his famous *Principles and Practice of Medicine.* Dr. Smith had in his hand my submission to the journal, the manuscript on theriac and mithridatium. He gave me a masterly demonstration of editorial skill, cutting a phrase here, bettering one there, deleting fancy passages; in short, making my article shipshape. Leaving with a compliment on what he kindly called a good piece of work, he carried the improved draft away, ready for the press. It appeared, my fifth paper and first historical essay, in the *Bulletin of the Johns Hopkins Hospital,* volume 26, June 1915, and was reprinted in the *University of California Chronicle,* volume 28, number 1, 1915.

A couple of weeks after the appearance of the article in the

Bulletin I received an envelope from my fiancée stuffed with a two-column clipping from the *Boston Transcript,* giving an enthusiastic account by a columnist of a remarkably interesting story of two ancient drugs written by a young doctor at Johns Hopkins. How that journalist (bless him!) found it I could not imagine. For me this was nothing short of an accolade. The Saturday *Transcript* was the nearest thing, in 1915, to the literary and artistic Sunday supplements of city newspapers today. In the Salmon Falls parsonage it was esteemed second only to the Bible. That Betsy's young man had won the *Transcript*'s august praise was final evidence to the elder Coppings that their daughter had made no mistake in choosing a mate.

As the year went on, I began to feel that Dr. Mall was right when he declared that gynecology needed stimulation from the anatomical and physiological sciences. In Dr. Kelly's operating room and classrooms I had observed that the technically skilled members of his staff had surprisingly little acquaintance with the physiology of the human female reproductive cycle. With all their competence in surgical excision and repair, they were unable to treat rationally the functional disorders of the female reproductive system—menstrual irregularity, dysmenorrhea, and sterility. Indeed, they did not understand the normal reproductive cycle, since (as I noted above) no one knew when in the human cycle ovulation occurs, what is the function of the periodically recurring corpus luteum, or just when an embryo implants itself in the uterus.

British zoologists had been writing on the ovarian cycles of the rabbit and the bitch. In St. Louis, Leo Loeb, a pathologist, was explaining the guinea pig's cycle. In French, German, and Austrian laboratories and clinics, evidence was appearing that there must be at least one and maybe two ovarian hormones that control the estrous cycle of animals and the human menstrual cycle. Yet little of this new and still partly confusing information had reached American gynecologists.

My studies of the past year had given me ideas as to how I might begin research on the human cycle. I asked Tom Cullen whether Dr. Kelly would consider giving me a special opportunity to combine clinical training with laboratory research, perhaps half-time for each. I put the same questions to Morris

Slemons, who was about to go from Johns Hopkins to the University of California as professor of obstetrics and gynecology, and I even wrote to William P. Graves, professor of gynecology at Harvard. To all these senior men my proposal evidently seemed preposterous. I suppose that in fact it was preposterous for a young man of twenty-five, and a mere intern, to propose himself as a scientific investigator.

One day in the late spring of 1915, while writing up some notes in my little office on Ward H, I had a visit from Herbert Evans, whom I had come to regard as one of the ablest and certainly the most brilliant of Mall's staff. During my year in his daily company he had been very friendly and encouraging about my research. He had come to tell me that he had been called to his native state as professor of anatomy in the medical faculty of the University of California at Berkeley and to offer me an instructorship in his department. When I replied that I had reason to think that I would be chosen to remain on Dr. Kelly's house staff as third assistant resident and ultimately chief resident, Evans said, "Why not come with me and do your gynecology on rats and rabbits?" This was obviously an answer to the problem I had been wrestling with, and to me a very tempting answer, with its combination of freedom to pursue research with the opportunity to see a distant and marvelous part of our country. When I sought Dr. Mall's advice, he was not enthusiastic. He did not think highly of the western universities and said that since I was eligible for an instructorship in the East, the University of California should offer me the next higher rank, an assistant professorship. Evans promptly wrote to Berkeley and was authorized to do just that, at a salary of $1,500 for the first year with an annual increase of $200 per year for four years.

For further advice I asked for an appointment with our austere professor of surgery, William S. Halsted, who was well acquainted with Herbert Evans. Dr. Halsted received me most kindly one evening in the study of his house on Eutaw Place. Telling me about his own desire as a young man for a career in research, for which there was in his day no opportunity in American medicine, he said that if at my age he could have had such a chance as I now had to join Evans at Berkeley, he would have accepted it without question.

Betsy Copping must of course be consulted. She had taken

it for granted that she was to marry a gynecologist; would she want a scientist instead? Her reply was prompt and definite; of course I should go to California. She would look forward to joining me there as soon as we could afford to marry.

As the time for decision neared, looking back over the past two years I knew that for me the call of the laboratory was stronger than that of the clinic. I had enjoyed the skillful teamwork of the operating room and the satisfaction of being directly helpful to ailing people, but I had enjoyed still more the previous year of intensive research and teaching. Whichever career I now chose would bring increasing lifetime responsibilities. I was not quite sure that I could carry happily and well the surgeon's burden of immediate decision and irrevocable action; I could more confidently undertake the no less weighty, though not so conspicuous, responsibilities of the scientist-teacher—unswerving devotion to the search for knowledge, faithful guidance of younger intellects. I accepted Evans's offer with a comfortable feeling that I had found the way to a career.

SCIENTIST
AND
TEACHER

7

ASSISTANT PROFESSOR

Until I went to Berkeley in 1915 I had never been west of the Allegheny Mountains. I therefore planned my railway journey to include interesting cities and scenery—a day in Chicago, a few days in Colorado, a day at Salt Lake City, passage through the Rocky Mountains by the Royal Gorge route and through the Sierra Nevada by the rugged canyon of the American River. During my three-day stopover in Colorado, after marveling at the fantastic rock formations in the Garden of the Gods near Colorado Springs, I took the mountain railway to the summit of Pike's Peak (14,100 feet). It was a cloudless late summer day, the air was warm but clear, and the famous view from the mountain-top, a hundred miles in every direction, was at its best. With a small-scale map of the region in my copy of Baedeker's U.S. guidebook, I could identify towns and villages far below me. Conspicuous to the southwest was Cripple Creek, ten miles away and 5,000 feet down. A trail from the rounded top of the mountain invitingly appeared to lead directly to it. I rashly decided to descend the mountain on foot. I was of course not dressed for mountaineering and wore ordinary low shoes, but the route looked so open that I felt sure I could make it safely to Cripple Creek. A hundred yards below the summit a drift of the last winter's snow covered the trail, but I trudged through it and went on. The path was rough but not really difficult; the southern slope of the mountain was not dangerously steep. I had at first a thrilling sense of solitary adventure and delight in the thin pure air, but as the trail widened and became a roadway, my head began to ache. By the time I reached Cripple Creek I was in the throes of a sick headache. At the railway station I was lucky enough to find a train about to depart for Colorado Springs, where I was staying for another night. The close air of the railway coach upset my stomach. I went out on the rear platform, sat on the floor and vomited intermittently during the swaying, rattling one-hour trip down to Colorado Springs. I spent the next day quietly getting over the effects of my reckless venture and was able to enjoy the magnificent scenery along the rest of the journey.

Arriving at the Berkeley campus on a bright September morning, I checked in at the faculty club, where I was to reside —a cozy-looking building half-hidden among live oaks in the Faculty Glade, a green oasis in the heart of the sun-baked campus. Storing my luggage there, I walked over to the nearby anatomical laboratory and reported to Professor Evans. The two-story frame building beneath tall eucalyptus trees, looking more like a little farmhouse than a scientific laboratory, contrasted oddly with its neighbors, the high, gawky Victorian Mechanic Arts Building and the handsome modern Hearst Hall of Mines. The laboratory had been the university's printing shop until 1906, when the San Francisco earthquake and fire of that year forced the removal of the preclinical laboratories to Berkeley. The interior had been partitioned into dissecting rooms, a class laboratory for histology, and a few private laboratory rooms and offices. It seemed, as I saw it with Evans, an incongruous setting for the handsome, intense, and ambitious young professor who had undertaken to make it a center of first-line research and modern teaching.

The department had limped along without a strong leader for several years. One or two junior members had left, and another was on sick leave from which he would not return. Only two qualified teachers remained, Robert Orton Moody, the acting head, a middle-aged man capable of teaching routine human anatomy and nothing more, and Philip E. Smith, a Cornell Ph.D. of 1912, who was to prove himself exceedingly able when freed from the burden of teaching in a shorthanded department under uninspiring leadership. Dr. Evans planned to have Moody and Smith carry on the teaching of gross human anatomy while he began building up the courses of histology and neurology under his own direction, with my help and that of another newcomer, Katherine J. Scott, a Johns Hopkins M.D. of 1915.

The entering class of medical students numbered forty, including two or three young women. The entrance requirements, as at most of the American medical schools in that period, were lower than those of Johns Hopkins, since the bachelor's degree was not required, but the level of competence was quite high, and some of our best students were outstandingly able. Among those with whom I formed special friendships during my four years at Berkeley were Elmer Belt, who became California's most distinguished urologist, very influential in the state's medical affairs, and Harry P. Smith, who became professor of pathology at Columbia University. These were both in the first class that Evans and I taught; later came Irvine McQuarrie, destined to be professor of pediatrics at the University of Minnesota. Two of our young men went on to be deans of the University of California's two medical schools, Stafford L. Warren at Los Angeles and Francis Smith at San Francisco and Berkeley.

Evans's histology course, which he based as much as possible on fresh tissues and physiological concepts, was to me even more exciting than Florence Sabin's at Baltimore had been. He delivered his weekly lectures in a fluent and somewhat high-flown style, as if he were conscious of his own brilliance. He told me that in his teaching he aimed at the most intelligent 10 percent of the class; he felt no obligation to cater to the rest. This suggested to me (though I did not say so to him) that Katherine Scott and I would have to look after the other thirty-six students. At any rate, Elmer Belt, one of the privileged 10 percent of that first class, wrote years later of Evans and his young associates:

> The effect of their scholarship and idealism upon the freshman class in medicine was electric. Each of us realized how great an opportunity it was to enter the study of medicine under their guidance and for us the study of medicine became an obsession. The routine work of gross dissection and histology was time-consuming but most of us, in addition, were stimulated to take up a separate problem in research. We were thus led to seek out and read recent contributions to the literature concerned with our special subjects. This pursuit inevitably led us to doubt didactic textbook statements unless verified by our own personal observations. This atmosphere of doubt and verification prevailed throughout the depart-

ment and led to intense application. For most of us this was our first taste of scholarly research.[1]

Departmental administration was for Herbert Evans a duty reluctantly borne. His compulsive urge to work intensively at research led him to put off administrative routine, the writing of articles against deadlines, and other less congenial tasks until the last minute. Thus the course of departmental affairs was interrupted from time to time by minor, or even major, crises. One of these in the early Berkeley days, somewhat mysterious to Evans's associates, evidently caused him deep concern. He and his secretary for several days were intently busy, occupied with account books and the adding machine. Evans's brother, a businessman familiar with accounting, was called in; there were urgent messages to and from the university bursar's office. Probably the professor had overrun his budget.

On another occasion he was overtaken by the deadline for an article long promised to an eastern scientific journal. In despair he retired to his study at home, sent for the secretary and her typewriter, and dictated hectically for three or four days. Typed sheets were sent up to the laboratory to be proofread by me. The manuscript was assembled at home as the last pages were being typed, while Mrs. Evans sat in the family car at the door, ready to dash to the Berkeley Southern Pacific station to get the parcel on the Overland Limited for Chicago and the East.

Under Evans's enthusiastic leadership the department was soon buzzing with research, although during the four years I was with him in Berkeley, Evans himself put out no such flow of scientific publications as later from 1920 on, when every year until 1950 saw the appearance of one to ten articles by him alone or with associates. Busy with administrative tasks, he published only one article between 1915 and 1919, and that one reported results obtained earlier in Baltimore. He was, however, working daily in his laboratory, on two important topics. Katherine Scott, to whom he had suggested an intensive comparative study of the two chief cellular components of areolar connective tissue, fibroblasts and macrophages, was making little progress until

1. Elmer Belt, "Medicine," in *There was light: Autobiography of a University,* ed. Irvine Stone (New York, 1970), p. 35.

Evans took over a share of the work, somewhat to her discomfiture. Their joint effort resulted in a distinguished monograph published in 1920. Another cooperative undertaking was even more fruitful. Joseph A. Long of the department of zoology, a Harvard-trained embryologist, had been working for some years on the reproductive cycle of the albino rat, using an ingenious but inadequate method which seemed to indicate that ovulation occurred every eleven days. Evans joined Long, introducing a new test for ovulation based on Stockard and Papanicolaou's work on the guinea pig at Cornell Medical School in New York city. The joint report of Long and Evans in 1922, "The Oestrous Cycle of the Rat" (Evans insisted on putting Long's name first), not only laid the foundation for Evans's massive future researches on vitamin E but also promoted the use of the albino rat for the investigation of endocrine and nutritional problems by scientists all over the world.

Philip Smith had for some years been struggling under an overload of teaching, trying to get ahead with an experimental study of the functions of the hypophysis (pituitary gland) using the larvae of a California frog. He was still only an instructor; although he was five years older than I, I outranked him. Evans gave Smith the relatively light assignment of assisting Dr. Moody in the dissecting rooms and, when his research in the ensuing years began to succeed brilliantly, got him promoted to assistant professor. Before long Smith, provided by Evans with facilities for using rats, had worked out a method for ablating the rat's hypophysis and was on the road to international recognition as an endocrinologist.

For me also Evans provided material help in getting a research program under way. I wanted to solve some of the problems of the female reproductive cycle that had baffled me in Baltimore, particularly that of discovering the time relation of ovulation to the external signs of the cycle in swine, namely estrus or "heat." Fortunately there was a small slaughterhouse in West Berkeley, easily reached from the university campus. Evans persuaded its manager to build a little shack for me on the killing floor, with a shelf for my instruments and a few bottles of reagents and a little space for handling uteri and ovaries. By sheer luck for me, local conditions in the pork industry caused the management to hold each consignment of pigs for a few days before slaughtering. One of the medical students, Archie Amsbaugh, volunteered to help me.

One of us went to the slaughterhouse pens every day and sat on the fence watching the sows. When one of them showed signs of estrus, nuzzling or riding other sows, we marked her by a device invented by me to avoid having to venture out in the muddy pen with the risk of being bowled over by the hefty swine. We had ready a can of white paint and a long pole with a wad of cotton waste at its tip. With this we could reach in from our post at the fence and rub the paint well into the hair on the sow's back. We also made a written memorandum of any individual markings such as a nicked ear, a lame foot, or a patch of dark hair, and we renewed the paint mark every day until that batch of hogs went to the killing floor. The management of the slaughterhouse was very helpful, even to the point of butchering a few sows out of the regular order to give us needed stages of the cycle.

In this way we collected a series of ovaries from each of the usual three days of estrus and up to a week after its onset. I found, more precisely than any previous investigator, that ovulation occurs on the first or second day of estrus, and is spontaneous, i.e., does not depend on coitus with a male, as in the rabbit. I learned what the ovarian follicles are like just before they rupture and shed their ova into the oviduct and obtained a dated series of ruptured follicles being converted into corpora lutea. By washing out the oviducts (Fallopian tubes) with physiological salt solutions, I recovered ova just discharged from the follicles, on their way toward the uterus. I preserved pieces of the lining of the uterus for future study of the uterine cycle.

Occasionally uncastrated boars were shipped for slaughter and some of our sows had mated with them in the pens. From the oviducts of two of them I obtained fertilized eggs with spermatozoa still clinging to them. The ova of the sow are just barely visible to the unaided eye if placed in a clear fluid in a strong light. I sectioned these recently fertilized ova with a microtome into slices 10 microns thick (1/240 of an inch) and found the egg nucleus and the head of the fertilizing spermatozoon in contact and two polar bodies present (embryologists will understand). This stage of development had never been seen before in any large domestic mammal. In fact, it had been seen only in a few small mammals including the rat, mouse, guinea pig, and rabbit. The process of maturation of the fertilized ovum in swine is thus similar to that in a few other mammals in which it had been observed. Two little papers in the *Anatomical Record*, one by Corner and Amsbaugh and the other by myself alone, made known these findings to fellow scientists. The chief object of my work, a definite description of the origin of the corpus luteum, would have to await the tedious preparation of thin sections of the ruptured follicles and newly forming corpora lutea for microscopic study.

I was fascinated by the life of the vast university, in which, unlike Johns Hopkins, the undergraduates were the most conspicuous element. It was amusing to see that the women students—a handsome lot they were—dressed more formally than the girls of Goucher College in Baltimore (the only college girls I knew), whereas the California boys tended to shabby corduroy trousers and open-necked shirts. And what numbers! The freshman class alone, men and women, was much larger than the whole student body of Johns Hopkins. I visited a history class one morning, just for the spectacle of Henry Morse Stephens lecturing to 1,800 students in the gymnasium because there was no other hall large enough to contain them all. The male members of the freshman and sophomore classes, in uniform for the military drill required at a land-grant college, mustered a full regiment. Even more spectacular was a traditional students' frolic called the pajamarino rally, in which all the college men paraded to the Greek Theater by torchlight, every man clad in pajamas. Our medical students had of course outgrown collegiate larks; they were a serious lot, but rather less awed by young faculty men like me than were the first-year medical students in Baltimore. One of the medical fraternities, to which Elmer Belt and Harry Smith belonged, made me an honorary member early in the fall.

At the faculty club also I was made to feel at home by friendships quickly formed with some of the bachelors who roomed there. Two men became special friends. George Boas, two years younger than I, trained at Brown University, was serving as an instructor in public speaking while working for a doctorate in philosophy at Berkeley. A critical scholar, widely read in the humanities and one of the best conversationalists I have ever known, he kindly tolerated what must have seemed to him my naive thinking and opened for me a wide range of thoughts about the fine arts and the history of ideas. When in 1917 the United States entered World War I, George volunteered for service in France, and I saw him no more until we were both at Johns Hopkins many years later. Another friendly resident at the faculty club, George McMinn, a few years older than Boas and I, was an assistant professor of English. His special intellectual interest was the cultural history of California, which made him an instructive companion for a newcomer like me. McMinn eventually became professor of English at the California Institute of Technology at Pasadena.

These friends introduced me to the lovely forest trails of Marin County, across San Francisco Bay from Berkeley. I needed no guide to the nearby Berkeley Hills, and soon found my way up Grizzly Peak, a 1,900-foot hill just behind the university campus, with a magnificent view of San Francisco and the Golden Gate. With Boas and McMinn I went on weekend walks by way of Muir Woods to Bolinas Lagoon, where my friends knew a lady, Miss Jessica Gilfillan, who with charming courtesy took in impecunious wanderers like us at a rate, if I remember rightly, of two dollars for a perfectly appointed room, dinner, and breakfast. On one of these trips we were joined by the physical chemist Richard Tolman, already on his way to national prominence in scientific circles. Chatting about his work as we strode along the trail beneath the redwoods, Tolman spoke of Albert Einstein's new ideas—the first time I ever heard the word "relativity."

With these friends and others I spent an evening or two in San Francisco enjoying a dinner at one of its famous restaurants. The journey from Berkeley to San Francisco, whether for pleasure or business, was always exciting—a fast run by electric train to the mile-long Oakland pier, then the twenty-minute ferryboat trip across the bay, with views of San Francisco, the Golden Gate, Mount Tamalpais and, looking back, Berkeley and Oakland against their hilly backdrop. The bay bridge, grand as it is, has taken away some of the joy of crossing to San Francisco.

The Panama-Pacific Exposition was held in the year 1915 on the site of San Francisco's old fort, the Presidio. I went to the fair once or twice on Saturday afternoons but came away with only confused memories of jumbled sights and sounds. Berkeley and San Francisco were giving me all the novelty and instruction I could assimilate; I needed no such added attraction as a world's fair. Berkeley, like other university towns, offered all sorts of lectures and concerts. During my first autumn there former president Taft gave a series of lectures on the problems of the presidency. One of the best American actresses of the time, Margaret Anglin, who had for several years been putting on annually one of the great Greek tragedies in English in the Greek Theater, produced in 1915 the *Iphigenia in Aulis* of Euripides. Beautifully staged at the open-air Greek Theater and acted by a large company augmented by students for crowd scenes and soldiery, the ancient drama affected me immensely.

That autumn of 1915 was a golden time for me, living amid new and beautiful surroundings, with my teaching and research going well, a growing sense of professional competence, and new friendships with colleagues and students. But my satisfaction could not be complete without Betsy Copping at my side. Her letters, arriving every few days, gave wistful hints that she too felt the pain of our separation. I began to ask myself whether it was wise to put off our marriage any longer. Anabel Evans, my chief's wife,—knowledgeable from her own experience, advised me that Betsy and I could manage, with care, on my monthly stipend of $125, and I wrote Betsy immediately.

We set the date of Betsy's twenty-seventh birthday, December 28, 1915, for the wedding. Her parents and mine were startled when the news reached them—Mrs. Copping in particular, for she had to get her daughter's outfit ready and prepare the parsonage for the ceremony; but by Christmas she and Betsy had assembled an adequate trousseau and a beautiful wedding dress. At Berkeley I went house hunting and found a pleasant little furnished apartment on a hillside a couple of blocks north of the campus, with a wide view over the Golden Gate and Mt. Tamalpais.

I let my twenty-sixth birthday pass without ceremony and started east a few days before Christmas, this time taking the fastest trains, reaching Baltimore in three days and twenty-one hours, in time for a happy Christmas with my family. Then I went on to New Hampshire, where I stayed at the hotel in Dover, near Salmon Falls. My parents and my brother and sister followed for the events of the twenty-eighth. Aunt Rena came, too, and even Aunt Laura, in spite of her great dread of travel on sleeping cars. Betsy and I were married by her father, in the parsonage sitting room, in the presence of my relatives and a dozen of Betsy's friends. The bridesmaid was Betsy's closest friend, Katherine Carlisle, who had been at the house all morning helping Betsy pack and dress and giving moral support to Mrs. Copping. My brother was my best man. Betsy had chosen to have her father use the Episcopalian marriage service, from which she struck out the promise to obey me. She was radiant during the ceremony and the informal reception that followed. I had a feeling, not uncommon, I believe, on the bridegroom's part, of being momentarily superfluous.

That night we took the through express from Bar Harbor to Washington, which made, on request, a special stop for us at Dover. I had reserved two rooms at the Willard Hotel. Although Betsy had never been to Washington before, we were both too tired to do much sight-seeing in the two days we were there. We returned to Baltimore for my parents' reception at the Ridgewood Road house, attended by dozens of my relatives and our family friends. Among all these cordial strangers Betsy, who, I thought, might be rather overwhelmed, was charmingly sociable. I had coached her about the guests to whom she should pay special attention. She won them by recognizing them at once— Uncle John King, for example, and Aunt Molly, Aunt Janie and Aunt Mary on the Corner side—and by knowing just what to say to old family friends whose names I had taught her. At her best socially when she was in some way singled out for favorable attention, Betsy was shy only with my mother, whose dignified reserve had overawed her. I must add that in Mother's old age the two women developed warmly affectionate relations.

We took the northern route to California in order to spend three days with Betsy's brother and his family at Bozeman, Montana; thence via Portland, Oregon, to Berkeley, where Herbert Evans brought the whole anatomy department to the railway station to meet us. We had used up my vacation leave; next day I resumed my duties at the laboratory and Betsy began the wifely work of making the apartment into a home.

Since that summer of budding friendship at Battle Harbor in 1912, we had been together only a few times, for periods of a few hours to three or four days, always under the strictest conventions of the Victorian era. Even after Betsy so willingly accepted my proposal of marriage, we were shy with each other when we were alone. The farthest we had ever gone in getting physically acquainted was at the Salmon Falls parsonage during my last visit before I went to California. One night when her parents had retired, Betsy consented, after some persuasion, to sit on my knees in an easy chair, with my arm around her waist. Thus cozily disposed we went on innocently chatting. She was comfortable and happy and, I believe, would have continued the tête-à-tête well into the small hours, but I got sleepy and rising from the chair with her in my arms carried her merrily upstairs to her room, deposited her on the bed and left that maidenly sanctuary, privately wishing that I could have stayed all night.

As to sexual activity I was as virginal as my bride but much better informed, and I was aware of the need for patience and a gentle, affectionate approach. At Berkeley, on our secluded sleeping porch, her sexual diffidence was soon happily dispelled. Betsy told me that before her marriage she had no explicit knowledge of what goes on physically between husband and wife. She knew that there was some sort of intimacy but not what it might be. Such ignorance was frequent among sheltered girls in that prudish era. Given an impetuous and inconsiderate bridegroom, this could result in serious emotional shock. Remembering what Betsy told me, when I wrote my little book for adolescent girls, *Attaining Womanhood* (1939), I included a brief description of sexual intercourse. I thought myself rather daring, but the times were already changing; I never heard of any objections to my frankness.

Circumstances had led me to bring my bride to the Pacific Coast at the beginning of the rainy season, something I would not now recommend to anyone. In such weather we could not spend much time out of doors. Betsy accompanied me twice a week to the anatomical laboratory, to attend lectures I was giving on human anatomy for nonmedical students, chiefly undergraduates majoring in physical education. I thought this a good way to acquaint her more fully with my field of science. She helped me by operating my lantern-slide projector and by useful advice on my style as a lecturer. I had done well to marry a New England schoolteacher.

On Sundays we went together to the local Unitarian church near the campus, wondering a little what our respective parents would think of this deviation from trinitarian practices. The very attractive Unitarian minister, Harold E. B. Speight, was, however, soon called to a New England pastorate and later to a professorship at Dartmouth College. After he left California we joined the local Congregational church, where near the end of our stay in Berkeley I was asked, to my intense embarrassment, to be a deacon, a lay officer who among other things assisted the pastor in the communion service. My Christian faith had by that time waned so much that to accept the diaconate would have been hypocritical. My timely call back to Johns Hopkins in 1919 saved me from having to decline the appointment.

When spring arrived and the straw-colored Berkeley hills were green once more under sunny skies, we enjoyed walking along hillside trails, once or twice climbing to the steep summit of Grizzly Peak. On one fine weekend we took the ferry to Sausalito and with knapsacks on our backs ascended Mt. Tamalpais, 2,600 feet high, staying overnight at the hotel on the summit to enjoy the grand view of the distant Coast Range, the whole Bay region, and the Pacific shore.

We spent the summer vacation, July and August 1916, at Carmel, on the seacoast near Monterey, about 135 miles south of San Francisco. Founded only about ten years before by a group of artists as a rural retreat beside one of the old Spanish mission churches, Carmel was still a village. We found a room in the cottage of a kindly Scottish woman, Miss Shiel, in the woods a quarter-mile north of the post office and the little hotel. For her two only guests, Miss Shiel provided excellent meals and harmless gossip about the landscape painters and young musicians who made up the summer colony. We spent our days quietly, for Betsy was three months pregnant and very happy about it. We enjoyed sitting by the sea at Point Lobos and strolling among wild flowers along the cliffs and in a verdant canyon that comes down from the mountains to the sea a little way south of Carmel Mission. In our botanizing, a pursuit delightful to two young people in love, I was again Betsy's pupil, for she brought to Carmel a love of wild flowers and a stock of information about them gained on New England hillsides.

I had with me a box of watercolor paints that I had used in medical school to depict tissues seen under the microscope, and I tried my hand at landscapes and floral subjects—extremely amateurish things that I showed to nobody but Betsy and later to Herbert Evans, both of whom were in a kind way unencouraging, but the effort taught me to look more appreciatively at serious painting and to feel more keenly the aesthetic effects of form and color in nature; my scientific training had already taught me to look for factual values. I had also a well-worn volume of Chaucer's poems which during our vacation I read from cover to cover, marking every passage of medical interest. A notebook full of my gleanings became the source of a lecture on medicine in the poems of Chaucer that I prepared later in Rochester. The lecture proved so popular that I never published it but kept it in reserve against future invitations to speak at academic gatherings. I gave it twenty times from Berkeley to Oxford.

Before we returned to Berkeley the owner of our apartment returned to live there, and we found another home, a little rambling frame house on the south side of Strawberry Canyon behind the campus, just to the west of where the university has since built a swimming pool. The owner was George M. Stratton, professor of psychology, who was widely known for a rather bizarre experiment. He had eyeglasses made that turned his field of vision upside down, and he wore them for a long time to learn whether his brain would adapt to the situation (it did). The house in the canyon, which he himself had designed and largely built, was also topsy-turvy; it stood on a steep hillside twenty-five steps above the road, with its kitchen at a higher level than the bedrooms. Its sleeping porch was roofless; in the dry season we slept under the stars, and when the moon was full we could hear a pack of coyotes baying up in the canyon. Betsy began to fit up a small room as a nursery. As the time approached for the baby's birth she longed so much for feminine support that I sent her mother an urgent letter backed by a railway ticket, asking her to come to Berkeley and stay with us for a while.

On December 22, 1916, our son was born at the Children's Hospital, San Francisco, under the care of Dr. Frank W. Lynch, my neighbor on Jackson Place, Baltimore, when he was a medical student. Ten days later the mother and child, both in fine shape, came back to Strawberry Canyon. Mrs. Copping had to return to New Hampshire in February but wanted to see her grandson properly baptized, so we had the ceremony performed at a morning service at the First Congregational Church when the child was only six weeks old. Of course the baby had to be named for his father, grandfather, and great-grandfather. As the Reverend Mr. Brooks, a man of ample size, took the tiny infant in his arms before a large congregation and solemnly began, "George Washington, I baptize thee . . .," a ripple of quiet mirth ran through the congregation.

My duties in the department of anatomy were the same in 1916–17 as in the previous year except that at the suggestion of Professor Evans I offered an elective course in the history of anatomy like that which I had conducted at Johns Hopkins. Again I had a dozen volunteer participants. To one of them, Elmer Belt, with whom I had formed a special friendship, I assigned a paper on Leonardo da Vinci as an anatomist. Belt, who always took up with enthusiasm any task that interested him, not only wrote an excellent paper but became a lifelong student of Leonardo and his period. As he went on to become the leading urologist in Los Angeles, he assembled in the library of his private clinic an unrivaled collection of books related to Leonardo's art and scientific interests, which by his generous gift is now the Elmer Belt Library of Vinciana of the University of California at Los Angeles. He has been made an honorary citizen of Leonardo's native town, Vinci, in Tuscany. As a token of my part in starting him on his career as a bibliophile, he has recently placed in the library a replica of the bronze bust of me displayed at the American Philosophical Society. I was at first rather bashful about this association with the great Florentine artist, but thinking it over I suppose that if the comparison be limited to our respective standing as anatomists, I may accept the honor. I could at least write a more accurate textbook of anatomy than Leonardo, even if I would not be able to illustrate it as well.

My systematic visits to the West Berkeley slaughterhouse, described earlier in this chapter, had won me a series of ovaries from sows that we had observed while in estrus, and the organs were therefore dated with respect to the time of ovulation. When

I sectioned them for study under the microscope, they revealed the whole process of maturation of the graafian follicles and their conversion to corpora lutea. The origin of the corpus luteum from the inner wall of the follicle had been discussed since 1840, when modern microscopes made possible detailed comparison of cell types. Since 1900 there had been twenty-five investigations on various species, with contradictory results.

The principal question was whether the cells of the corpus luteum were derived from the inner layer of the follicle (granulosa) or from the underlying layer, the theca interna (see figure 1, in chapter 6). The question was not trivial, for the corpus luteum was evidently an organ with special functions, even though these were not yet clearly understood. My specimens gave a definite answer to the problem, at least for swine; both layers contribute to the cellular substance of the corpus luteum. Because there had been so much confusion in the literature on this problem, I worked hard on my report of results, striving to produce a clear and definitive account. The sixty-six-page article, covering the history of the subject as well as my own observations and beautifully illustrated by Ralph Sweet, an artist skilled in microscopical work, appeared in the *American Journal of Anatomy*, volume 20, in September 1919, under the title "The Origin of the Corpus Luteum of the Sow from Both Granulosa and Theca Interna." Its conclusions, so far as I know, have never been challenged. While it was in press I made an unsuccessful attempt, with Felix Hurni, an instructor in our department, to test the hypothesis that a hormone of the corpus luteum inhibits ovulation. Using only aqueous extracts of corpora lutea we obtained a negative (and incorrect) result. Fortunately for my self-esteem, the correct answer was obtained a dozen years later as a result of my joint work with Willard Allen at Rochester, N.Y., and led to the development of the birth control pill.

Also while at Berkeley I made a chemical study of the phosphatides in the corpus luteum in various stages of pregnancy, with correct but unimportant results. With a very able student, Stafford Warren, later the founding dean of the University of California's medical school at Los Angeles, I confirmed by experiments on rats Leo Loeb's discovery of 1907 that the corpus luteum is responsible for the formation of decidual tissue in the uterus in pregnancy. After F. P. Mall's untimely death in 1917 I published in a memorial volume (number 29 of the Carnegie *Contributions to Embryology*) a short paper, with handsome illustrations by Ralph Sweet, in which I demonstrated by a rather difficult technical method (Bielschowsky-Maresch silver impregnation) that the exceedingly thin cells forming the walls of blood capillaries (endothelium) in the pituitary, thyroid, and adrenal glands produce reticular connective tissue fibrils. The observation was significant because for the past eighty years histologists had been trying to distinguish the various cell types, partly by their products; for example, connective tissue cells (fibroblasts) had been distinguished from endothelial cells because the former produced connective tissue fibrils. My demonstration showed that the distinction had been carried too far.

I found, somehow, a little time for private reading in the history of anatomy, following up, among other topics, a passage that had attracted my attention, when I was a medical student, in the *Anatome corporis humani* of Isbrand van Diemerbroeck (1685), in which he discusses the location of the soul in the body. I had compiled some notes on this fascinating subject; at Berkeley the Bancroft Library provided sources for further study, and I wrote an essay that I read to a club of young faculty men with broad interests, of which I had become a member. The article, "Anatomists in Search of the Soul," appeared in *Annals of Medical History* in the spring of 1919. Its style, unlike that of anything else I ever wrote, reflects my admiration of Sir Thomas Browne's *Religio Medici* and a rash effort on my part to attain something of his grandiloquence. Reading it now, sixty years later, I see that in the final paragraph I was hiding under a cloud of fine words my own growing doubts about an immaterial soul, whose temporary place of residence in the body many anatomists had sought to discover. In defense of this reticence, if it needs defending, I refer to my guide in such matters, *On Compromise*, by John Morley. My own views were not critically relevant to my historical narrative; there were those near and dear to me to whom avowed skepticism on my part would have given grievous pain.

The entrance of the United States into World War I on April 17, 1917, raised a question as to my duty, to my family and my country, which I was not in a position to solve for myself.

Professor Evans decided my problem without consulting me. The army had directed the university to draw up a list of members of the medical faculty who were needed at home to keep the school in operation, training doctors for service in a war that might last a long time. Evans put my name on the list and that was that, though ever since I have been troubled by a feeling that I did not really deserve so easy and comfortable a solution.

I offered my time during the summer of 1917 to the Public Health Service to help fight an epidemic of smallpox then threatening to get out of control in the Southwest, but summer volunteers were not wanted. The nearest I could come to patriotic service that summer was to find some sort of essential work that was going undone because of the departure of young men for military service. Sending Betsy and the baby to Carmel to spend the summer with Miss Shiel, I joined a surveying crew on the Northwestern Pacific Railroad, which runs from Sausalito on the northern side of the Golden Gate to Portland, Oregon. I was one of a three-man maintenance-of-way party, a surveyor and two assistants serving as rodmen and chairmen as needed.

Our boss, Mr. Miller, had a high-school education; he had learned his trade on the job. There were some pleasant days, in cool canyons or near the ocean, but the work was mostly hard, often uncomfortable, and without stimulating companionship for me. Miller was a decent man but dull; my fellow assistants (they changed several times during the summer) were deplorable, the kind of people the army would not take. One was a numbskull; one (I thought) a drug addict; and one burly rascal could talk of nothing but his sexual achievements. The outdoor work, however, was healthy; I felt that I was serving the war effort, and the pay eked out my university salary as wartime inflation cut down its purchasing power. The country was charming—prosperous modern farms, well-tended vineyards in Napa County, and near the sea primeval groves of the coast redwood, *Sequoia sempervirens*. Betsy, too, and young George had a healthy summer at Carmel. We rejoiced in being together again after the summer-long separation.

We moved again that fall, renting a small unfurnished house north of the campus. Young George was learning to walk; a conventional house would be safer than the Stratton cottage perched on a steep hillside. When we were married my father told me that when we wanted to furnish a house, he would give me five hundred dollars for the purpose. Betsy and I had an amusing time for a couple of weeks visiting San Francisco auction rooms to bid for a bed, a dining table, and chairs. The house had a wide view to the west. I remember the baby, just beginning to talk, looking down at a streetcar moving along a downtown street and saying "cah! cah!" in his mother's New England speech. About this time I had my first call to a full professorship. Theodore Hough, dean of the University of Virginia's medical school at Charlottesville, wrote offering me the headship of its small department of anatomy at a considerable increase in salary, but he was careful to point out that the facilities and help would be limited. I might have to wash my own laboratory dishes, he said. The thought of living on the historic campus was mildly tempting, but not enough to take me away from Berkeley's opportunities for research.

By the fall of 1917 the entry of our nation into the world war had begun to create visible changes on the Berkeley campus. All able-bodied male college students were in army or navy uniforms. Temporary barracks were going up on vacant areas between academic buildings. Younger faculty men were going to war; sadly for me, George Boas, my best friend at the faculty club, was on his way to very useful staff service on the French front. The medical departments did not lose many members because of the army's need to keep medical classes going, but our department lost its embalmer to the infantry, and for the duration of the war I had to prepare all the bodies for dissection— a routine task involving slow and careful injection of preserving fluid into the arteries. I had to do this work mostly at night. I was not superstitious; I did not expect dead men's ghosts to trouble me, but I must confess that to be alone in the building with a stark and staring corpse set up a quite irrational mood of apprehension: a creaking joist or the sudden cry of a nocturnal bird outside the window could make me shudder in spite of myself. I was glad when the job was done and I could lock the door behind me and go home. I begrudged the time spent in this task, but the experience stood me in good stead seven years later when I undertook to organize a brand-new anatomical department of my own at Rochester.

The work of preparing cadavers for storage and dissection

is a routine in anatomical laboratories, but Professor Evans, with his urge for perfection in teaching as well as in research, once set for his staff an even more gruesome task. For classes in microscopic anatomy it was, and I suppose still is, customary to provide the students with sections of selected organs and tissues permanently stained and mounted on glass slides, ready for study at leisure. This can readily be done with animals killed for the purpose, so that the healthy tissues can be preserved at once. Normal, healthy human tissues are, however, hard to come by. Post-mortems are seldom done immediately after accidental death, and tissues from the operating room are of course mostly in abnormal condition. Evans hit upon the idea of obtaining healthy tissues from an executed criminal and arranged with the warden of San Quentin prison to allow us to autopsy in our own way the body of a man, a brutal murderer sentenced to death by hanging who had no relatives to claim his corpse for burial.

On the appointed day Evans, Katherine Scott, and I went to the death house of the prison with our instruments, bottles, and a demijohn of picro-acetic-formol fixing fluid. When the warden asked Evans to be one of the official witnesses required by law, he accepted the duty without any visible qualms. Dr. Scott and I declined the honor and waited in a room next to the death chamber until the prison doctor pronounced the man dead and the body was brought out and laid on a table. Once we went to work my emotional stress disappeared. His carcass might have been that of a sow at the slaughterhouse or a dead rat in the laboratory. We rapidly cut down on a femoral artery, injected the warmed fixing fluid throughout the body, and proceeded on a planned schedule to excise portions of the various organs and tissues. Enough was stored away to supply the classes at Berkeley for years to come with sections of normal, superbly preserved human tissues.

In the autumn of 1917 Evans assigned me to assist Robert Moody in teaching gross human anatomy instead of microscopic anatomy, which meant that I worked under much less stimulating leadership than before. The first-year medical students were under the command of a brash young man just out of college who had won his silver bars only a few weeks before at a reserve officers' training school. His notion of command was to pull rank on every occasion. Once he came to the anatomy building during the morning hours of study, bawled out his orders in the corridor, and took the entire class away from the laboratories to march up and down the campus and practice the manual of arms.

Fatigued by their redoubled duties, and harassed by their petty tyrant, the soldier-students finally grew desperate. One of them, Stafford L. Warren, a mature, sensible young man destined for high responsibilities in later life, came into my office one day and in confidence told me that some hotheads in the medical company were planning to get rid of the captain by shooting him from the ranks. Warren's deep concern persuaded me that the situation was serious. I urged him to get his colleagues to postpone action until I could get something done about it. Professor Evans, admitted to the secret, got word to the commandant of the students' battalion. In a few days the obnoxious captain was replaced by a sensible older officer.

The worldwide epidemic of influenza in 1918 gained in virulence as it crossed the continent from east to west and struck the Berkeley campus with violence. Army barracks became hospital wards, and the medical students, even those of the first and second years with no clinical experience, served as orderlies. To their duties in classrooms and wards was added the grief of seeing fellow students, often their own friends, gasping and dying from the uncontrollable flooding of their lungs with virus-induced exudate. One of these student orderlies, unsung heroes who braved a disease as murderous as bullets, came to my office for a talk and released his strain by breaking into tears. I did not contract influenza, but my wife fell ill toward the end of the epidemic at Berkeley, fortunately with only mild pulmonary symptoms.

We enjoyed the comfort of our new quarters, and our life ran on uneventfully. My teaching and research continued to go on well during the rest of 1918 and the spring of 1919, but I found my mood darkening because of financial worry. The salary increase of $200 a year promised me by Dr. Evans had been met, but postwar inflation had given my prospective $2,300 income for 1919–20 less purchasing power than $1,500 in 1915. My small savings had been used up; I foresaw no likelihood of a greater increase through academic promotion; I was the third man in a small department and fourth in age. Betsy's influenza had been followed by chronic arthritis of the hips and knees, mild at first but getting no better. Only exuberant young George was free from pain or worry. I tried not to let this growing worry show in my letters to my parents, but perhaps they sensed it; at any rate they invited us to come east for the summer and stay with them in Roland Park while Betsy's arthritis was studied at Johns Hopkins Hospital.

When the Overland Limited pulled out of Berkeley station one day late in May, I could not know that I would not return to Evans's laboratory. He had been kind and generous to both of us. Betsy, like all the women in his circle, liked and admired him. If our next child had been another boy, she would have wanted to name him after Dr. Evans. I, too, at that time felt unalloyed liking for him—more than the other members of his staff I could appreciate the respect for artistic and literary values that characterized his whole career and made him a distinguished bibliophile, and I was grateful to him for encouraging me in my studies of medical history. I thought him then, and still do, the most brilliant American anatomist and endocrinologist of our time. I could smile at his pride of intellect expressed in haughtiness to pretentious or stupid people and an ostentatious show of learning to his peers. I knew nothing then of a rift that led in a few years to Philip Smith's grave discontent and departure, nor of divagations that broke up his marriage with Anabel Tulloch. I saw only the beginnings of a craving for recognition and honor that became uncomfortably evident in his later life. I have put on record in the *Biographical Memoirs* of the National Academy of Sciences my personal estimate of his scientific ability and leadership as I saw him close at hand in 1915–19 and from a distance during the rest of his life. For me at a critical age he was a kind friend and inspiring leader. I leave it to some future biographer (I understand that one is now at work) to tell what others saw of the flaws in his complex character and to balance them against his great scientific achievements.

8

ASSOCIATE PROFESSOR

Toward the end of May 1919, Betsy and I with little George, now almost two and a half years old, were on our way to Maryland for the summer. We did not go at once to Baltimore, for my aunts, Laura Evans and Irene Evans Gorsuch, had invited us to come to them for a week or two in the country before going to my parents' home in Roland Park. This could be arranged quite conveniently, for our sleeping car from Chicago was to be set out at Harrisburg from the Pennsylvania Railroad's New York express and attached to a Washington-bound express train on the Northern Central line. The latter railroad, in response to my request telegraphed from Chicago, kindly ordered the train to be stopped at the rural Glencoe station, twenty-five miles north of Baltimore, where we were greeted with affectionate warmth by the two aunts and our uncle by marriage, Dickinson Gorsuch. The ladies, I knew, were curious to see what Betsy was really like, for they had met her only at our wedding and my parents' reception in 1915. Betsy, grateful for their generous hospitality, became at once a member of the family, and little George rejoiced in the novelty of life on the farm—the barn bigger than the farmhouse, Dick's prize-winning Ayrshire cattle, Aunt Rena's handsome Rhode Island Red chickens, a brook so tiny that he could wade safely in its clear, cool water. I, fatigued by our preparations for the journey and four days of railway travel, was at peace in the loving atmosphere of the Glencoe household. To me, coming from California's hillsides, half-baked by the summer sun, the woods and fields of northern Maryland, greenest of all our states, seemed blessedly homelike. On the Gorsuch farm I could lie in the same hammock, under the same trees, where in college days I had first dreamed of a career in biology.

Soon after we settled in at 212 Ridgewood Road in Roland Park, Betsy was examined at the Johns Hopkins Hospital. The verdict was that her arthritis was probably caused by chronic tonsillitis. I asked the head of laryngology at the hospital, Dr. Samuel J. Crowe, to operate, and a date was set for mid-June.

In the meantime, my father informed me that Dr. Lewis Weed of the Johns Hopkins anatomy department had called to speak with me, having attempted unsuccessfully to reach me in Berkeley. As it turned out, Lew Weed had exciting news for me. He had just been appointed to succeed the late Franklin P. Mall as head of the Johns Hopkins anatomy department and wanted me to join him in the fall with the rank of associate professor. The salary would be $3,000. The dean of the school, J. Whitridge Williams, knew of Weed's plans for reorganizing the department and would do all he could to further my researches. I was surprised by the university's choice of Weed to head the department, as were anatomists around the country. Only thirty-three years old, he had not previously held a teaching position. After graduating from Johns Hopkins Medical School in 1912, second in class standing only to Alan Chesney (both of them became deans of the school), Weed passed up the usual choice of an internship in internal medicine or surgery and went to Harvard as a research fellow with Harvey Cushing, newly appointed to the Harvard faculty as chief surgeon of the Peter Bent Brigham Hospital. Within two years Weed completed a brilliant study of the origin and absorption of the cerebrospinal fluid. When the United States entered World War I in 1917, he was commissioned lieutenant in the army medical corps and was detailed to direct an army neurosurgical research laboratory at the Johns Hopkins Medical School—in fact, in Mall's former private office and workroom. In this task he achieved conspicuous success, under the same roof with Warren Lewis, who as acting head of the anatomy department since Mall's death was having an unsatisfactory time that ruled him out of consideration for Mall's post.

Weed told me that George L. Streeter, who had been appointed by the Carnegie Institution to head its department of embryology in Mall's place, had averted an embarrassing situation by inviting Lewis to join the Carnegie staff. Dr. Sabin, the next in rank, was ineligible for the headship in those days because of her sex. She would remain in the department, however, suppressing whatever resentment she might feel at such discrimination. I would rank third in the department, a very different matter from third place at Berkeley because under the circumstances I would be first in line for a call to a full professorship in some other high-ranking school of medicine. Furthermore, Johns Hopkins University would provide better support than Evans could get for an ambitious research program that I had in mind.

I knew Weed well enough to feel that I could work happily with him. I would have accepted his offer then and there if I had not been obligated by common courtesy to discuss it with Herbert Evans, and above all I had to consider my wife's inclinations. The time was rather late for Weed to get his department together for the start of teaching in the first week of October. He asked me to give him my decision on a day he designated, which happened to be the day set for Betsy's tonsillectomy.

Betsy in fact was not happy about this sudden threat of change in our family affairs. She was not sure that she would like Baltimore as well as Berkeley, and she dreaded another change. For the next few days we discussed over and over again the merits and demerits of the proposed move. She was hoping, I believe, that Evans would make a counteroffer, but I received from him only an earnest plea to return to Berkeley. His hands were probably tied by budgetary considerations. As the time for decision drew near, I thought it undesirable to keep Betsy in a state of indecision and agitation on the eve of a surgical operation that would add further strain; Sam Crowe's tonsillectomy procedure was drastically thorough.

It has never been easy for me to impose my judgments on other people close to me—wife, children, friends—or anyone else, for that matter. In this case, however, I felt my judgment was sound, and I could not abandon it. On the day of Betsy's operation I spent the morning hours with her in the hospital room, not mentioning our problem, but just before she was wheeled away to the operating room, she said to me wistfully that she knew how much Weed's offer meant to me; she hoped that I would not accept it, but she was in no mood to argue any longer. I must do as I thought best. There she left the matter. When the nurse and orderly had taken her away, I walked across Monument Street to the anatomy building, feeling almost like a traitor to one I had sworn to love and honor, and told Weed that I would join him in the fall. When Betsy was able after her operation to talk about our affairs, she bravely accepted my decision. In good time she came to realize that it had been a wise one and to love Maryland even more than California.

My parents were delighted to have us in Baltimore. My father, with characteristically practical generosity, solved our housing problem by buying for us a comfortable suburban house at 4509 Maine Avenue in Forest Park, a western suburb of Baltimore, which he rented to me at low cost. The house had three bedrooms—barely enough, for in February 1920, the birth of a daughter, Hester Ann (named for my maternal grandmother), increased the family to four, and later that year Betsy's parents came to live with us, Mr. Copping having retired from the ministry. The next problem was how to bring our household effects across the continent. When I hesitated to ask for an advance of salary, Betsy astonished me by proposing to see Dean Williams about it. I was weak enough to let her go. She returned triumphant; Williams had promised her $500 outright, for moving expenses. In August I took the train to Berkeley and during a week's stay packed and shipped our furniture and personal effects and my scientific materials. My return trip to Baltimore was my third crossing of the continent in 1919.

When in late September I reported to Weed for duty, he had completed his assignments of the staff. Dr. Sabin—who had been promoted to a full professorship in 1917—would continue to conduct the histology course; Weed planned to take an active part in teaching gross human anatomy and wanted me with him in the dissecting rooms. Dr. Sabin would have an able helper, Robert Sydney Cunningham, who had joined the anatomy department immediately after taking his M.D. at Johns Hopkins in 1914, was now raised from instructor to associate. A Southerner, courteous but rather moody and a very competent histologist, he remained in the department until in 1925 he was called to the professorship of anatomy at Vanderbilt University. In 1920 George Bernays Wislocki returned to the department from Harvard, where he had been a research fellow on Harvey Cushing's surgical staff. He remained in Baltimore until he was called in 1931 to the chair of anatomy at Harvard. Cunningham chiefly studied the embryonic development and identification of the blood cells, Wislocki the microscopic structure of the endocrine glands.

Thus Weed had with him, besides Dr. Sabin, three juniors, all Johns Hopkins graduates, who were active in research. I think that no other department of the medical school at that time, except possibly surgery under W. S. Halsted, had a staff of such quality. At the same time as I, another former assistant in the department, Eben Clayton Hill, rejoined the staff. Thirty-seven years old, he had been a captain in the army medical corps doing radiology. He brought some x-ray equipment of his own and worked in a desultory way on anatomy as seen by x-rays. He entertained us all, staff and students, by his audacious clowning. Once he sauntered through the corridors ostentatiously brandishing a huge 100cc syringe, pointing it at his arm with gestures and muttering in pretense that he was giving himself a shot of morphine. I never saw evidence of a morphine addiction, but he may have been high on some kind of stimulant. One day he came strutting to the staff lunchroom arm in arm with Dr. Sabin—middle-aged, serious, dignified, plain looking, and plainly dressed Dr. Sabin—loudly whistling the wedding march, to her obvious pleasure.

In the fall of 1921 we had another recruit, Eben Hill's complete opposite, Ernst Huber, a gentle, serious little Swiss M.D. from Zurich, was an expert on the muscular system. Ernst always seemed a little puzzled and troubled by American ways. Once he came to my room almost in tears. "The professor was teasing me. I think he does not like me. Does he think I am a stupid child?" I tried to explain that Weed had merely been kidding him in a friendly way—a concept that Ernst could not understand. If a Zurich professor talked to an instructor like that, he said, the younger man would know that he was not wanted. He never got over his insecurity, made an unsuitable marriage, and one day several years later I heard that he had ended his life, in the laboratory, by a dose of bichloride of mercury.

We had almost every year visiting anatomists from other

institutions or other countries, who came on fellowships of one sort or another to spend a semester or a year working with us. One of these guests whom I recall with affection was Randolph Shields, a very agreeable and intelligent medical missionary on leave from a medical school in China. With the help of an old Chinese scholar Shields had accomplished what seemed to me a stupendous feat, a translation of *Gray's Anatomy* into Chinese. He had fascinating tales to tell of the introduction of Western medicine into China. One was of an elderly practitioner of the old school whose knowledge of human anatomy had been acquired by memorizing the words of his teacher and gazing at diagrams in antique books. Some of Shields's modern students had persuaded the old fellow to visit their dissecting room. Shown a dissected cadaver, he was delighted. "Yes," he said, "it is just as the books told us. There I see the heart, and there is the liver; he has two kidneys; there is his spleen, as we learned from the books."

Another visitor, from South Africa but trained in a British school, was quite supercilious about our admittedly less exacting demands upon our students' memory of anatomical detail. At lunch one day, to show his superior knowledge, he said, "Give me an imaginary arrow passing through a human body; if you tell me the points of entry and exit I will name in order every structure through which it passes." "Hell," said Eben Hill, "in this country we don't fight with arrows any more."

Lewis Weed, our chief, continued at first his anatomical and physiological studies of the cerebrospinal spaces and the fluid that fills them. Walter Dandy's sharp criticism of Weed's hypothesis that the absorption of the cerebrospinal fluid is carried on exclusively by the arachnodial villi that jut into the great cerebral venous sinuses of the brain had irked Weed and impelled him to further study of the evidence. In the course of his experiments he developed a physiological method for temporarily reducing the size of the living brain that has been widely used by surgeons in operations on that organ. Weed was a skilled executive and leader; the daily routine of teaching and laboratory service ran smoothly. He constantly encouraged and supported his juniors in their research and promoted their future careers. A certain chilly hauteur he sometimes showed to people he disliked never appeared within his own departmental circle.

In 1923 he was appointed dean of the Johns Hopkins medical faculty and thereafter devoted himself entirely to executive duties in many capacities. I published in the *Year Book of the American Philosophical Society* for 1953 an account of his career of distinguished service to the school, to American medical science, and to the nation.

Teaching gross human anatomy in a first-class professional school, to students of the kind we had at Johns Hopkins, is not a matter of recitations and assigned readings in textbooks. These highly selected young people have learned to study for themselves. They perceive the problem, which is to make the complete structure of the human body clearly visible by careful dissection and to understand as far as possible the relation of one part to another. If anything is puzzling or obscure they have their textbooks and anatomical atlases close by the dissecting tables. All that an instructor can do is to explain difficult points or advise as to sources of information and add helpful comment from his knowledge of zoology and embryology. If he is historically minded, he can bring up stimulating information from the work of bygone anatomists; in short, he tries to surround this complex and often tedious subject with inspiring scientific interest. This is better done, as Franklin Mall had taught us, by informal comment over the dissecting table than by lectures. Weed did not revive lecturing on gross anatomy, but he introduced a few set talks in the dissecting rooms, on themes of particular interest to the instructors who gave them. His own talks of this kind, for example, on the mechanics of joints or the fluid-filled cerebrospinal spaces, were very clear and instructive.

One obvious contribution the teacher can make is to point out how one or another anatomical structure bears on the practice of medicine and surgery, but this pedagogical method led me once into an embarrassing situation. When the students of my section were dissecting the spinal region, I undertook to show them the anatomical factors involved in doing a lumbar puncture to collect spinal fluid for diagnosis or to relieve pressure on the spinal cord. It seemed a good idea to let the students know that I was not without clinical experience. So I got a lumbar puncture needle and began to demonstrate the procedure. Halfway through the brief demonstration one of the students, Charles Doan, politely remarked that the step I was taking at the moment was usually done differently. Surprised that a first-year student should speak so confidently, I said, "Mr. Doan, I have done this procedure twice on patients; how many times have you done it?" "About fifty," he said. "I was a medical corpsman in the army." I handed him the needle, asked him to continue the demonstration, and left the room. I never felt that I had lost face with the eight students, men and women of the highest quality, who were present. For Doan and me the episode provided an amusing recollection when we met in later years. He became a professor of internal medicine at Ohio State University.

A few weeks after school opened in the fall of 1919 Curt Richter of the Phipps Psychiatric Clinic at the Johns Hopkins Hospital came to see me. I knew about Richter, an experimental psychologist of my own age who had taken his Ph.D. under my teacher of college days, John B. Watson. He had gained a reputation for ingenious experimental methods, in particular in a study of food preferences of the albino rat. He had provided a number of rats, each in its separate cage, with a "cafeteria" of bottles and little dishes containing the essential ingredients of a balanced diet—pure fat in one dish, proteins and carbohydrates in others, the essential salts and trace elements, and the necessary vitamins. Richter's remarkable finding was that the rats voluntarily chose an optimum amount of each ingredient, obtaining for themselves a balanced diet on which they grew as well or better than control animals on standard rat food.

When Curt appeared at my door, accompanied by a young Chinese fellow worker named Wang, he turned out to be a delightful person. He was now studying, he said, the motor activity of albino rats by keeping them in individual cages, each of which gave access to a wheel in which the rat could exercise as much and as often as it liked. The amount of running by each animal was recorded by a cyclometer on its wheel. What had brought Curt to me was a surprising discovery, that female rats exercised much more actively every fourth or fifth day. Since his male rats showed no such cyclic pattern, he naturally thought of an ovarian factor, but when he looked up what was known about the rat's reproductive cycle he found no definite information about its length. He had heard that Herbert Evans was studying the rat cycle in Berkeley and had just learned that I had come from Evans's laboratory.

When I gave him the as yet unpublished news that Evans and Long were finding the duration of the cycle to be four or five days, he and Wang almost leaped out of their chairs. Then, to show them how Evans and Long detected the day of estrus, I picked up some little instrument that could serve as a vaginal scraper and a few glass slides and went with Richter and Wang, almost on the run, to their laboratory, where they had a couple of dozen female rats merrily running in their wheels. Richter handed me one whose cyclometer showed a high rate. I gently scraped a few cells from the vaginal lining and under the microscope showed Richter the desquamated epithelial cells that told us the rat was in the estrous phase and must have ovulated that day.

There is no thrill quite like that which a scientist feels when two previously unrelated facts suddenly snap together to teach him something new. We fairly chattered with excitement as I examined other rats, some in high activity, some low, and I showed Richter that I could tell one from the other by looking at the vaginal spreads as well as he could by reading the cyclometers. This episode started a friendship between Curt and me that has lasted through the years. As it has continued I have come more and more to appreciate his scientific enthusiasm, his breadth of knowledge, and his warm heart, and to admire his charming wife, as my Betsy also did.

Our little household in Forest Park on the whole enjoyed our four years' residence in Baltimore. With two very young children we were tied closely to home until the Copping parents came to live with us. After that Betsy and I could now and then get away for evening diversions. A favorite one was to have supper at a plain little oyster house on north Howard Street, well known to impecunious Baltimore gastronomes, and then see a play from the upper gallery of one of the Howard Street theaters. George IV was soon old enough to enjoy with us an afternoon excursion by steamboat to Tolchester or Love Point, across the Chesapeake Bay. Once Betsy and I managed to have a long weekend on the York River, a Virginia estuary of the Bay. I had developed curiosity about the geology of the tidewater area and especially about the fossils found in the low cliffs along the Western Shore; so we spent that hot summer weekend collecting Miocene shells from the sandy York River cliffs. At home I identified most of our finds from the publications of the Maryland Geological Survey and actually sold some of our best shells to a biological supply house. One or two specimens that defied my amateur identification I took to the Maryland Academy of Sciences, then on Mount Vernon Place, to match them with the huge collection made years before by Johns Hopkins geologists. The academy was at the time in a low state; in its dusty rooms an aged curator looked after occasional visitors like me. He was so much impressed by my interest in the Miocene mollusks that he begged me to accept a subcuratorship of paleontology. Considering my zero knowledge of the field, I begged off. I hasten to add that in recent decades the academy has flourished again and has a new house on Baltimore's rehabilitated inner harbor.

The matter of church attendance was a problem for me, with two sets of pious parents watching over us in Baltimore— mine devotedly Methodist, Betsy's somewhat more open-minded denominationally, in spite of Mr. Copping's long career in the Congregationalist ministry. My parents would have liked me to take an active part in the observances and social work of the Broadway Methodist Church, the family's spiritual anchorage for a hundred years, but I had no interest in church work and could not face the evangelism. Betsy was slower than I to drop the religious customs of our forefathers, but her views were shifting, too. Before the Coppings came to live with us we went occasionally to the only Unitarian church in Baltimore—a choice somewhat less shocking to my parents than it might have been because an artist cousin, Tom Corner, deeply admired in the family circle, was a member there, thus conferring a certain worth on Unitarianism even in Methodist eyes. After the Coppings joined us, we went to the Congregational church, whose pastor, Dr. T. Sturges Ball, a likable and liberal man, was an old friend of the Coppings.

In the summer of 1920, an unusual call to scientific service provided a pleasant vacation for Betsy and a stimulating season for me. Charles B. Davenport, a prominent geneticist who headed the Long Island Marine Biological Station at Cold Spring Harbor, was studying problems of inheritance in sheep and was selectively breeding a strain of sheep whose ewes were bearing a high proportion of twin lambs—very interesting scientifically and possibly of practical value because of this increased rate of reproduction. Davenport, wishing to know whether his twin lambs were of the identical (single ovum) or fraternal (double ovum) variety, wrote to George Streeter of the Carnegie embryological laboratory for advice. As a sort of test he sent Streeter a pair of human ovaries from a post-mortem examination in a New York hospital, from a woman who had died about a week after giving birth to triplets. Davenport gave only these bare facts; he did not tell what the obstetrician and the pathologist had learned from the placentas and fetal membranes. He asked Streeter and his colleagues to deduce from the ovaries alone what was the type of triplet formation. This was a kind of challenge from the Carnegie Institution's Department of Genetics to the Department of Embryology, as if to say "You M.D.'s down there in Baltimore, show us how much you know." Streeter turned the ovaries over to me. The corpora lutea of pregnancy (there were only two of them, one in each ovary) had retrogressed so much that Davenport and even the pathologist had probably not recognized them (human ovaries can be rather humpy). I had thin sections made through the two corpora lutea; the cells of both were similarly retrogressive to a degree compatible with the history of parturition a week before death. I concluded that two of the three infants were single-ovum twins, the other a single sibling. There would have been two placentas, one with two umbilical cords and a single chorionic sac, the other with a single umbilical cord.

This was a routine task for me with my eleven years of studying ovaries, but Davenport thought it almost magical that I had the correct answer. The result was an invitation to me to spend the summer at Cold Spring Harbor to work out the problem of the twin lambs. We packed up in June and went to that picturesque village on Long Island's north shore. For years Davenport had conducted a summer school of biology there, and the Carnegie Institution of Washington had established on the same grounds, under his direction, a department of genetics housed in solid brick buildings alongside the ramshackle old wooden houses of the Long Island Biological Laboratory, relics of whaling days. Davenport housed us on one floor in a big mansion up the hill from the laboratories that had been bequeathed to another of his enterprises, the Eugenics Record Office. Our rooms were utterly bare but clean and airy and the house was surrounded by a beautiful wide lawn. Davenport and I gathered together from various sources the necessary beds, a breakfast table, and a few chairs. Thus housed in relative luxury we lived well, taking our lunches and dinners down the hill with the summer students and scientists. Davenport bred a couple of his ewes for me. When they were butchered two weeks later I found two corpora lutea in the ovaries of each ewe, and in the uterus of each two separate embryos. So the problem was solved and we all had mutton chops for dinner.

During the summer I made friends with the Carnegie staff, all well-known biologists—Albert Blakeslee, botanical geneticist, E. Carlton McDowell and Clarence C. Little, animal geneticists, and Oscar Riddle, physiologist and biochemist. The last I got to know quite well, for he was then working on the reproductive physiology of pigeons, and in later years his research bordered even more closely on mine. He had good command of quantitative methods in his field, sufficient to win him election to the National Academy of Sciences, but his hypotheses ran away with him, notably in his lifelong espousal of a theory that sex is determined by metabolic factors.

When I first met him in Long Island he was a jolly bachelor and the most continuous chain smoker I ever knew. Once a few years later when I happened to be briefly at Cold Spring Harbor alone, he took me to dinner at a nearby beach, and we had a nocturnal swim in Long Island Sound. He swam on his back to avoid quenching his cigarette. When he was far out on the dark water, all I could see of him was a glimmer from the still lighted cigarette in his mouth. In spite of his incessant smoking, he lived to the age of eighty-six with no obvious signs, as long as I knew him, of emphysema.

The staff of the Department of Genetics conducted a weekly seminar all summer to which I was invited, so that I had a three-month course in advanced mammalian and botanical genetics. The problem of the twin-bearing sheep having been solved so quickly, I was free to work on anything I chose. Dr. Davenport generously provided me with an assistant, an enthusiastic youth from a midwestern college who was willing to commute to New York City daily to a large slaughterhouse to pick up a milk can full of sows' uteri at various stages of pregnancy. My aim was to study the prenatal mortality of the embryos and fetuses. Franklin Mall, in an impressive monograph on human prenatal mortality written in 1908, had declared that the death of human embryos in utero usually results from an unfavorable uterine environment caused by infection or some physiological inadequacy of the uterine lining that makes it unfit for the developing embryo. I had some reason, from my observations at Berkeley, to doubt Mall's conclusion, and I was prepared to test it in swine.

My assistant brought me during the summer 1,000 pregnant uteri. I carefully examined the fetuses of the late pregnancies and compared their number in each case with the number of corpora lutea in the ovaries. I also prepared samples of the uterine lining for microscopical study. When the ovaries contained recently ruptured follicles, I searched the oviducts and uteri for segmenting ova and early embryos and likewise sampled the uteri for microscopical examination. In this laborious way I studied the thousand pregnancies, finding a prenatal loss of about 30 percent; that is to say, the number of embryos or fetuses in a given uterus was on the average less by one-third than the number of ova that had been shed, as shown by the corpora lutea. This loss occurred mostly during the first week, before the attachment of the embryos to the lining of the uterus (endometrium). A few more embryos disappeared after attachment. Most of these were resorbed and were not to be found, but in a few later pregnancies there were dead fetuses to be seen among an otherwise healthy litter. In almost all my specimens the endometrium (uterine lining) was in healthy condition, even over dead fetuses, and on microscopical examination I found that the endometrium was not only free from disease but had been brought by action of the corpora lutea to the correct physiological state for attachment of the embryos. Studies of other species, by myself and other embryologists and obstetricians, have shown a curiously similar rate of prenatal loss.

If the bulk of prenatal loss is therefore not caused by uterine pathology, as had been thought, and not by malfunction of the corpora lutea, the only other available explanation is that the germ cells—the ova or the sperm cells that fertilized them— must in one-third of all pregnancies have carried some inherent deficiency. This hypothesis was tentatively accepted by the eminent geneticists at Cold Spring Harbor when I presented the evidence from swine at their seminar. Other genetic observations, for example, those of Cuenot's yellow mice, in which one-fourth of all fertilized ova fail to develop, reinforced my conclusion, which is now a part of current genetic theory. My report on this study, done largely at Cold Spring Harbor, appeared in the *American Journal of Anatomy*, volume 31, 1923, under the cumbrous title, "The Problem of Embryonic Pathology in Mammals, with Observations on Intrauterine Mortality in the Pig." Incidental to this study I published in the Carnegie *Contributions to Embryology*, number 60, a brief article illustrated by James Didusch on three abnormal pig embryos of the seventh to the eleventh day, all of them found in healthy uteri among normal siblings. These are among the earliest abnormal mammalian embryos ever reported; they were not yet attached to the endometrium (attachment occurs later in the sow than in the rodents and carnivores and our own species) and certainly had not been subjected to an unhealthy uterine environment. One of them, with a wildly atypical embryonic disc, may be regarded in a technical sense as a true monster. It is the earliest mammalian monster ever to be described.

I had told Lew Weed, when in 1919 I first discussed my research program with him, that I had two major projects in mind, each of which would involve some expenditures from his departmental budget. I wanted first to finish my study of the reproductive cycle in swine and then go on to the primate cycle with the hope of understanding the puzzling phenomenon of menstruation, which occurs only in the human species, the higher apes (chimpanzee, gorilla, and orangutan), the gibbons, baboons, and Old World monkeys. Weed was enthusiastic about these plans and promised his support.

The reader will recall that in my study of estrus and ovulation in the sow, narrated in the preceding chapter, I had been able to follow the events of the estrous cycle for only about a week after ovulation. Since the sow's estrous cycle averages twenty-one days from one period of "heat" to the next, I had not been able to discover how long the corpora lutea persist, nor when a crop of follicles for the next ovulation begins to enlarge and mature. It was necessary somehow to follow the cycle through the whole period of three weeks.

If I had remained at Berkeley, I suppose it would have been

possible to interest the university's agricultural school at Davis, California, in helping me, but Davis is sixty miles from Berkeley; the travel would be expensive and time-consuming, and I would need, besides at least twenty sows, the labor of two or three farm hands for three weeks and the use of a large pen. Paradoxically, I could do the work far more easily and less expensively on the outskirts of urban Baltimore than on the university farm. The high cost of proteins and fats during World War I had caused several eastern cities to encourage the establishment of piggery farms on which swine were fed on city garbage. Householders were induced as patriotic service to keep separate the kitchen and table refuse that could be fed to pigs. At the Baltimore establishment of the American Feeding Company on the lower Patapsco River twenty miles southeast of the center of the city, large numbers of pigs were kept from an early age until they attained a profitable weight for slaughter. The company's local manager, Mr. Walter M. Cooper, a college-educated man whose brother was a professor in an agricultural school, understood my project and generously offered assistance.

I visited the piggery farm every third day for three weeks; at each visit I selected three sows that were actively rutting; Mr. Cooper's men captured them, marked them with numbered ear tags, and placed them in a special pen reserved for my use. At the end of three weeks I had twenty-two animals, representing all stages of the twenty-one-day cycle. The Johns Hopkins University then went into the pork business, with me as its agent, by purchasing the sows for $800. I had them hauled by truck to Hohman's slaughterhouse on Monument Street near the medical school, where I had arranged to have them butchered. The transaction was relatively inexpensive. The American Feeding Company had upped the price a little over market rates to compensate for their extra labor. Hohman's in turn reduced their payment a bit for the same reason. The university lost a hundred dollars or so in the deal, but Weed had expected that and paid it from his departmental funds. Hohman's butchered the lot at the end of a morning's run, slowing the pace of the killing floor routine so that I could collect the ovaries and uteri systematically.

Sydney Cunningham of the anatomy staff volunteered to help me, and Weed let me have two of the technicians. With this competent crew, I got all the ovaries and samples of the uteri, properly labeled, into separate bottles of Bouin's picro-acetic fixing fluid. The specimens from days 3 to 10 of the cycle, which might contain unfertilized ova in the oviducts or uteri, were carried to my laboratory, where I spent the rest of the day washing them out with salt solution and searching the washings for ova.

I had acquired considerable skill in recognizing these tiny precious objects under a low-power wide-field microscope. Dr. J. Whitridge Williams, dean of the medical school and professor of obstetrics, visited me once when I was washing ova from a sow's oviducts. I showed him some of them. It was the first time he had ever seen a mammalian ovum, although he had mentioned them often in his lectures and his textbook. He was so deeply impressed by the sight and by my ability to find and handle such small objects that he sometimes brought an important visitor over from his clinic for a demonstration, saying, "Corner is a wizard with eggs."

It took me months, of course, to have thin sections made of the follicles and corpora lutea and uteri and to study them. But

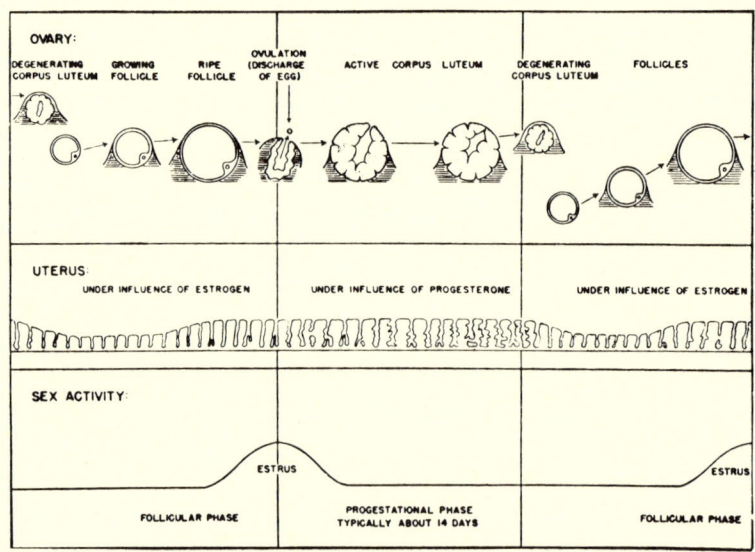

Figure 2. Diagram illustrating the sequence of events in the typical reproductive cycle of mammals. From G. W. Corner, The Hormones in Human Reproduction.

finally putting together what I had learned in Berkeley and Baltimore, I had the whole story of the sow's cycle before me, as in the diagram above (figure 2). As shown by the straight horizontal line, immature follicles up to five millimeters (1/5 inch) in diameter are always present in mature sows. At intervals of about twenty-one days, several follicles suddenly enlarge to a diameter of eight to ten millimeters. On the second day of estrus, they rupture and discharge their ova into the oviducts. On the fourth day after ovulation the ova reach the uterus, where if they are not fertilized by mating with a boar, they degenerate and disappear. I could find no ova later than six days after ovulation. Meanwhile the discharged follicles are converted into corpora lutea which, reaching full development about ten days after ovulation, put forth progesterone to condition the endometrium (uterus) to receive and nourish the embryos.

The preparation for pregnancy is characterized by a great increase in complexity of the endometrial glands. I have called this changed state "progestational proliferation." As seen in women, gynecologists have named it the premenstrual stage. If the ova are not fertilized, the corpora lutea degenerate, beginning on about the fifteenth day. The endometrium, no longer supported by progesterone, reverts to its original state, and another estrous period soon sets in. If the ova are fertilized,

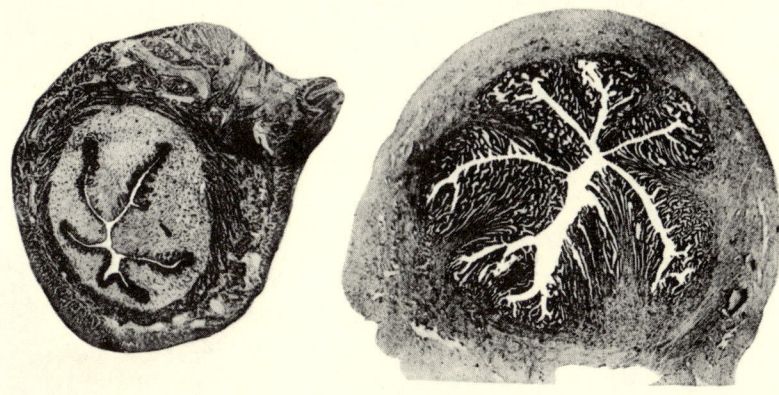

Figure 3. Sections of two rabbit uteri, illustrating (right) progestational proliferation from the corpus luteum. This is equivalent to the premenstrual state of the primate uterus.

however, the corpora lutea persist, maintaining the progestational state of the uterus until the end of pregnancy.

I reported these findings in number 274 of the Publications of the Carnegie Institution of Washington (*Contributions to Embryology*, volume 13, number 6), 1921. I was much pleased by the smooth course of the research and its clear results; it seems to me now that the monograph marks my appearance as an authoritative scientific investigator. Certainly it shows a great advance over my first study of the corpus luteum of pregnancy, published six years before. That had been the work of a promising beginner; this work of 1921 is thoroughly professional. As to its place in the history of research on mammalian reproductive cycles, I am perhaps not a disinterested judge. A number of workers in Europe, Australia, and the United States had during the past thirty years been slowly arriving at a concept of the female cycle, estrous in most mammals, menstrual in the higher primates, which sees the cycle as basically a means of producing egg cells at suitable intervals, getting them fertilized, and preparing the uterus to take care of the embryos (see my "Oestrus, Ovulation, and Menstruation" [1923]). Facts supporting the concept had been found by study of several species by workers I have already mentioned in chapter 7, but none of their accounts, I think, had covered as completely as I was able to do with the sow the schedule of estrus, ovulation, the fate of the unfertilized ovum, the rise and fall of the corpora lutea, and the progestational change in the uterus.

Furthermore, the pattern of the cycle in the sow is so simple and well defined that it provided me and, I believe, other workers with a basic scheme to which all of us could try to fit the confusing diversity of detail in various species, for example, ovulation only at special seasons of the year (many wild animals); widely spaced ovulation (dog, cat); inconspicuous estrus (guinea pig, rat, mouse); no discernible estrus (rabbit); and above all the strange phenomenon of menstruation, peculiar to Old World monkeys, apes, and our own species. My diagram of the sow's cycle, and later those similar ones in which I related the primate cycle to the basic mammalian pattern represented by the sow, have been widely reproduced or imitated in textbooks of physiology and gynecology.

For me, at least, what I had learned from the sow was essential to my next effort, which was to analyze the cycle of a menstruating animal, the rhesus monkey. Where in the diagram are we to place the monthly periods of vaginal bleeding of the human female and her simian kin? This problem had been attacked chiefly by German, Austrian, and French gynecologists, beginning in the 1880s. Those able surgeons and pathologists knew little about the cycles of other animals. Their findings from the operating room and pathological laboratory differed widely. Some thought that menstruation corresponds to estrus, a view supported by the fact that in the bitch and cow a little vaginal bleeding sometimes occurs at estrus. Others could find no temporal relation at all between ovulation and menstruation. Since about 1900 a few experienced gynecologists, R. Schroeder at Kiel, Ludwig Fraenkel at Breslau, R. Meyer and Carl Ruge at Berlin, utilizing as far as possible information gained from other species, conjectured that menstruation corresponds to the stage of degeneration of the corpus luteum, at which in other animals (e.g., the sow) the progestational stage of the endometrium reverts to a less active state without breaking down, whereas in primates it breaks down and bleeds. This supposition seemed to me plausible. I wanted to test it, not by opportunistic studies of operating-room and autopsy-room specimens, but by controlled observations on healthy females of a menstruating species.

Obviously the best prospect was to use the one species, the Indian monkey *Macaca rhesus*, that could be purchased at moderate cost and was readily kept in American zoos. I learned that at the National Zoo in Washington and the Philadelphia Zoological Society's zoo, rhesus monkeys were being bred successfully. I went to Philadelphia to talk with the superintendent of the zoo, Mr. Ned Hollister, his head keeper, Mr. Blackburn, and the zoo's pathologist, Dr. Herbert Fox. They showed me a large colony of rhesus monkeys living to my surprise out of doors in a converted bandstand the year round. With such animals I could work at my home laboratory with all the necessary facilities for experimental study ready at hand.

Dr. Weed found the money to buy eleven female monkeys. Six of them arrived in April 1921 and the rest in March 1922, and I had them under observation from one year to two years and one month. We housed them in a wooden shack built to my specifications on the fifth-floor balcony of the Hunterian Laboratory building, just behind the anatomy laboratory. They had ample outdoor space in which to climb and jump and swing on hanging ropes. This was the first monkey colony in the United States for long-term physiological experimentation.

Our methods of caring for and handling the animals would now seem crude to workers in the handsomely equipped centers for primate research that have sprung up in several U.S. scientific centers. We caught them for daily observation with a long-handled net that I made from light rope. To detect the first sign of menstruation, I washed out the vagina daily with salt solution from a medicine dropper and examined the washings under the microscope for red blood cells. For months I did not dare to entrust the observations to anyone else and went to the laboratory every day during the summer of 1921 and the winter of 1921–1922, on weekends, and even on Christmas Day, once trudging the five miles each way from Forest Park through an eighteen-inch snowfall that stopped all the streetcars and automobiles. When the medical students were at work in the dissecting rooms I was in full view catching the monkeys and often got a jolly round of applause from my pupils.

The monkeys were young, just reaching sexual maturity, and their menstrual cycles were somewhat irregular, but I observed each one through 8 to 17 cycles, 125 cycles in all, and found the modal (most frequent) interval to be twenty-seven days. Because of the variability of cycle length I decided to terminate observations on each animal when she exhibited 3 cycles of fairly uniform length, varying not more than three days on each side of the modal number of twenty-seven days. The first step was to test the working hypothesis that ovulation occurs about the middle of the interval between two menstrual periods. After this was done with a few of the more regular animals, the remainder were to be killed during menstruation or shortly thereafter, to see whether menstruation was associated with the degeneration of the corpus luteum.

With these aims I killed my animals in a regular sequence beginning about the middle of the interval between two menstrual periods. An animal autopsied on February 21, 1923—a great day in my life—fourteen days after the onset of the last menstrual period and twelve days before the probable date of the next had, exactly as predicted by the working hypothesis, a ruptured follicle, characteristic of the first or second day after ovulation. I recovered the ovum from the left oviduct. This was the first primate ovum ever found on its way down the oviduct at a known stage of the menstrual cycle.[1] In another animal killed seventeen days after the onset of the last menstrual period and seven days before the next expected period, I found a degenerating ovum in the uterine cavity, again as predicted by the hypothesis. Three other monkeys killed in the latter half of the intermenstrual period each contained a recent corpus luteum. Thus the primate cycle as seen in the rhesus monkey could tentatively be diagrammed as it is shown in chapter 11 (figure 4), resembling that of the sow with the exception that the higher primates do not exhibit an estrous phase at the time of ovulation and undergo a phase of menstrual bleeding when the corpus luteum degenerates. This interpretation, since then amply confirmed for the human female as well as other primates, is now standard doctrine. As I write these pages, in August 1978, the world is agog with the news of the first "test-tube" baby. I hardly need to point out that the success of that procedure and similar methods such as artificial insemination *in corpore mulieris* depends basically upon the knowledge of the primate cycle that has been worked out since the beginning of the century by a few embryologists and gynecologists in Europe and America, of whom I am one.

My five cases constituted, of course, a very small statistical sample but were sufficient to give me confidence for future work; it took many years before I could present a complete account of the ovarian and uterine cycle of *Macaca rhesus*.

A second aim of the observations, to relate the onset of menstruation closely to the state of the corpus luteum was, to my disappointment, not fully realized at this time because of the astounding fact that the remaining six females of my colony, each killed after three or more fairly regular menstrual cycles, had not ovulated at all. In their ovaries I found neither maturing

1. The Hubrecht embryological collection at Utrecht, Holland, contains two specimens of the fertilized (segmenting) ovum from Javanese macaques, recovered from the oviducts of animals shot in the jungle.

follicles nor corpora lutea, and they were bleeding not from a premenstrual uterine lining but from endometria of the interval type. In my report of this research, published in the Carnegie *Contributions to Embryology* in 1923, I had to conclude that when ovulation occurs in the primate cycle it takes place at a definite time, about the middle of the interval between two menstrual periods, but menstruation may occur without a previous ovulation and therefore without a progestational phase of the cycle. I called the attention of physicians to this puzzling fact in 1927 in "The Relation between Menstruation and Ovulation in the Monkey," in the *Journal of the American Medical Association*, backing up my evidence from monkeys with three reports of anovular menstruation in women that I dug out of older literature and one clear-cut case I saw at Rochester. A young girl who had been having regular twenty-eight-day cycles died of heart failure from an attack of diphtheria that did not disrupt the cycle, menstruation having been observed on schedule when she was in the hospital, nineteen days before her death. I was given the ovaries and found no corpus luteum in either, nor any old corpora from previous cycles.

My paper was sharply criticized by several British and German gynecologists, notably by Robert Meyer, who had promulgated the dictum "ohne Ovulation keine Menstruation" ("without ovulation, no menstruation"), but it has been fully confirmed for both monkeys and women, and is accepted by gynecologists everywhere. I know now that the high frequency of anovulatory menstruation in my first little colony was due to the relative youth of my animals; the same phenomenon sometimes occurs in girls during the early years of adolescence.

During these four years in Baltimore from 1919 to 1923 several medical students asked me to let them work on research problems in my laboratory, in the free time provided in the school's schedule for elective courses or independent work. I set them to work on problems arising in my own study of the reproductive cycle. One of these concerned the way by which the ova find their way along the oviduct. Are they propelled by cilia, tiny brushlike waving fibrils on the surface of the lining cells of the oviduct, or by peristaltic contractions of involuntary muscle in its walls, just as the contents of the intestine is moved? Both possibilities had been put forward. Franklin Snyder at my suggestion studied these cilia and found no evidence for transport of the ova by them. When he wrote up his report for publication it was so badly put together that I had to revise it drastically. Snyder, a stubborn Pennsylvania Dutchman, would not let me publish it unless I would put myself down as coauthor, but he learned so much from the editorial process that a second paper he wrote a year later needed no such revision.

When Alan and Manfred Guttmacher, a handsome pair of identical twins, applied to work with me I had them check an idea I had, that the collapse of mature ovarian follicles at ovulation, when they shed the ova into the oviduct, may be brought about by involuntary muscle fibers in the outer layer of the follicle wall (theca externa). I thought that I had detected such muscle fibers, but it was difficult to distinguish them from connective tissue fibers, and I wanted a physiological test. I showed the twin brothers how to cut a ring out of a sow's ripe follicle, suspend it in a bath of physiological salt solution, and attach it by a silk thread to a lever made of a long, light straw whose tip was pressed against a revolving smoked drum, or kymograph (nowadays an electronic recorder would be used). When they added to the bath a muscle stimulant such as adrenalin, the resultant contraction of the ring, if there were muscle fibers in it, should show on the drum. Some of the first experiments, done with adrenalin from a drugstore, worked well and others failed. I went over to Pharmacology to get advice from Prof. John J. Abel, who had been the first to untangle the chemical structure of adrenalin. He suggested that the drugstore preparation the Guttmachers were using might contain a preservative that could affect the response of the very delicate tissue. Unlocking a cabinet in his laboratory he produced a small vial containing pure crystalline adrenalin left over from his chemical work of some years before. With a few milligrams of this precious material, the Guttmachers' experiments worked perfectly. I never had the time to follow up this discovery. To show that muscle fibers actually function to empty the follicle would require experiments on the whole animal under anesthesia, but animals with follicles large enough to work with, such as the pig or cow, are not convenient for laboratory experiments.

The Guttmacher brothers, charming companions, intelligent and high-minded, became my friends for life. Manfred became a psychiatrist, remembered for valuable services as physician to the criminal courts of Baltimore. Alan went to Rochester with me in 1923–24 and then returned to Johns Hopkins for postgraduate training in obstetrics. Of his distinguished career I shall have more to say later. A few experiments Alan did as a sideline to the follicle study suggested to me that the involuntary muscle in the walls of the oviduct and uterus behaves differently at different stages of the cycle and must therefore be influenced by the ovary. So I entrusted that promising new idea to the next two students who sought research experience, John D. Keye and Daniel L. Seckinger. My former chief at Berkeley, Herbert Evans, had hit on the same idea and had a student named Blair try it with rat uteri. Strips of such tissue placed in warm, oxygenated physiological salt solution undergo spontaneous rhythmic contractions, almost as regular as the swing of a pendulum. Hitched to a kymograph lever they write beautiful undulations on the smoked drum. Blair had published some records of these contractions ahead of my two young colleagues, but the rat's cycle is peculiar, and Blair's tracings had not the remarkable regularity of Keye's tracings from sow's uterine tissue and Seckinger's from the oviduct, both showing striking changes in rate and amplitude of the contractions at different stages of the ovarian cycle. Thus began a long story of subsequent important research to which I shall return in a later chapter.

I presented Keye's and Seckinger's findings at a national meeting of physiologists, showing their beautiful tracings. In the audience was one of America's most experienced physiologists, A. J. ("Ajax") Carlson of the University of Chicago. Rising to discuss my talk, he astonished me by saying in his blunt and emphatic way that he and his pupils could get no such regular tracings with intestinal muscle. This came close to calling Keye and Seckinger fakirs, or me a liar, or both. I was about to reply angrily when Carl Hartman from Texas (of whom much more in later chapters) jumped to his feet and rebutted the great Ajax by declaring that he had witnessed the recording of some of our data. Carlson, rebuked, sat down. I must add that a couple of years later, when I presented some of my own work in Carlson's presence, he again entered the discussion, this time congratulating me on the soundness of my work. He and I had many friendly meetings after I was elected to the National Academy of Sciences.

People who try to be helpful to others sometimes find that they have taken on more than they intended. A notable example of this kind was the chain of circumstances that led to my presiding over a surgical operation on a full-grown Siberian tiger. Gentle, melancholy Ernst Huber was an expert on the comparative anatomy of the facial muscles—an intriguing subject, I think. It is interesting to consider, for example, that the same set of facial muscles, suitably modified, has to serve the needs of the elephant, the English bulldog, and a Hollywood star. Huber wanted to dissect all varieties of facial muscles. Zoos are excellent sources of dead or discarded animals for dissection. A cousin of mine, Leroy Nichols, was superintendent of Baltimore's Druid Hill Park and as such was in charge of a small zoo. I got a few specimens for Huber by asking Nichols to save for us any animals that died. Since the zoo was too small to have a resident veterinarian, I gradually became an informal medical adviser to the head keeper. One day Leroy called me up to say that his Siberian tiger was ill. At the zoo I found the handsome beast completely prostrated on the floor of his cage, his eyes glazed, so sick that I did not hesitate to enter the cage with the head keeper, or to take the tiger's pulse and palpate his swollen abdomen. Since the animal was worth a thousand dollars, I advised sending for Dr. Herbert Fox of the Philadelphia Zoological Society. In three hours Fox arrived, made a tentative diagnosis of intestinal obstruction, and suggested an exploratory operation. Fox was not a surgeon, and Nichols did not want to entrust the patient to a local veterinarian. The only thing I could suggest was to take the tiger over to the medical school, where I could try to arrange an operation. I went back to East Baltimore while the keepers put the beast into a strong portable cage and loaded him on to a truck. Dr. Weed permitted me, somewhat reluctantly, to stage the operation in the basement of the anatomy building. Finding that Professor Halsted and his chief of the surgical staff, Dr. Finney, were both out of town (I have often wondered what Halsted would have said if I had reached him), I called the surgical resident, Emile Holman, who promptly brought his two assistant residents, William F. Rienhoff and Cecil Bagley, all three quite enthusiastic about the adventure and equipped with sterile sheets, gowns and masks surreptitiously lifted from the hospital stores. The arrival of the tiger at the Wolfe Street side of the anatomy building attracted a crowd of bystanders, including the policeman on the beat. I got him to come in and stand by with his revolver ready in case the patient should awake from coma when we took him from the cage, a duty that evidently did not appeal to the cop, who remained close to the door. Meanwhile I was called on the telephone by Dr. James F. Mitchell, acting head of surgery in the absence of Dr. Halsted and Dr. Finney. Mitchell said to me that being responsible for the welfare of the surgical house staff, he had forbidden Holman and the others to take part in the operation, but since they could not be found in the hospital, he supposed that they had disregarded his orders, so he was going home and would leave them to their fate.

At this stage the eminent Dr. Hugh Hampton Young, professor of urology, arrived uninvited and appointed himself to be the anesthetist. Since he was the senior M.D. present, I let him have the job. The cage was dragged in, the keepers removed the bars, and we lifted the tiger out and onto a dissecting table draped with sterile sheets. He made no sounds or defensive movements. The surgeons draped him for operation. Hugh Young poured some ether on a broom borrowed from the janitor and held it over the patient's nose. When Holman opened the abdomen we were shocked to see that the tiger had a general purulent peritonitis, quite inoperable. There was no intestinal obstruction. The patient was dying and there was nothing to be done. When he expired, the surgeons picked up their equipment, Professor Young put down his broom, and everybody departed, leaving only me, with Ernst Huber at my side quietly weeping over the corpse but ready to begin dissecting the facial muscles. I had to tell him that Nichols had directed me not to let the tiger be dissected, because the skin was to be given to a member of the city council for a rug.

This is the first time that I have told the story in print, but Hugh Young has it (in *A Surgeon's Autobiography,* pp. 209–10) wrong in almost every detail. The lapse of eighteen years and Young's love of a good story turned our pitiful tragedy into a Hollywood farce. Dr. Young says that somebody from the anatomy department asked him to come over and help (I certainly did not). He has the tiger ferociously growling and breaking up several brooms before he could be gotten under the ether. Lew Weed, like Jim Miller, had discreetly stayed away; Young has him come in and set a ventilator in action, alarming the tiger, whose sudden rage, he says, frightened Cecil Bagley so much that he jumped over the operating table; and finally he states that the tiger had multiple abscesses in its chest, which was not even opened. Historiographers, take note: old doctors' autobiographies are not always reliable.

At the end of the day's work in the laboratory, Lew Weed and I often started for our respective homes by walking a mile together westward along Monument Street to St. Paul Street, where we parted, he continuing on foot to the apartment house where he and his mother resided, I taking a streetcar to Forest Park. We talked about school and departmental affairs, gossiped about our colleagues, and sometimes took advantage of the opportunity for confidences best divulged outside the laboratory.

On one of these walks in the early spring of 1923 Weed told me that I was being considered for appointment to head the anatomy department of the new medical school being planned by the University of Rochester. This news was exciting but not a surprise. I knew something about the university at Rochester in upstate New York, which began in 1850 as a Baptist institution, but had long since shed its denominational connection. To its two colleges, for men and for women, George Eastman, the Kodak magnate, had recently added a sumptuously modern school of music. Abraham Flexner, secretary of the General Education Board, which administered large Rockefeller funds for the advancement of medical education in the United States, had picked Rochester as the site of a new medical school of the highest quality and had secured from George Eastman a gift of $5,000,000, to be matched by Flexner's board. Rochester, he had told his trustees, was a prosperous, self-confident city of 250,000 population, with a thoroughly sound college headed by an able and universally respected president. "Dr. Rush Rhees," he said, "belongs to the small group of eminent administrators who have carefully defined their objects and who have by substantial educational success won the confidence and esteem of all critical students of higher education in America." Dr. Rhees had persuaded my former teacher George Whipple to accept the large task of organizing the new school.[2] Early in 1923 Mr. Eastman and Dr. Rhees made a tour of some of the leading medical schools, which I suspect Dr. Rhees had arranged to educate his patron as to the ways and needs of a first-rate medical school. At Johns Hopkins they spent a morning in the anatomy laboratory. We of the senior staff, well aware that this was a significant occasion, behaved with appropriate reserve when introduced to our distinguished visitors, except the irrepressible Eben Hill, who seized the opportunity to complain that his last supply of Kodak x-ray films was unsatisfactory, to which Mr. Eastman, a businessman for the nonce, drew a notebook from his pocket and, while Weed scowled at the brash offender, took down from Eben the date and batch number of the box of film, to be passed on to the proper department at the Kodak works when he returned to Rochester. I was invited by Dr. Welch to attend that evening a formal dinner at the Maryland Club in honor of Mr. Eastman and Dr. Rhees at which, besides our genial host and Dr. Weed, other guests included, if I remember correctly, Dr. William H. Howell and Dr. John J. Abel. The fact that I was the only guest of less than full professorial rank, confirmed what Weed had told me. I had wondered, before dinner, whether my table manners were to be observed, as William Osler's were (according to Harvey Cushing's biography of him) when he was under consideration for a professorship at the University of Pennsylvania, but the food was so good and the conversation of my eminent companions so interesting that I forgot to be self-conscious. I was fully prepared by this occasion for a letter from George Whipple a few weeks later saying that he and Dr. Rhees were coming to Baltimore in a few days and asking me to dine with them at the Belvedere Hotel.

There was no reluctance, this time, on my wife's part. She had learned to love Maryland, but the postinfluenzal depression that had made her fear a move four years ago had long since cleared away. She was ready for another step up the academic

2. In my biography of George Whipple, I have discussed at length the period of reform and progress of American medical education following the publication of Abraham Flexner's shattering report, *Medical education in the U.S. and Canada* (New York, 1910). See also Flexner's circumstantial account of his dealings with George Eastman in his autobiography, *I remember* (New York, 1940).

ladder and was as eager as I to know what the Rochester president and dean had to offer us. Anxious that I should make a good impression on them, she would not let me start for town until she assured herself that my dinner jacket was brushed, my tie straight, and my shoes well shined.

After a good dinner Dr. Rhees led the way to his room, where he and Whipple told me about their great plans for the new school. Laboratories of ample size, teaching quarters, and a 300-bed hospital were to be housed under one roof in a building of many wings, to make communication convenient in the long northern winters. The promised endowments totaling $10,000,000 had been paid in by Mr. Eastman and the General Education Board; Dr. Whipple would see to it that the income from the fund would pay for the building. The city of Rochester was to build a new municipal hospital to be staffed by the school, alongside the university's Strong Memorial Hospital (named for Eastman's first partner Henry Strong and paid for by Henry Strong's daughters). A medical library was already being assembled under expert guidance. The dean had his eye on some of the ablest young men in the nation to head his departments. Research facilities would be ample. A first-rate man, Nathaniel Faxon, assistant superintendent of the Massachusetts General Hospital, had accepted the directorship of Strong Memorial Hospital. I was the first prospective professor invited to join the faculty; the president and dean hoped that I would accept and help to pick my colleagues. My salary would be $6,000. I would choose my own staff and share in designing my laboratory. Since the building would not be ready for more than a year, the president hoped that I would spend the academic year of 1923–24 abroad, on the Continent or in Britain, at the school's expense.

The breadth and scope of these plans deeply impressed me, all the more because of the men who laid them before me. George Whipple's solid character and great abilities I had known for a decade, ever since I had been a student in pathology at Johns Hopkins. Rush Rhees won at once my deep respect and, on longer acquaintance, my affectionate regard. He had been at first a Baptist pastor, then a professor at Newton Theological Seminary, and for twenty years president at Rochester. He combined lightly borne dignity with warm friendliness. He had evidently been studying the current problems of medical education quite thoroughly and was ready with liberal responses to my questions about his plans for the curriculum and for choosing and admitting students. I felt confident that I would make no mistake if I entrusted my career to his leadership and that of George Whipple. I was almost ready to accept the chair of anatomy then and there, but in order not to appear overeager, I proposed that I should visit Rochester in April to see the university and the city for myself. After they had gladly accepted this response, I took my leave and went home to Forest Park, where Betsy and I talked long into the night about the happy prospect that was opening before us.

My chief, Lewis Weed, was not distressed by the thought of losing me; indeed, he had done all he could to secure the new post for me because success for him in the executive career he was consciously heading for would be measured in part by the number and quality of the younger men he sent out to other schools. I wanted, however, the official blessing of my alma mater on my leaving and went to talk it over with Dean Whitridge Williams. When I said that I would be sorry if my departure on rather short notice caused Weed any difficulty in filling my place, Dr. Williams, a kind but blunt man, said: "You must go; you're getting to be a bigger scientist and teacher every year. Pretty soon the anatomy department won't be big enough to hold both Weed and you. Better go while you have this great chance."

My trip to Rochester in April satisfied me completely. George Whipple drove me around the city, which I found attractive, showed me the magnificent Eastman Theater at the school of music, and introduced me to the city's extraordinary health officer, Dr. George W. Goler, of whom I shall say more later. Dr. Rhees listened kindly to my simple stipulations, the most important ones being that I should be guaranteed a departmental staff member for every ten students. The president was rather amused, I thought, when I asked him whether there was a large pork-packing plant in the city because I would want to continue my study of the sow's reproductive cycle. He smilingly rang up the president of the Rochester Packing Company and passed on to me the assurance of willing cooperation. Before I left his office I had accepted the professorship of anatomy in the new school.

PROFESSOR

9

A YEAR ABROAD

I began to serve the school of medicine at the University of Rochester before my last trimester at Johns Hopkins came to an end. Dean Whipple had given me the bare outlines and square footage of the space on the fifth floor of the new building to be occupied by my department, and had given me, quite literally, carte blanche to lay out the histological laboratory, the dissecting rooms, staff offices, research laboratories, technicians' space, and seminar room, and to list the equipment for fifty students and a staff of five—laboratory tables, stools, chairs, and cabinets; special lighting for the dissecting rooms and lamps for the microscopes (at Johns Hopkins we had lighted the students' microscopes by daylight from the windows, but Rochester has many cloudy days in the winter). Having heard that Henry Knower, one of Mall's former associates, had some new ideas about dissecting-room equipment at his laboratory at the University of Cincinnati, I made a special trip there, and after consulting a lighting engineer about the strength of illumination, in foot-candles, required for the dissecting tables, I went to Jersey City to see some adjustable lamps, designed for close work in factories. With Weed's consent, I equipped a table in a Johns Hopkins dissecting room with one of the lamps, to test it in actual use. These and other tasks of planning kept me busy in all the time I could spare from teaching and writing. In addition, Whipple had me return once or twice to Rochester (in those days an overnight trip by railway) for consultations about building plans, the assembling of a library, and above all the choice of the other department heads. Whipple found my layout acceptable, with a few modifications, and even adopted some minor features in his own plans for the pathology department. At home Betsy and I also had planning to do, to get ready for a year abroad with the two children, George IV, now seven years old, and his lively sister, Hester Ann, aged four.

So the spring of 1923 went by quickly, and on June 9 we sailed from New York for Southampton aboard *Orbita*, a small but very comfortable ship of the Royal Mail line. I had, of course, given serious consideration to the choice of a base for research and scientific contacts during the year to come. I had thought of going to Robert Schroeder's clinic at Kiel, Germany, if he would have me, to learn from his experience with the human reproductive cycle. With his facilities for observation in the operating room and pathological laboratory and the skill I had acquired in handling mammalian ova, Schroeder and I might have been the first to recover human ova in transit through the oviducts (Fallopian tubes), instead of Edgar Allen and his colleagues of St. Louis, Missouri, who succeeded in that effort in 1930, but my exploratory letter to Schroeder brought only a discouragingly grudging acceptance of my tentative request to work with him. On the other hand a similar approach to Ernest Starling, professor of physiology at University College, London, brought a much warmer reply. Starling and his senior colleague, Sir William Bayliss, headed one of the world's leading centers of physiological research. I could hope to gain there some background of experience with the physiology of involuntary muscle, to equip me for intensive study of the remarkable cyclic variation of contractility of uterine and tubal muscle, then very much on my mind, that my students Keye, Snyder, and Seckinger had observed. A year in London, furthermore, offered many advantages for my family.

The ship *Orbita*, which carried us to England, had been in the Far Eastern trade, but the Royal Mail Steam Packet Company was trying to break into the New York–Southampton run. She afforded us at second-class rates the first-class accommodations she had been built to provide. To increase the enjoyment of the voyage, a report of icebergs in the north Atlantic caused our captain to take a southern route through warmer waters and sunshine on the ten-day crossing. There were several Johns Hopkins people aboard, including Arthur O. Lovejoy, professor of philosophy. An agreeable bachelor about fifty years old, he was fond of children, and mine took an immediate fancy to him. With his bright eyes and little beard he looked like anybody's uncle. It was amusing to see four-year-old Hester Ann gravely conversing with the professor.

Dr. Lovejoy happened to be in a jam. With the absent-mindedness that professors are thought to display, he had sent his luggage to the New York docks too late to be put aboard *Orbita.* His travelers' checks were in his trunk; he had only a few dollars in his pocket and would have to stay somewhere near Southampton for a week, awaiting the next ship of the same line. Professor Felix Morley, a mathematician, lent him some money; I could spare twenty-five dollars, and other shipmates chipped in enough to stake him for a week. He decided to pass the time in Winchester and suggested that we break our journey to London by joining him there. This was an irresistible opportunity to see the historic city with a distinguished guide. Taking his advice we stopped at the ancient God-Begot Hostel and happily saw the cathedral and other sights with our learned friend. Scholars remember Arthur Lovejoy for his famous book *The Great Chain of Being;* I remember him for his kindness to two little children.

Bidding farewell to the gentle philosopher after a couple of days, the Corners went on to London and found temporary rooms in a boardinghouse on Primrose Hill, a good base for exploring London and its surroundings by bus. We were planning to go somewhere on the seashore for a summer vacation before I began laboratory work in September, but there were some people for me to meet at once. A brief call on Professor Starling was sufficient to let him know that I was in England and looked forward to the year ahead in his laboratory.

George Whipple had asked me to see Professor Charles Sherrington of Oxford, then at the top of British physiology, as well known for his work on the role of the nervous system in motor activity and postural reflexes as Starling was for his studies on the physiology of digestion. Whipple had concluded that we could not find in America a rising young physiologist good enough for our new faculty, and he wanted Sherrington's advice about the possibility of finding someone in England. I made the mistake of going to Sherrington's laboratory and asking to see him without advance notice. Nobody had told me not to bother an eminent English scientist without first sending a letter of introduction. Sherrington received me, but he kept me waiting a long time and though formally polite was not cordial. His reply to our request for advice was almost a rebuke for our thought of taking away someone who would be needed in the homeland. America, he said, should produce its own scientists, not raid another country for them. I thanked him for the interview, feeling inwardly that I, and Whipple by proxy, had been slapped on the wrist. Never again did I ring an English professor's doorbell without a proper introduction. I must add, however, that thirteen years later, when I was Vicary Lecturer at the Royal College of Surgeons, Sir Charles came to hear me and afterward at tea chatted with me in a most friendly way.

I had met Sir Arthur Keith, conservator of the Royal College of Surgeons and the most widely known British anatomist of the time, a year or two before when he lectured at Johns Hopkins, so my name was familiar to him, and I was cordially received. I asked permission to attend one of his regular lectures, intended to prepare candidates for the anatomical part of the rigorous Conjoint Board examination for the license to practice medicine. His discourse dealt with the complicated relations of structures in the neck; it was superbly clear and instructive. Keith, a Scot from Aberdeen, then fifty-seven years of age, was a handsome figure, tall, blond, with boldly regular Nordic features. The distinguished sculptor Malvina Hoffman, who had Sir Arthur's advice when doing for the Art Institute of Chicago her grand project of sculptures representing all the races of mankind, chose Keith as her example of the Anglo-Norman physiognomy and modeled a portrait of him that stands out vividly amid more than a hundred portrait statues and busts in the impressive exhibit of anthropology and art.

Sir Arthur invited us to join him and Lady Keith for lunch in the fellows' restaurant at the London Zoo. We left Hester Ann with a baby sitter and took young George, who put on his best manners for the occasion. After lunch Sir Arthur led us past the cages and corrals and the imposing Mappin monkey terrace and all the other wonders of the place, mingling technical comments for me on zoological features with suitably entertaining and instructive remarks for young George, winning the admiration of both of us for his vast knowledge. When finally at the zoo's gate we took leave of our host and hostess, George wanted to add his bit to his parents' expression of thanks. Looking up at Sir Arthur, who was wearing what Americans call a derby hat, the British a bowler, he politely said, "Sir Arthur, do you who you remind me of?" "I can't guess," said our host. "Who is it?" "Charlie Chaplin," George replied. Lady Keith was obviously not amused, and Betsy was horrified, but Sir Arthur kindly said, "Well, George, perhaps my head looks like Charlie's, but I hardly think my feet do." The incident must have lingered in his memory, for in his *Autobiography* (New York, 1950, p. 432) he mentions a happy day at the zoo with George Corner, the American anatomist, and his young son. In spite of his great experience, Keith was one of those scientists who were deceived in 1912 by the faked Piltdown skull. On a later visit I made to his rooms at the Royal College of Surgeons, he showed me his own hypothetical reconstruction of that fictitious creature's cranium.

We took the opportunity also, before going to the seaside, to visit Betsy's distant cousin, Harold Copping, and his wife at their little home in the country near Shoreham in Kent. Betsy had known of this relative for years, for his work as an artist was familiar to everybody in English-speaking lands who attended a Protestant Sunday school. People of my generation will remember the sheaf of large colored posters that hung on an easel on the platform, one of which was turned over each Sunday to show the "golden text" for the week, illustrated by a graphic scene from the Bible, showing prophets or apostles or Jesus himself in appropriate costume against the background of the Holy Land. For years Mr. Copping, a talented illustrator, had been painting these scenes with careful attention to historical detail. He had even made a trip to Palestine to see the country for himself. Betsy had written to him from Baltimore, expressing a wish to meet and talk over family history, and had been invited by the Coppings to come down to Shoreham.

When our train arrived at the station, Mr. Copping was there to lead us a quarter-mile along a road beside the Darenth, a quiet canal-like stream perhaps thirty feet wide, a river by British rating. His cottage stood to the left of the road, across the stream, with no bridge, but there was a little flat-bottomed boat, a punt, tied to a post on the bank, in which we all sat and were poled across by our host, to the immense delight of the children. Hester Ann, who took a great liking to Mrs. Copping, always thereafter called her "the grandma with a punt." The Coppings had anticipated our visit with such pleasure that they provided an expensive treat for us, a fine luncheon of Scottish salmon. While Harold and Betsy talked family history, Mrs. Copping entertained the children and me.

Betsy had another distant cousin, Olive Copping Smith, who had taken a degree in French literature at King's College, London, and then married a London schoolmaster. Olive came to see us and began a friendship with Betsy and me that brought us together many times during our subsequent visits to England. During World War II the Smiths moved with their three young daughters to the country in Kent. Horace Smith became head of a consolidated rural school in the Isle of Thanet.

George Whipple, not daunted by Sherrington's admonition that I reported to him, wrote directing me to see Edgar Douglas Adrian, lecturer in physiology at Cambridge, tell him about the plans for a first-rate medical school at Rochester, and ask whether he would be interested in the chair of physiology. I wrote at once to Adrian, of whom I knew only that he was about my own age and had been doing fine work on the transmission of nerve impulses. He replied to my request for an interview by inviting me to come and have a look at Cambridge University and stay overnight with him. I found him a man of impressive personal quality, combining social grace with aristocratic bearing and obviously keen intelligence. He had recently married a young woman of equal charm, Hester Pinsent. After a tour of Trinity College, of which Adrian was a fellow, a visit to the magnificent fifteenth-century chapel of King's College, a view of the lovely Backs along the Cam and a pleasant dinner *à trois*, Adrian listened attentively to my tale about Rochester, into which I tried to put the enthusiasm I truly felt for our venture. He said that after discussing the matter with his wife he would tell me in the morning whether I might advise Whipple to proceed with a definite proposal. The outcome was that as much as he appreciated Whipple's interest in him, and attractive as Rochester's prospects seemed, both he and Hester felt that they should not leave England. He gave as the reason that they both had elderly parents who would soon need their presence. I was not surprised, for during the evening's earnest conversation I had begun to feel that to move to America these admirable young people, utterly English, bred to the high traditional culture of an ancient university, might be as inappropriate as to set down King's College Chapel on the banks of the Genesee River. This visit was the beginning of a friendly acquaintance with Edgar Adrian in which I watched him go on to the chair of physiology at Cambridge, to the presidency of the Royal Society of London, to the Order of Merit, highest of Britain's official honors to civilians of distinction, and the House of Lords as Baron Adrian of Cambridge. My disappointment at his decision that early summer morning in 1923 would have lasted a lifetime if we had not soon found an American physiologist of comparable worth and intellect—but that story comes a bit later.

For our summer vacation English friends recommended the little seaside town of Broadstairs, a quiet family resort on the Isle of Thanet, the northeast corner of Kent. Broadstairs had no historic distinction except that Dickens's Betsy Trotwood had lived there; they show her house to prove it. Few of the families on the beach at Broadstairs had the intellectual curiosity to seek acquaintance with strangers from overseas. George and Hester Ann, however, struck up an acquaintance with a family of gentlefolk named Quilter, who posted themselves daily near us on the beach. The father was a London insurance man of considerable standing. He, his wife, and two adolescent daughters took a fancy to the bright American children. The parents, cordial folk, later that year invited us to Sunday dinner at their home in Wimbledon.

Before returning to London we had a week at Canterbury, long enough for a good look at that entrancing city and the surrounding villages. We also visited Oxford for a week, taking lodgings in Walton Street and getting a first acquaintance with a city we were in after years to know intimately.

Returning to London at the end of September, we looked for lodgings in the northern suburbs and found comfortable rooms in a modern house at 22 Temple Fortune Lane, in the Hampstead Garden Suburb, near Golders Green. We chose that location not only for family reasons but also because I could get to work at University College quickly by the Underground from Golders

Green to Gower Street tube station. Hampstead Garden Suburb was one of those residential areas created in the first decade of the twentieth century, when planners hoped that garden cities and suburbs combining wholesome housing with good schooling and facilities for adult self-improvement could solve some of the problems of sprawling English and American cities. Our surroundings were really quite attractive and well suited to our needs. In the parklike town center was the excellent Henrietta Barnet School, to which our son went on weekday mornings, proudly wearing a little brown cap and his brown uniform jacket with the school's emblem, a golden sunburst, embroidered on its breast. Next door to the school was the Hampstead Institute, containing a hall for town meetings, lectures, and music, and workrooms for several kinds of art work and domestic economy. Betsy, for the fun of it, enrolled in a pottery class and during the winter turned out a couple of creditable vases that were awkward to take home to America. They perhaps still adorn a Garden Suburb mantelpiece. For little Hester Ann there was a supervised playground.

As soon as we were comfortably settled in Temple Fortune Lane, I hastened to execute another commission from Rochester. Dean Whipple had learned, through Walter Cannon of Harvard, of a promising young American physiologist, Wallace Fenn, who had been working with A. V. Hill at Manchester and had accompanied Hill to London in 1923 when he was called to the medical school of University College. When Whipple's letter arrived, Fenn was in London, finishing his work before returning to the States, where he was to take up a fellowship at the Rockefeller Institute in New York. Whipple, assuming that Fenn knew nothing about the plans for Rochester, asked me to get acquainted with him, form an opinion as to his suitability for our professorship of physiology and, without commitment, find out whether he would be interested in joining us. I wrote to Fenn inviting him to Temple Fortune Lane for an evening's talk. He unexpectedly brought his wife along, so Betsy Corner, who liked Clara Fenn at once, joined us by the fireside, and the occasion became a social one rather than the professional tête-à-tête I had intended. Nevertheless I carried out my instructions, discoursing at length about the great project and the eight carefully chosen young men who by this time had accepted professorships in all departments except physiology.

I had no difficulty making up my mind about Fenn's suitability for the still vacant post; although the evening's talk was hardly more than a monologue by me, the few words he said, his quiet reflective manner, and his obvious intelligence assured me that he would be an agreeable and more than competent colleague.

Wallace Fenn was then only thirty years old. He had Yankee genes and Yankee reticence but not strongly characteristic New England speech like his wife's, for he was born in Chicago and spent his childhood there, where his father was a Unitarian pastor. Fenn senior moved in 1901 to Cambridge, Massachusetts, to be dean of the Harvard Divinity School. Wallace went to Harvard College and on to a degree in botany under W. J. V. Osterhout. This was not the botany of wild flowers and mosses, of pistils and stamens. Osterhout was a physiological chemist and physicist, studying the cellular physiology of plants, basically like that of animal tissues. Fenn, in fact, had had a postgraduate year in medical physiology with Walter Cannon at Harvard Medical School, where his brilliant work won him a fellowship at the Rockefeller Institute for Medical Research.

I put into my story of the rich resources and bright hopes of the Rochester enterprise all the force I could assume. When I finished, Wallace was silent for a few moments and then with a smile said, "I suppose you don't expect me to say anything definite now?" I learned later that Walter Cannon had told him about the Rochester plans and had let him know that he was being considered for the professorship of physiology. I might as well have saved my breath, except that I had given him some idea of the kind of associates he would have in the new school. In his own good time Fenn accepted the post, which he held for life, winning the affection of colleagues and students and by his front-line research bringing distinction to the school.

At University College I found that a change had occurred in the eminent physiology department. Sir William Bayliss, the senior professor, had retired and seldom came to the laboratory. I was introduced to him one day, and still remember his stocky little figure, his white hair, close-cropped beard, bright smile, and exceedingly crooked teeth; he looked like a hobgoblin or kobold from the medieval forest. His successor was Archibald Vivian Hill (who always cut his gaudy name to a plain "A.V."), one of the rising stars of British medical science, already well known for brilliant experimental study of the energetics of muscle contraction. Handsome and self-possessed I thought him then, and later, when I met him in America, rather distant and cold.

Some weeks after I began work in his department I heard one day a sudden great shouting and trampling in the corridors. A crowd of students, excited by a news bulletin just received, burst into Hill's office chanting: "Who won the Nobel Prize? Hill won the Nobel Prize!" They set Hill upon the shoulders of a burly youth and marched him triumphantly out into Gower Street, down to the British Museum and back, bawling the great news to all the passersby. There was of course much excitement in the college and a send-off dinner for the Hills when they went to Stockholm in December.

Besides Starling, holder of the second full professorship of physiology, Hill's department included A. J. Clark, a pharmacologist soon to be promoted to a chair at Edinburgh, and two outstanding Russian émigrés, Boris Babkin and G. V. Von Anrep, a concentration of talent that could have provided professors for five ordinary medical schools. Ernest Starling was a tallish, well-built man of Nordic type like Arthur Keith, smooth-shaven, rather quiet-spoken, reserved but quite friendly with me. I think that an incipient serious illness was beginning to cut down his physical energy. Before telling about his suggestions for my research, I must add something about another department of University College, that of anatomy under Sir Grafton Elliot Smith.

Being myself rated as an anatomist, I saw a good deal of Elliot Smith, and I also renewed my acquaintance with his colleague, Henry H. Woollard, who had spent a year with us at Johns Hopkins in Weed's department in the early 1920s. Elliot Smith, an Australian by birth, had won wide recognition by long and sound research on the comparative anatomy of the brain but in recent years had interested himself in the cultural history of mankind and had not only studied the anatomy of primitive man but, with more valor than caution, had developed an imaginative theory of human culture that brought together all the megalithic monuments of the world, from Stonehenge to Yucatan and Easter Island, as the work of one worldwide cultural epoch. Other anthropologists were sharply critical, but Elliot Smith's enthusiasm had attracted followers, and because of his earlier work he retained a respected position in British science. I found his informal colonial manners delightful and his conversation stimulating even when I doubted the validity of his ideas about the makers of the great stone monuments.

University College had broken away from the English practice of having histology (microscopic anatomy) taught as a branch of physiology, and as in Germany and America placed it in the department of anatomy. The professor in charge was James Peter Hill, a Scot whose fourteen years in Australia had not worn away the accent of his native land. Like A. V. Hill, to whom he was not related, J.P. was known by his initials rather than by his full name. With Walter Heape and F. H. A. Marshall, he was one of the British pioneers in the modern study of the physiology of reproduction, upon whose extensive if incomplete knowledge of the ovarian-uterine cycle of mammals a younger group, of which I was a member, were building their research. Hill had done his work with some of the Australian marsupials, among them the kangaroo and the marsupial cat *Dasyurus.* He had described the peculiar type of ovulation by which these animals shed twenty or more ova at one time, although only a small number of the embryos can find room in the marsupial pouch. The rest of them die a few days after ovulation.

Short of speech and cautious, J. P. Hill was not the man to receive a newcomer from America with open arms. He was quite dubious about the two ova of *Macaca rhesus* that I had recovered from the reproductive tract; I had to go into great detail before he accepted my evidence. Nevertheless I liked him because he was so learned and so honest, and we became friends. I joined his class of thirty or forty students from various colleges of the University of London who were aiming at a degree in biology and hoped that Hill's lectures on advanced vertebrate embryology would help them pass the universitywide examination. He limited his talks to the embryology of birds, chiefly the domestic fowl and the sparrows, describing the earliest stages in almost endless detail in his droning nasal voice and strong

Lowlands Scottish accent. As the course wore on, it became obvious that J. P. was not going to get beyond the stage of the primitive streak, a few days after the beginning of incubation. I heard grumbles from my fellow listeners who had paid their fees and came twice a week, some of them from the other end of London; but to me, having no examination to face, the course was an instructive example of professional specialization.

A dozen years later, in December 1936, I attended a dinner of the Anatomical Association of Great Britain and Ireland, a few days before the abdication of King Edward VIII. As the time approached to end the meal with the usual toasts before the after-dinner speeches, I wondered what we would do about the customary "royal toast" to the king; none of us knew whether the United Kingdom had a king or not. But the chairman, Professor J. E. W. Frazer of St. Mary's Hospital School of Medicine, followed precedent by rising, glass in hand, and declaiming, "Gentlemen, the King!" We all rose and according to protocol replied, "The King, God bless him!"—all but J. P. Hill, who waited until everyone else had responded and then in fervid tones cried out, "The King, God grant him sense!" We all, dumbfounded, took our seats and sat for a while in silence, touched by the solemnity of J. P.'s prayer.

I had not been at University College long before I learned that Charles Singer, England's leading historian of medicine, was offering a course in the history of anatomy. I called at his office and was cordially granted the privilege of attending the lectures. Singer, then forty-seven years of age, was the son of a London rabbi. He held the Oxford degree of bachelor of medicine and master of surgery and the supplementary degree of M.D. After some years as a physician in the colonial service in Singapore, he had returned to England, married a learned wife, and entered upon a career as medical historian. His lectures that I heard in 1923 were scholarly, very well organized, and interestingly phrased. We rapidly became friends. When I told him that while in Berkeley I had begun to study the early medieval anatomists, he with great generosity put into my hands a file box containing a collection of his own notes and a half-dozen German dissertations on such misty figures of the eleventh and twelfth centuries as Copho of Salerno, Ricardus Anglicus, and the author of the second Salernitan anatomical dissertation. He told me to keep these papers as long as I liked, for he did not expect to return to studies of that period. His kindness encouraged me and helped me greatly in research that culminated in my first book, *Anatomical Texts of the Earlier Middle Ages*, published by the Carnegie Institution of Washington in 1927. Singer's wife was a medievalist, at that time engaged in compiling a catalogue of all the Greek and Latin medical manuscripts in British libraries. The Singers extended to us the hospitality of their home, and Betsy Corner and Dorothea Singer became warm friends.

Charles Singer was a jolly, humorous man of informal manners. He was, I think, disappointed that he was never called to a university chair, rising only to a lecturership at University College, London. There was no chair of the history of medicine in Great Britain at the time, and nobody with the money and inclination to endow one; nor was Charles ever knighted, an honor he deserved and would have accepted with zest. One evening in the 1950s when we were guests of the Singers at their home in Par, Cornwall, Charles appeared at dinner in a brightly colored waistcoat. His plump form, his round rosy face above a turned-down collar, gave him a hearty English look; I would have said like Mr. Pickwick, but Betsy thought the picture was that of a country squire and laughingly called him Sir Charles. I was alarmed; he might have taken the appellation bitterly, considering that he had been passed over for the honor, but actually he was pleased and took it as a compliment.

Charles Singer was in demand as a lecturer in British and American universities and medical societies. In the 1940s, on a tour in the United States that I had helped to arrange for him, he left Dorothea with us in Rochester while he went to give a lecture in Columbus, Ohio. I had observed that he was impractical in daily affairs and depended on his wife to manage his travels, and I was interested to see her in action when she and I accompanied him to the train. "This is your railway ticket, Charley; put it in your wallet and don't lose it. Don't forget to give the colored man in the sleeping car a dollar when you leave the train at Columbus; don't forget to set your watch back an hour when you go to bed." Charles got there and back safely, much amused about his reception in Columbus, where a committee of doctors with civic pride took him to see a new penitentiary. Later in his career Dr. Singer was engaged by the great science-based corporation, Imperial Chemical Industries, to direct the compilation of the five-volume *A History of Technology*, eventually published by Oxford University Press. He astonished me and other friends by handling the assigned task with notable efficiency, organizing a competent staff and bringing out on time the successive volumes of a valuable work. One of my numerous regrets for good deeds not done is that I never tried to get him elected a foreign member of the American Philosophical Society. He would have appreciated the honor, and both he and Dorothea would have contributed to the scholarly sociability of its meetings; but by the time that I acquired some influence in the Society, the Singers were growing old and no longer came often to the States.

The most enduring friendship I made while at University College was with Solly Zuckerman, then prosector at the London Zoo. A South African, he had come from Cape Town to London to study medicine. Solly was tall and good-looking, with strong Jewish features, highly intelligent and ambitious. I know of nobody else who in a long life has made so many wide-ranging and influential acquaintanceships. On my subsequent trips to England I saw him go from London to Oxford, where he was reader in anatomy with Professor W. E. Le Gros Clark, then to Birmingham as professor. For some years, while he was studying reproduction in baboons and other primates, our academic careers and research projects ran parallel, but in World War II Solly by sheer persistence and ability gained a position of great influence as scientific adviser to the air force on the problems of strategic bombing, as he has told in his vigorous autobiography, *From Apes to Warlords* (London, 1978). He was raised to the peerage in 1971 as Baron Zuckerman of Burnham Thorpe. Solly married a charming and intelligent woman who was a lady before he was a lord, for she was a granddaughter of the eminent lawyer and judge, Rufus Isaacs, Lord Reading, and as the daughter of the Second Marquis of Reading was called by courtesy Lady Joan. My wife met the Zuckermans on one of our later visits to England, and the two ladies became friends.

I have not yet discussed the research that I carried on at University College because as things went it was of little consequence. When I talked over my program with Professor Starling I told him about the discovery made by my students, mentioned in the preceding chapter, that the behavior of the involuntary, or "smooth" (meaning "not striated") muscle in the walls of the uterus and oviducts varies with the stage of the reproductive cycle and is therefore under the control of the ovary, presumably through hormonal action. I hoped that by carrying on some sort of experimental study of smooth muscle under his guidance I might gain background experience that would help me to investigate further the endocrine control of uterine and tubal muscle. Starling replied that nobody knew much about the physiology of smooth muscle; he had no clear idea as to how I might begin my inquiry. On the other hand, an apparently fundamental discovery about cardiac muscle had been announced in 1921 by Otto Loewi of Graz.[1] Heart muscle has one characteristic in common with smooth muscle, its spontaneous contractility. To study that might give me a lead. Loewi's findings had not yet been confirmed and were open to criticism. Why not spend my time in Starling's laboratory by checking Loewi's experiments? To this suggestion Starling added a practical argument: "You have got your professorship; you no longer have to prove yourself and can afford to risk a little time on something that may or may not be relevant to your major interest."

Of course I accepted Starling's advice, as courtesy required. There is no need to go into detail here about Loewi's discovery, which has been amply confirmed and led to basic advances in neurophysiology. In brief, what he found is this: it was well known that the spontaneous beating of the heart is to a considerable degree under the control of the vagus (tenth cerebral) nerve. Stimulation of the vagus slows or stops the heartbeat. How this control is exerted was not known until Loewi discovered that the nerve impulse acts upon the heart muscle by releasing into it at the manifold nerve endings a chemical substance (not then identified) that affects the contraction of the muscular tissue. The method by which he observed this mechanism—the humoral control of nerve action—was in principle simple but required apparatus and a kind of dexterity with which I was unacquainted. The experiments were done on frogs because

1. Otto Loewi, "Über Humorole Übertragbarkeit der Herzenerwirkung," *Pflüger's Archiv für die gesamte Physiologie* 189 (1921): 239–42.

their hearts go on beating for hours after they have been rendered insensitive to pain.

After a couple of weeks of clumsy beginnings, I was able to conduct more or less satisfactory experiments, some of which clearly repeated Loewi's findings; others were indecisive. When word got around the laboratory that I was getting somewhere, staff members—A. V. Hill, Clark, Anrep, and Babkin—came to look on and comment. These experienced men, who were unconvinced by Loewi's report, offered all sorts of theoretical explanations of my results that did not involve the hypothesis of humoral transmission. I did not have time to test their various suggestions. The upshot was that I never published my tentative findings.

I think now that if Starling had been younger and in better health he might have found for me some way of attacking the problem of uterine contraction. There was, in fact, a physiologist in London, C. Lovatt Evans of St. Bartholomew's Hospital medical school, who was beginning to make progress in the study of smooth muscle. If I had known of Evans and had gone to work with him, my pathway might have opened up. As I look back, however, the outcome seems unimportant. I had other lines of research awaiting my return to Rochester that were to win a rich yield of discovery. Two decades later associates of mine, S. R. M. Reynolds and Arpad Csapo (as I shall mention in later chapters) brought to the study of uterine muscle much broader experience than either Starling or I had in 1923–24. In any case University College afforded me far wider contacts with eminent scientists and scholars than I could have had at one of the hospital schools or even at Kiel with Schroeder.

I wanted while in England to make the personal acquaintance of two biologists whose work on the physiology of reproduction was fundamental to the research of investigators of my generation. Both were at Cambridge. Walter Heape had preceded me by almost thirty years in studying the cycle of female macaques under laboratory conditions. His work, begun in India and continued in Cambridge, was handicapped by illness, first his own and then that of his animals; he did not get very far, but his studies of other, more accessible animals had been very useful. My request to meet him brought a courteous reply saying that he was seriously ill and could not receive me.

Francis H. A. Marshall, author of *The Physiology of Reproduction* (1910), an indispensable handbook for workers in the field, invited me to visit him in his rooms at Christ's College. On a cold day I found him at his tea table by the fireside. A bearded, friendly man of forty-five, he treated me like a long-lost nephew. He talked about his work of many years and listened with interest to my report of my studies, but when I hinted that I would like to see his laboratory at the farm of Cambridge University's school of agriculture outside the city, he said that his successor, John Hammond, was in charge and did not offer to take me there or to give me an introduction to Hammond, whose work I knew about. I did not meet Hammond until a later visit to England. Evidently, Marshall had retired to the quiet life of a bachelor college don.

During our year in London, Betsy and I, with the aid of baby sitters (how vociferously bright George and self-sufficient Hester Ann would have resented the implication that they were babies!), managed to see many of the capital's major buildings and beauty spots from Greenwich to Hyde Park. We saw some memorable plays and three of the greatest English actresses of the time—Edith Evans in *The Merry Wives of Windsor* (the best performance by the leading lady I ever saw in a Shakespearean comedy); Beatrice Lillie at Golders Green in the revue in which she introduced Noel Coward's famous song "Mad Dogs and Englishmen," and Sybil Thorndike in the second performance of Bernard Shaw's new play, *Saint Joan.* We missed the premiere because of a minor illness that kept me from getting to the box office in time. The children enjoyed with us a lively performance of Barrie's *Peter Pan* with Gladys Cooper in the title role. The Blue Bird Theater company from Petrograd introduced us to the Russian stage, putting on a suitably mournful dramatization of the "Song of the Volga Boatmen," some boisterous Cossack dances, and a series of skits taking off the characteristics of various peoples. The American episode was danced by a quartet, two tall handsome blond young men and two tall beautiful girls, all stylishly dressed, the men in full evening dress with tails and white ties, the girls in *haut ton* evening gowns and fashionable coiffures, promenading round and round each other, stiffly erect, with mechanically regular steps, singing a song whose staccato refrain went "Telegraf, telefon / Henry Ford, Edison / Time iss money / Time iss money." I was prepared for the emphasis on American mechanics, inventiveness, and business zeal, but not for the depiction of sartorial perfection and social rigidity as American traits.

On several Sundays Betsy and I went to hear some of London's famous preachers, a diversion not unrelated to theater-going but perhaps odd for a scientist who was shedding his orthodox beliefs. Betsy was the daughter of a parson who took his homiletics seriously; I had and still have a perverse interest in the clergy and their various ways of expounding and exemplifying their faith. We heard the Bishop of London in St. Paul's Cathedral; in Westminster Abbey, thoughtful Ronald Knox, Anglican turned Roman Catholic; Maude Royden, Anglican, preaching in a Nonconformist auditorium; and to Betsy's astonishment, a high-church Congregationalist, wearing a little cross on his ample chest, gold buckles on his patent leather shoes, preaching a neatly polished sermon. At the Roman Catholic Westminster Cathedral I was so taken by the grand Romanesque architecture and gorgeous mosaics that I scarcely heard the preacher.

In April 1924, we set out to see more of what Londoners are pleased to call the provinces. We chose to sample Norwich, Lincoln, York, Whitby (The Corners' ancestral home), Edinburgh, and Glasgow, not stopping at hotels but taking lodgings in small boardinghouses or private homes.

In Glasgow I had arranged to meet John H. Teacher, professor of pathology in the University of Glasgow. With a colleague, the anatomist Thomas H. Bryce, Teacher had in 1908 described a human embryo about fifteen days old, believed to be the youngest ever seen up to that time. Dr. Teacher invited us to stay a couple of days at his home. We took the popular tourist route from Edinburgh to Glasgow, by rail to Callander, then by motor coach into the mountains and through the rugged gorge of the Trossachs, then by steamboat on lovely Loch Katrine to Stromachlachar; and by motor coach again to Inversnaid on Loch Lomond. From there a steamer took us to Balloch, whence we reached Glasgow by rail. The all day journey was beautiful but fatiguing to both parents and children. We arrived at the Teachers' front door in the late afternoon, tired and hungry and a bit frazzled.

The house was large and elegant. (I found out later that Teacher belonged to the family of distillers who produced

Teacher's Highland Cream.) After a cordial greeting by Mrs. Teacher the children were taken in hand by two maids in caps and frilly aprons. Professor Teacher arrived and added his courtly welcome. After a glass of sherry we sat down to an excellent meal accompanied and followed by good talk until about 10:00 P.M. I was beginning to think how good it would feel to lay my head on a pillow when our host said, "I know that you are eager to see the embryo. You will not have to wait until tomorrow; I keep the slides here, and if the ladies will excuse us we can get at it at once."

He set up a microscope in his study and we sat down to a three-hour session. Teacher knew that some other embryologists, including George Streeter, with whom I had been closely associated in Baltimore, were inclined to think that the Teacher-Bryce embryo was not normal. He wanted me to bear witness that the illustrations in his book were accurate. They were indeed quite faithful; to that I could agree, but for courtesy's sake I managed to avoid giving a verdict as to the state of the embryo. In the following three decades the Carnegie embryological laboratory, under Streeter's direction and later under mine as his successor, acquired largely through the work of John Rock and Arthur T. Hertig of Boston normal specimens of every day from the two-cell cleaving ovum through the first weeks. The Teacher-Bryce embryo has now been clearly seen to be abnormal and has faded from the textbooks.

The next day Professor Teacher took me to the site of a little brick building that had stood in a courtyard of the Glasgow Royal Infirmary, in which Joseph Lister in 1860 did the first operations under antiseptic conditions. Shortly before my visit Teacher had led a group of the medical faculty in protest against the demolition of the Lister ward, making himself, he told me, persona non grata with the hospital's board of managers. After they tore it down, he and his chauffeur went there in the night and smuggled out a dozen bricks as souvenirs. I made bold to ask him for one of them to set in the walls of our new operating suite at Rochester. This he willingly granted. After my return I had our medical illustrator, Nat Jacobs, model a little bas-relief portrait of Lord Lister in plaster, which we attached to the brick when it was laid into a corridor wall between the doors of two operating rooms. Our hospital director, Nathaniel Faxon, thereupon went to Massachusetts General Hospital to wangle a tile from the room where William T. G. Morton first demonstrated the use of ether as an anesthesia in 1846. Jacobs made another portrait, of Morton, and the tile was placed next to the Lister brick. Finally, our young chief of orthopedic surgery, R. Plato Schwartz, went all the way to the island of Cos in the Aegean Sea, where Hippocrates lived and taught, and brought home a small fragment of ancient marble which, he said, he picked up in the ruins of the temple of Aesculapius. The three relics remained for a quarter-century where we set them, and when in the 1950s the surgical area was altered, they were placed in the north wall of the medical library's reading room, where I trust they will stay as long as the building stands, as a reminder of the universality of the healing arts.

Early in June 1924, we settled our affairs in London and started for the Continent on the night boat from Harwich to Antwerp. After a day there we went on to Liège to stay a couple of days with the Firkets, whom we had known and liked when they were in Baltimore. Their children and ours somehow solved the language problem and played together while Betsy and I saw the city with Jean Firket. Our ultimate destination was Strasbourg, for a stay of two months to give me a taste of a European laboratory. We found excellent accommodations in a pension. Strasbourg's charming park, the Orangerie, provided a playground for the children. A private school accepted George as a temporary pupil and a nursery school for girls was equally ready to have Hester Ann. Not many Americans visited Strasbourg; our children were objects of curiosity to the teachers and pupils alike and were made much of.

G. Schaeffer, professor of physiology in the University of Strasbourg, had kindly consented to let me carry on some experiments on uterine motility. He provided a couple of kymographs and the services of a technician, and sent daily to an abbatoir for a pailful of sows' uteri. I wanted to see whether there was a reversible gradient of muscular activity along the tubular uterine horns that might help to explain a curious phenomenon I had reported (in "Internal Migration of the Ovum" [1921]) in sows, internal migration of early embryos from one uterine horn to the other to even up the number when one ovary had shed more ova than the other. As in London, research was hampered by my unfamiliarity with the facilities of the laboratory. I obtained no significant results but learned enough to turn the problem over some years later to a guest investigator in my own laboratory in Rochester.

It was for me a great pleasure to become acquainted at Strasbourg with the professor of histology, Paul Bouin, and his immediate colleague Paul Ancel, the embryologist; their beautifully clear and decisive monograph of 1910[2] had been a major landmark in the search for understanding of the corpora lutea. My French was barely sufficient for the occasion, but Bouin had a knack for leading the conversation with a foreigner, and we had a good talk. Then about fifty-three years old, he was plump and jolly. I fancy that his students must have called him Papa Bouin, just as we Johns Hopkins men spoke of Popsy Welch. Ancel, Bouin's contemporary, was lean and morose. He would not take me to his laboratory because, he said, the Ministry of Education had not seen fit to give him decent quarters.

The anatomy department at Strasbourg had, besides the two older men, a rising star of French science, Robert Courrier, a man of my own age. He and I had mutual interests, for he, too, was working on the reproductive cycle. His English was, to say the least, no better than my French, and he would not use what he had of it, but we had a technical vocabulary in common. As we sat together at his microscope he conducted both sides of the conversation in clear, textbook French. Putting a slide under the lens, he would describe what he was showing me and say, "Vous comprenez, M'sieur Corner?" to which I could generally reply, "Oui, vraiment." If now and then I did not agree with his interpretation, he would politely say in French, "Then your opinion must be so-and-so," stating my contrary interpretation for me. In this way we conversed with mutual comprehension. Courrier was called to Paris, became a leader in French endocrinology, and was elected permanent secretary of the Académie des Sciences. We met again in 1941 when we both addressed the Medical Society of Santiago, Chile, following an international congress of endocrinology at Montevideo. He was as keen as

2. P. Ancel and P. Bouin, "Recherches sur les fonctions du corps jaune gestatif, 1. Sur le déterminisme de la préparation de l'uterus à la fixation de l'oeuf," *Journal de Physiologie* 12(1910): 1–10.

ever and very popular with the Latin-American doctors.

Strasbourg, since 1917 once more French, is a handsome city and its surroundings in the Vosges Mountains equal the Black Forest for walking tours. In mid-July the four Corners took to the mountains with rucksacks on their shoulders. For five or six days we wandered through the forests and ancient villages, stopping to see ruined castles and passing also the remains of earthworks and campsites of World War I. Our rate of travel was set by the children. George could do ten miles a day. Hester Ann trudged gaily along, a mile or two at a time, then rode for a spell on my shoulders. We covered some of the same ground that I had been over in 1911 with Grover Powers and the Freiburg schoolmasters. The grand restored castle of Hoh-Königsburg was the climactic point of the tour, which the children enjoyed as much as Betsy and I. In a little list I carry in my head, of the happiest hours of my life, one of the most cherished items is a stop for rest on a grassy mountain slope, where we enjoyed our lunch in happy companionship, finishing the simple feast with wild strawberries that nature had provided for our dessert. We were at Ribeauville on the eve of Bastille Day, July 14, and slept in the dormitory of a girls' school whose concierge gained an honest penny by renting rooms to holiday tourists. The good woman, noting my bad French, asked if we were foreigners, and when I said we were Americans exclaimed with astonishment, "Vous avez traversé la mer avec les enfants?" At the fine old city of Colmar, we took the rucksacks from our shoulders and returned to Strasbourg by railway.

At the end of August we left for Paris, stopping one day at Nancy because Betsy, keen about the eighteenth century, wanted to see the palaces and plazas created by the city planner Stanislas Leczinski, last duke of Lorraine. I do not remember much about the few days we spent in Paris; my thoughts must have been centered on getting home. George IV of course wanted to ride to the top of the Eiffel Tower; we had a boat trip on the Seine, and I suppose we took the children through a wing or two of the Louvre. Betsy and I traveled one day to Chartres, leaving the children in charge of a temporary nursemaid. I had written to the Bibliothèque Municipale for permission to see a thirteenth-century manuscript of *Anatomia Ricardi Anglici* ("Anatomia vivorum"). The librarian, M. Huet, welcomed us kindly and in a few minutes produced the precious book, remarking that not every French library could find a manuscript so promptly.

We sailed from Le Havre on the immense Cunarder *Berengaria* in third class ("college cabin"). Our friend George Boas from Berkeley days was aboard with his wife and infant daughter. We had arranged to cross the Atlantic with them so that Betsy could help Simone Boas, who was subject to seasickness even in good weather, to care for the baby—a willing service that cemented our friendship with those fine people. From New York we returned to Baltimore, where I stayed for a fortnight. Leaving Betsy and the children to the hospitality of my parents, I went on to Rochester to report for duty and find a home for the family.

I have given a whole chapter to this one year abroad, because it meant much for each of us. It had brought me the friendship of eminent scientists and redoubled my zeal for teaching and research; to my wife, love of her father's homeland and knowledge of English ways that flowered years later in her two fine books. Young George had stored away memories of people and places that half a century has not dimmed. Hester Ann—her horizon, too, widened by foreign travel—would tell her new playmates in Rochester about a little river in Kent and the grandma with a punt, Belgian children chattering in French, and a green Alsatian hillside dotted with wild strawberries.

10

ROCHESTER: THE SCHOOL OF MEDICINE

Arriving at Rochester on a cloudy morning in September 1924, to enter upon the professorship of anatomy that I was to hold for seventeen years, I stepped off the sleeping car from Baltimore, booked a room at the YMCA, and took a taxi to Elmwood Avenue on the southern edge of the city. Before me as far as I could see to the south was level, open country dotted with handsome trees, through which to the right (westward) I could glimpse the quiet Genesee River flowing toward the city. Immediately before me a muddy, rutted lane ran from Elmwood Avenue, itself hardly more than a country road, into a wide field, until recently a pasture for horses. Here stood the concrete frame of a huge five-story building that was to house the Strong Memorial Hospital and the University of Rochester's school of medicine and dentistry. Dean Whipple had first put up a small square brick building, the future animal house, in which he had installed forty dogs he had brought from California, plus two professors, himself and our biochemist, Walter Bloor, and also Nathaniel Faxon from Massachusetts General Hospital, our hospital director-to-be. There was a room for me, with a bench for my microscope, a drawer for my papers and instruments, and a couple of chairs.

The site was a half-mile from the nearest letter box on Mt. Hope Avenue, where our incoming mail was deposited each morning. The dean told me that as the latest comer, it was my duty to pick up the mail every morning, and this I did for many weeks until Stanhope Bayne-Jones, our bacteriologist, arrived from Johns Hopkins. The pasture lot, already scarred and rutted by trucks and bulldozers, became on rainy days a wide pond that the medical students, when they came, called Lake Faxon. In the long winter of 1924–1925, the lane from Elmwood Avenue was so often blocked by snow that Karl Wilson, our professor of obstetrics and gynecology, and I carried a couple of shovels in my car every morning to open up the way. We all lunched together with the construction crew in a wooden cookhouse beside the lane.

The dean saw to it that I was promptly introduced to two eminent Rochester doctors whose goodwill he considered essential to our undertaking. Dr. Edward W. Mulligan, chief surgeon of the Rochester General Hospital, was an elderly man of large frame and heavily jowled face who was beginning to be shaky with age and a mild diabetic condition. He was a close friend of George Eastman and, as such and because of his own rugged honesty, was the most influential medical man in the city. Whipple depended upon him for advice on dealings with the local physicians, choosing a few of the best of them for appointment to our faculty as visiting physicians and fending off less suitable people whose disappointed ambition to join the school was already beginning to create jealousies. Dr. Mulligan's wife, younger than he, conducted at their home on East Avenue, near George Eastman's big house, a kind of salon of socially elite Rochesterians, to which the Corners were admitted when Betsy came to town. Betsy was duly introduced to Mrs. Mulligan by the dean's wife, Katherine Whipple. Betsy and Mrs. Mulligan liked each other, and we became frequent guests at the Mulligans' house.

The other influential medical man to whom Dr. Whipple introduced me for political reasons was George W. Goler, the city's health officer. Dr. Goler was the opposite of Dr. Mulligan, slight of build, outgoing, enthusiastic, and a belligerent guardian of the city's health. He had won a secure position of authority among the local politicians, who were rather a better lot than their kind in other American cities. George Aldritch, the Republican boss, had learned not to meddle with the public schools and the health office. He left Goler alone and supported his plan to build a municipal hospital adjacent to Strong Memorial, to be staffed by the university's medical faculty. The university has recently acknowledged its debt to Dr. Goler for his help in the early days by naming after him a large residence hall on the medical campus.

Dr. Goler—to test, I suppose, my interest in clinical medicine—took me to his small hospital for infectious diseases to see a case of smallpox. There cannot now be many people left in the United States who have seen that once common disease. Goler's patient, a woman whose face was one horrible swollen mass of confluent purulent vesicles, died a few days later.

Important as it was that the medical professors should win the regard of Dr. Mulligan and Dr. Goler, it was even more important that Mr. Eastman should be apprised of our arrival and (the dean hoped) look upon us favorably. He had met me in Baltimore when I was being looked over as a possible member of the faculty, so no formal introduction was needed. Betsy and I were invited three or four times a year to Mr. Eastman's Sunday evening musicales. He was then, in 1923, sixty-nine years of age, of medium height, with a rather pale, squarish face, shrewd eyes, and a straight firm mouth. He stood sturdily erect but walked with the unhurried steps of a man of his years. He said little to guests like us, with whom he was not intimate, but his manner was easy and friendly.

Entering his large and handsome residence at 5:00 P.M. on one of these occasions and turning over our coats and scarves to deferential servants, we found ourselves among a party of fifty or seventy-five men and women representative of Rochester's business, social, and educational enterprises and the civic government—the president of the university, perhaps a dean or two, and top professors; the pastor of St. Luke's, maybe the mayor or the local congressman; leading industrialists, business and professional men. In the course of a year we met there everybody that our host looked upon as an asset to the city's culture and political governance, of course with their ladies; Eastman, though a bachelor, well understood the power of feminine influence and enjoyed the company of intelligent women who were safely married.

From five to six o'clock we were seated in the music room to hear the Kilbourne Quartet, named for Eastman's mother and composed of professors in the university's school of music. Then followed a light supper at tables for four (carefully assigned by place cards) in the sitting room and in the trophy room under the trophies of our host's hunting expeditions from Alaska to Africa —great mounted heads of superb beasts, bears, lions, deer of many lands, and an elephant. After supper Eastman's personal organist, Harold Gleason, played for us another hour on the built-in pipe organ. We left with gratitude for a pleasant evening and flattered by the feeling that we had been included in a hand-picked coterie of influential Rochesterians.

One of my first concerns as professor of anatomy was to secure a supply of unclaimed human bodies for my dissecting rooms. The city and state officials with whom I had to deal had no previous experience with such a sensitive business. Dr. Goler gave me his moral support. So also did Dr. Floyd Winslow, the politically minded coroner's physician, but in Rochester, a well-ordered and prosperous city of medium size, most of the unfortunates who died under the coroner's jurisdiction were claimed by relatives. My chief resource would have to be the large state hospital for the insane, in whose care many lone paupers ended their lives. I was warned that its director, Dr. Eugene H. Howard, would probably not be cooperative, and I therefore asked President Rhees to accompany me to Dr. Howard's office.

In later years I had many opportunities to observe Dr. Rhees's diplomatic talents, but never was I more impressed than when I sat beside him watching those two politically skilled old gentlemen fight it out. Dr. Howard argued that his superiors at Albany required post-mortem examinations on all patients who died in the state hospital. Dr. Rhees pointed out that the laws of New York State compelled all persons in charge of unclaimed bodies to deliver them on request to a chartered medical school, and he gently warned Dr. Howard that the University of Rochester was chartered by the state and had friends in Albany. Dr. Howard capitulated, and I never had any trouble from that source.

An unexpected event recalled me briefly to scientific endeavor quite soon after I set up my microscope in the animal house. In Rochester at that time most abdominal gynecological operations were done by general surgeons. I had told not only Dr. Mulligan but also Dr. Thomas Jameson, chief surgeon of the Highland Hospital, that I would like to receive materials of embryological interest from their operating rooms. One evening about nine o'clock Dr. Jameson had me called to say that he was operating on a woman for a ruptured tubal pregnancy. By that time I had my own car, and hastening to the hospital I found the patient still on the table. Dr. Jameson was closing the abdominal incision. The specimen he had saved for me, a small blood clot, was in a basin on the steam radiator, where he had ordered it put to keep it warm. I had arrived just in time to save it from cooking. I took it out to my room in the animal house, to which the night watchman admitted me. Putting the clot in a small dish of physiological salt solution under the beam of my microscope lamp I went to work with needles and fine forceps, carefully picking away at the clot until I saw the white outer (chorionic) layer of the embryonic sac. The chorion was about fifteen millimeters in diameter. Within it I could vaguely see the embryo. An embryologist with more experience of early human embryos would have placed the unopened sac in fixing fluid, opening it a day later when the tissues were fixed, but I opened it at once under my dissecting microscope with fine scissors, fortunately making only a small nick in the umbilical vein, and had before me a beautiful sight, a perfect embryo 3.0 millimeters (⅛ inch) in length, with ten somites—the first human embryo of precisely ten somites ever recorded.[1] It was about twenty-five days old. With a medicine dropper I gently flooded it with Bouin's picro-acetic fixing fluid, thus getting prompter fixation than if I had waited for the fluid to filter through the intact chorion. I sat for a while in the dark room, where only the embryo was brightly lighted, admiring this gem of nature's making.

Since we had as yet no facilities for photographing the embryo nor for sectioning it, I took it to Baltimore to the Carnegie Institution's Department of Embryology at Johns Hopkins Medical School, whose director, Dr. George L. Streeter, had it photographed. James Didusch, the skilled Carnegie artist, made preliminary sketches. A technician, C. H. Miller, imbedded it in paraffin and cut it on the microtome into a perfect series of sections ten microns (1/240 inch) thick. Under the microscope its

1. The somites are pairs of elevations in sequence along the back of the embryo, formed by masses of cells below the embryonic skin, that will give rise to the muscles of the trunk and limbs. Before the limb buds develop, the number of somites gives a convenient indication of the stage of development of the embryo.

cellular structure proved to be excellently preserved. From the sections Osborne Heard, Streeter's modeler, exactly reproduced its external form and internal structure, magnified 100 times, in plaster by a special method developed by the Carnegie laboratory. Didusch's final drawings based on the photographs, his own sketches, and the models, are among the finest depictions of a human embryo ever made. They are reproduced in my article "A Well-Preserved Human Embryo of Ten Somites," in the Carnegie *Contributions to Embryology*, volume 20, number 394, 1929. Some of them appear also in various textbooks. For my technical description of the embryo I needed enlarged photographs of many of the sections. With the goodwill toward the medical school that I was finding to be characteristic of Rochester's industrial scientists, Dr. C. E. K. Mees of the Eastman Kodak Company asked an expert on his research staff, Mr. A. P. Trevelli, to make the photomicrographs for me. The sectioned embryo on glass slides is still preserved as no. 5074 of the Carnegie collection of human embryos. I still shudder when I recall how near I came to cutting it in two.

A month or so after I arrived in Rochester Betsy came from Baltimore and we went house hunting. Katherine Whipple, feeling her responsibility as the dean's wife to advise newly arriving professors' wives about the social conventions of the intellectual elite of the city, gave Betsy a map on which she had circled a residential area to the south of elegant East Avenue and eastward from Oxford Street with its long aisle of magnolia trees. To live outside this region, she hinted, would impair our social standing. We took the hint and found a modestly comfortable house for rent at 115 Barrington Street. We lived there three years and then, disregarding conventionality, moved to a less prestigiously situated but charming cottage at No. 1 Castle Park, just off Mt. Hope Avenue, on the grounds of a large nineteenth-century castellated mansion covered with wistaria vines, the former home of a prominent old Rochester family. Here the children had more room for outdoor play. We were near the medical school and Highland Park with its superb collection of lilac trees, in May a scene of heavenly beauty. We were not troubled by proximity to the large Mt. Hope Cemetery; we had no personal ties to those who lie there, and its quiet dignity was restful to contemplate.

Our children entered school at once, George at Allendale, a private preparatory school in the suburbs, Hester Ann at first at a nearby public school, then at the Harley School for girls, also in the suburbs. Betsy and I thought it advisable to form a church connection, largely out of consideration for our devout parents. After trying a Methodist church and St. Luke's (to whose Episcopalian ritual Betsy inclined) we surprised both sets of parents by going more or less regularly to the downtown Brick Presbyterian Church because we liked its intelligent and liberal pastor, Justin W. Nixon, and also because it had a reputedly excellent Sunday school (both children found this dull and balked at attending it). Toward the end of our residence in Rochester we were falling away from church attendance.

Betsy soon found an appealing opportunity for social service. At the Rochester General Hospital, where Dr. Mulligan reigned supreme, his enterprising wife had created a library service for patients, something of a novelty at that time, which brought to the bedside a choice of light and serious reading to while away the weary hours of a stay in the hospital. Nat Faxon, director of Strong Memorial Hospital, discovering that Betsy Corner loved books and had some library training, invited her to organize a similar service. To prepare herself for the task, she volunteered to work with Mrs. Mulligan for several months, and when the doors of our hospital opened for patients in 1926, Betsy was ready with a little cartful of books to trundle through the wards and private rooms. Soon she had her own corps of volunteers who made a daily service possible.

My own introduction to the best element of Rochester's masculine society came through my election to membership in the "Club." Rochester had several little groups of intellectually inclined men of importance in the community, who met fortnightly in the homes of the more affluent members or at the Genesee Valley Club for dinner followed by the reading of a paper by one of the members. The Club, jocosely called the "Pundits" by the members' wives, was the oldest of these clubs; it claims, indeed, to be the oldest existing group of the kind in the United States. Its members, in my day, included President Rhees, Dr. Mulligan, two professors of the university (Dexter Perkins, American history, and Ryland Kendrick, Greek); two professors of the Rochester Theological Seminary (a Baptist divinity school); a couple of bank presidents and a lawyer or two; E. G. Miner, head of a technical industry and a keen bibliophile; Raymond Ball, treasurer of the university; and Marion Folsom, treasurer of the Eastman Kodak Company. George Eastman had been a member, but after reading one paper, on price fixing in the photographic trade, he resigned on the ground that preparation of a paper every few years was too great a burden. George Whipple had also been a Pundit, but resigned for a different reason from that of the Kodak magnate. We met in black tie dress every second Thursday evening in the season, drank cocktails, ate a rich dinner, and listened to a serious essay, after which it was our custom for each member in turn, beginning at the right of the host of the evening, to discuss the paper, no matter how far it was from his own field of interest. It was this rule that caused George Whipple to resign; he saw no fun or value in talking about something he could not expertly comprehend. To me it was useful practice in marshaling my thoughts. I remember some of my Pundit Club papers, one on medicine in the poems of Chaucer, another on the discovery in my laboratory, by Willard Allen and myself, of the ovarian hormone progesterone. The latter, of course, had to be adapted to the membership, in which I was the only scientist, but to air ideas hatched in a laboratory in that environment of mahogany and old silver could be a wholesome corrective of scientific brashness.

One winter after being a Rochesterian for several years, I wrote from the depths of my heart a bold essay, "The Place of the Scientist in the Rochester Community," in which among other things I spoke of the pressure of routine duties and routine social demands upon men engaged in advanced scientific investigation. Ryland Kendrick, steeped in the humanist way of life (his father had been professor of Greek before him), in his discussion of my remarks implicitly accused me and my fellow scientists of inhuman coldness and philistinism. To my astonishment Dr. Mulligan, that rugged old surgeon, came to my defense with a sharp reprimand of the humanist who could not see behind the rigor of such research as mine a love of learning and a respect for humanity equal to his own.

We were not always so serious; now and then comedy broke in. One autumn evening it was Kendrick's turn to entertain the club at his old family home north of town, halfway to Lake Ontario. He was a teetotaler; we could expect neither cocktails nor wine. Three or four members, including Tom Spencer, a quiet-spoken businessman and trustee of the university, and Dexter Perkins, professor of history, plump and vocal in a high-pitched voice, a weighty intellectual of the college faculty, stopped at a bar in town to fortify themselves against the evening's drought. When we took our seats on Kendrick's antique mahogany chairs at his heirloom table decked with the family silver and chrysanthemums from his garden, Perkins and Spencer, still warmed by their martinis, began a mock argument over some remark of Spencer's. "That's not true," shouted Perkins. "What!" cried Tom. "Do you, a professor in the University of Rochester, dare call one of your trustees a liar?" Perkins stiffened in his chair, about to launch a retort, and at that very moment the rungs of his chair gave way. With a crash he landed on the floor, sitting on a pile of disjointed mahogany, his black tie askew, his legs under the table, his flushed face a map of discomfiture and chagrin. The chair, fortunately, was not beyond repair, but the Pundits' dignity was shattered. We laughed and laughed until we had to stop for breath. At intervals while the essay of the evening was being read someone would start laughing again and all of us, Perkins included, joined in. As I drove homeward three hours after the debacle, the thought of our learned friend on the dining room floor hit me so hard that I couldn't drive straight and had to pull over to the curb until I recovered my composure.

But I have wandered from the theme of this chapter, the founding of a front-rank school of medicine. During the fall of 1924 Whipple, Bloor, and I had plenty to do, planning for the beginning of instruction in a year's time. Stanhope Bayne-Jones, Southern gentleman and all-around master of microbiology, came next to set up his office in the animal house, and Wallace Fenn soon followed. With their arrival the preclinical departments were all represented. John Murlin was ready to bring his department of vital economics (nutrition) out from the college campus to join us. The four clinical chiefs came during the next year as they finished their commitments elsewhere—my classmate at Johns Hopkins, John J. Morton (surgery), William S. McCann (internal medicine), Karl M. Wilson (gynecology and obstetrics), and Samuel W. Clausen (pediatrics). Old John Abel, my former professor of pharmacology, said to me, "You boys are just starting a Johns Hopkins country club up there in Rochester," but that was an exaggeration. Only five of the nine (not counting Faxon) had studied medicine at Johns Hopkins. Every one of us except Bayne-Jones had had experience in other schools, and he had wide European contacts during World War I. We brought together experience gained in a dozen of the foremost medical and biological institutions in the United States, Canada, and Great Britain.

Not long before this time the nation's newspapers had been full of the famous trial of John Scopes for teaching the theory of evolution in a Tennessee high school. One day the Rochester expressman brought out from town a crate of rhesus monkeys consigned to me. Setting it down outside the animal house, he bawled out, "Here's a bunch of professors from Dayton!"

I was ready for the monkeys. Dean Whipple had built open-air cages for them and a workroom for me on top of the animal house. A young man named Frederick Kesel who had been working with the construction crew applied for a permanent job with the school, and I took him on as my animal caretaker. Fred worked for me with intelligence and perfect reliability during the seventeen years I was in Rochester. With his help I began in the summer of 1925 a long series of observations and experiments on the menstrual cycle of *Macaca rhesus* that will be described in the next chapter.

Under the extraordinary modular building plan that Whipple worked out with the architect and the contractors, the concrete frame of the building was being bricked in at one corner of the structure while the concrete workers were pouring the other end of the frame two or three hundred feet away. By the spring of 1925 the northwest corner, where my department was to be housed on the fifth floor, was ready for us. I was working there at my desk and my microscope bench before the carpenters had hung the doors of my office and private laboratory. The interior construction was utterly plain—unplastered brick walls, unpainted concrete ceilings, naked cement floors, exposed pipes for water and drainage. At this stage Dr. Goler brought to see me a well-known German zoologist. On the way to my office they happened to meet Wallace Fenn, the youngest member of the new faculty, and William McCann, our professor of internal medicine, who was the same age as myself. On leaving my office, Goler told me afterward, the visitor exclaimed: "What kind of place is it? The building is a barn, the professors are all boys!"

Once we were established in permanent quarters my department began to take shape. Fred Kesel added to his duties those of embalmer of cadavers for dissection, an art that I was able to teach him because of the experience I had reluctantly acquired in Berkeley in 1917–19. For the microscopical technique Dr. Whipple transferred to my laboratory a capable high school graduate, Bessie Bodine, whom he had been training for several months. I acquired also a departmental secretary, Cornelia Clark, just graduated from a secretarial school, who handled my clerical work admirably for several years until she married a medical student. I had plenty of work for her, for besides my teaching, research, and historical studies, the dean called on me quite often to serve the school as a scribe. I drafted at his request the first catalogue of the school, setting forth our aims and program, the courses offered, admission policy, and the roster of the faculty. With a little revision by the president and the dean, this went to press early in 1925 to announce our readiness to receive in October our first class of medical students.

Newspaper publicity and hearsay among the colleges had begun early to bring applications for admission. Whipple appointed a selection committee consisting of himself, Walter Bloor, William McCann, and me. We four continued to act as the committee on admissions during my seventeen years at Rochester. In the busy spring season when applications were coming in, we met weekly in the dean's private office, sitting on laboratory stools around a table piled with application papers. We looked first of all for men and women with high college records in biology or (at that period somewhat less important) chemistry. We were impressed by evidence of special achievement in non-scientific subjects, especially English, but also in out-of-the-way fields. We accepted a woman who had majored in music, a bachelor of divinity, and a young man who had worked his way through college as a skilled bartender at a country club. Whipple, a doctor's son and in college an athlete, was keen on doctors' sons. They were prepared by observation of their fathers, he said, for a career of hard work and responsibility. He also favored college athletes, especially captains of teams, who, he thought, were likely to carry sturdily the physical and mental burdens of our profession. Looking back at our decisions, I see that the others—Bloor, the biochemist; McCann, the internist; and I were also looking unconsciously for applicants after our own respective images. Since there were four members of the committee, we probably averaged our selection reasonably well.

Out of about one hundred candidates for the first class we chose twenty-two, twenty men and two women, seven of them from the University of Rochester, the others from a dozen colleges from Lund, Sweden, to Berkeley, California. They were all good students; there was no dullard nor dawdler among them, and they have all been useful practitioners of medicine. As I think about the first class, two stand out especially, Fred Metildi and Jack Goldstein, because of their long service to their medical alma mater as members of the visiting faculty.

To help me teach gross human anatomy, histology, and neurology, I tried first to get Elmer Belt, my best friend among the students I had taught in Berkeley, then working in Baltimore, but he was bent on returning to Los Angeles, his native city, to begin his brilliant career in the practice of urology. Two recent graduates of the Johns Hopkins Medical School who had done research with me there, as I mentioned in chapter 8, joined me—Alan Guttmacher and Franklin Snyder. Guttmacher, a young man of superior quality, found himself less interested in research than in practice. He left me after one year to return to Baltimore for an internship in obstetrics and went on to become chief of obstetrics at Mt. Sinai Hospital in New York. He ultimately rose to international leadership of the family planning (birth control) movement.

Guttmacher was the first of three outstanding leaders in the practical application of scientific thought to problems of human sex behavior who were students of mine in medical school. The three included Guttmacher at Johns Hopkins and at Rochester Mary Steichen Calderone, founder and head of SIECUS (Sex Information and Education Council of the United States), and William H. Masters, who now leads his own Masters and Johnson Foundation at St. Louis. Detlev Bronk once humorously introduced me to a visiting scientist as "the man who made sex respectable." If there is any truth in his greatly exaggerated characterization, such influence as I have had rested upon the work of those pupils, for I never carried on research on human sex behavior. Yet I did have to face lingering taboos when I began my research on sex physiology. I think that Guttmacher's career was influenced to some extent by my stand. Masters has acknowledged that my advice helped him with the strategy of finding moral support for his daring work; I told him to get a post in a strong university department of obstetrics and gynecology and start from there—which he did through the backing of another of my former students, Willard Allen, at Washington University, St. Louis. I do not think I had any direct influence on Mary Calderone's well-informed and high-minded efforts for better understanding of sexual relations, except perhaps for the example of scientific interest evinced in my teaching.

Franklin Snyder was a Pennsylvania Dutchman, stubborn and argumentative, with critical rather than constructive talent. The students liked him because he joined their bull sessions and philosophized with them whole evenings at a stretch. I liked him, too, but I could never get him to finish a solid piece of research. George Wislocki thought I underrated Snyder, even though I got him promoted to assistant professor. Wislocki took him to Harvard in 1928 but never promoted him beyond the rank he had held at Rochester.

A year before Snyder left I recruited Wilfred Copenhaver, who had just taken his Ph.D. in zoology at Yale with Ross G. Harrison. A quietly cheerful man, he was a careful teacher and a dexterous experimental embryologist, working, like most of Harrison's pupils, on frog and amblystoma tadpoles. I enjoyed driving him in early spring to Mendon Ponds Park, fifteen miles south of Rochester, to collect amblystoma eggs for his experiments. In the spring after he came to join me the Rochester newspapers, eager for sensational news from the new medical school, found out that Copenhaver was transplanting hearts from one tadpole to another—not mature beating hearts, as they assumed, but pinhead-sized bits of embryonic tissue that would develop into a heart. After a lurid news story, a disgruntled citizen wrote to the *Rochester Herald:*

Has the new Rochester Medical School gone into the advertising business, or have they simply employed the best advertisers to be had in the country?

The daily reader of the local press reminds us old timers of Kilmer's Swamp Root, Piso's Cough Cure, Hood's Sarsaparilla, good old Peruna and other highly advertised cure-for-alls. Who are these wonderful doctors that no one has ever heard? Who are these wonderful surgeons who operate so successfully on tadpoles? Who are these wonderful men who have never had even a private practice?

Is Rochester about to be deluged with an avalanche of quacks?

Copenhaver remained with me for two years until Samuel Detweiler enticed him to Columbia University, where he ultimately became head of the anatomy department of the College of Physicians and Surgeons and is now emeritus professor.

To replace Snyder as my senior associate I was fortunate in securing Robert Kyle Burns, another of Ross Harrison's students, who had been instructor at the University of Cincinnati. He came to us as assistant professor and was soon promoted to associate professor. Burns is a cultivated Virginian, widely read in literature and American history and a skilled field naturalist. His research on experimental embryology was aimed at analyzing the development and differentiation of the reproductive organs, particularly the testis and ovary and their respective ducts. His subtle and thorough work, carried out with great technical skill, brought much credit to our department. Thoroughly devoted to teaching and research, Burns had no desire for executive burdens. He remained at Rochester as long as I was there and then went with me to Baltimore as a member of the Carnegie Institution, a post equivalent to a full professorship. At Rochester he took over the leadership of the course in gross human anatomy. More than any other of my staff associates at Rochester he became my personal friend and intimate adviser in departmental affairs.

In 1930 I put our course in anatomical neurology on a firm basis by securing from Johns Hopkins Wilbur K. Smith, a medical graduate in the class of 1927. Thoroughly acquainted with the human nervous system and a student particularly of the brain cortex, he has remained at Rochester throughout his career, first in anatomy, then in clinical neurology.

As the classes grew in size, reaching fifty men and women

in the 1930s, Burns needed help with the gross anatomy course. I took on another Yale Ph.D., Charles E. Tobin, an ardent gross anatomist—a rare species nowadays. He did some good work on the adrenal gland, but his chief interest was in gross and surgical anatomy. He spent long hours in the dissecting room, increasing his own knowledge of the human body and passing it on to the students, who loved him for his friendly ways and careful teaching. Tobin remained with the school long after I left. The University of Rochester, recognizing his devoted services, created for him in 1960 a professorial chair of human biology in the department of anatomy. Dr. Elbert B. Ruth, who came to us from the University of Wisconsin in 1931 as an instructor and was promoted to assistant professor in 1935, helped effectively with the gross anatomy course. He was called to Georgetown University in 1937. Another member of my department, though he really served the entire school, was our medical illustrator, Nat C. Jacobs. Trained first at the Art Institute of Chicago, then in medical illustration under Max Broedel at Johns Hopkins, Jacobs was a versatile draftsman especially skilled in pen-and-ink line drawing. Those I have named were the senior members of my department. As the school grew larger there were others who served for a year or two as teaching associates and fellows or came as guest investigators. In all, during my seventeen years as professor in charge, thirty-five men and women were listed in the school's catalogues as attached to the department of anatomy. Several of the fellows took part in teaching.

With two of the three major anatomical courses in the hands of permanent teachers—gross anatomy under Burns and neurology under Wilbur Smith—I could devote myself to the histology course. In many medical schools this subject had been taught entirely from prepared sections of the various organs and tissues. From Franklin Mall, Florence Sabin, and Herbert Evans I had learned how the subject could be made alive by introducing as much as possible the study of fresh tissues such as fresh blood smears, areolar connective tissue spread out on the slide, and nerve and muscle fibers teased out with needles, all studied under the microscope in comparison with the fixed and stained permanent slides. I tried to go farther than my teachers in this respect. I had the school's carpenter shop make up simple "warm boxes" to place over the microscopes with only the eyepiece projecting at the top, heated by an electric lamp bulb which the student turned on and off to keep the interior at body heat. With this equipment the student could watch his own white blood cells moving about on the slide, and by adding some india ink he could see them ingest the fine carbon particles just as if they were hostile bacteria. The then wholly mysterious mitochondrial cell inclusions were made visible in the living state by placing bits of tissue in a highly dilute solution of the aniline dye nile blue. On the afternoon designated for study of the lymphatic vessels I had a bucketful of sows' uteri sent up from a slaughterhouse. In that organ and its supporting membrane, the mesometrium, lymphatic vessels are very large and easily seen; each student could draw off a drop of peripheral lymph with a hypodermic needle and see for himself that lymph contains no lymphocytes until it passes through the first lymph nodes on its way to join the blood stream. I immodestly cherished the thought that this was the best histology course in the country; it certainly was the most boldly physiological.

I seized the opportunity to let the students know that microscopic anatomy has a history. On the lecture table in the laboratory I placed at almost every session a book or journal volume containing the first description or illustration of something in the day's teaching—Paul Langerhans's discovery of the pancreatic islets, announced in his doctoral dissertation in 1869; Regner de Graaf's first clear pictures of the ovarian follicles (1672); Aselli's illustration of the intestinal lymphatics (1627).

As long as the classes were small, our teaching could be informal. With an assistant or two, I moved about the room looking through the students' microscopes, helping them to see the important details of their preparations. A student who saw something particularly well would call his neighbors to have a look. If a knotty point baffled the students, we could all adjourn to a blackboard for an extemporaneous five-minute lecture. Nobody went to sleep in our histology sessions.

When the first class in the fall of 1925 came to the salivary glands, I put on a nice little experiment. Two white rats were brought into the class laboratory. One had not been fed for a couple of days, and the other had been given injections of pilocarpine, a salivating drug. My assistants killed the rats, rapidly exposed the submaxillary glands, and distributed a pinhead-sized bit to each student on a glass slide. The students flattened their samples under glass cover slips for examination under their microscopes. The cells of the unfed and dry-mouthed animal's salivary gland were certain to be full of unused zymogen granules; those of the salivated rat were certain to be drained of the granules.

After a few minutes, one of the men, Olan Mecker, came to me and said that he could see no difference between the two specimens. He offered to bet me five cents that I could not tell the two glands apart. We each slapped down a nickel and named two stakeholders who took the rats out of my sight and made up fresh slides marked *A* and *B*. The other students had by this time all left their places and gathered behind me as I bent over the microscope. I overheard some of them whispering. They were betting on the outcome and the odds were two to one against me—poor judgment statistically, for by merely guessing I had an even chance, and if I knew my business the odds were totally in my favor. I identified the specimens correctly, and collected my easily won nickel.

Amused by this sporting brand of pedagogy, I told the story to the two leaders of the local profession I have mentioned earlier in this chapter. Both had studied medicine in the old didactic days. Dr. Mulligan was shocked. Dr. Goler was charmed. Gleefully slapping his thigh, he cried: "Good, good! If you young professors and your students are going to challenge each other like that, we'll have a great medical school here!"

Informality, not often as extreme as that just narrated, was indeed characteristic of the school while we were all young together. I think there never was a medical school where good students could get so close to good teachers, at work and at play. Every spring and fall some of us, students and teachers, played softball on the open lawn just west of the J wing, where the rear of the psychiatry clinic now stands, in full view of the dean's office. Dr. Whipple, who had been a semipro baseball player in the Panama League for a season when he was a pathologist at Ancon, heartily approved our getting outdoor exercise. He had a backstop built for us and benches for the teams. He could not play ball himself because of a trick knee, but Fenn and I often took part in a lunch-hour game with William Bradford, who later succeeded Clausen as professor of pediatrics, and Sam Stabins, the surgeon, who is now a leading citizen of Rochester and a trustee emeritus of the university. As a member of the committee on admissions I used to ask every applicant why he wanted to study medicine at Rochester. One young man replied, very sensibly, I thought, that he had heard that the professors played softball with the students.

Of course we had a few problems with students, and some of them had problems of their own. Because I was the first senior member of the faculty to meet the entering class each year, new students generally brought their personal troubles to me. The dean seemed rather formidable until, in the second year, they got to know him better. The first year was a time for adjustment, sometimes difficult. I could fill a chapter of this book with human-interest stories of young people with acute homesickness, sudden doubt of their competence, girl trouble, a quarrel with a termagant landlady. One young man tried to abate his distress with whiskey, another developed a desperate state of claustrophobia. Our psychiatrist, Andrew Akelaitis, rescued them both with professional skill compassionately applied. Another young man was on the verge of suicide because he knew that he was about to be dropped from the school for failure in his studies. I asked two friendly classmates to stand by him night and day until a member of his family could be summoned, which they did with efficiency and kindness boding well for their future as physicians. A fine young woman was in medical school because her father, a friend of mine and a successful physician, having no sons, was trying to make a doctor of his daughter. She found in the course of her first year that she hated medical study and in her distress laid upon me the burden of relaying this heartbreaking news to her father. She later did the next best thing; she married a promising surgeon. I hope she produced for her father's satisfaction a grandson or two for the profession.

When, as occasionally happened, I had to discuss one of my problem cases with the dean, he was always helpful. He was tolerant of every youthful peccadillo except laziness and public misconduct unworthy of the profession. Student problems caused me deep concern, but they were few. It was a joy to watch the great majority of these men and women (and some of the troubled ones, too) grow in knowledge and judgment as they passed through the four years of hard work and emerged as clear-headed, competent young M.D.'s.

Besides the medical students, we had in the anatomy department candidates for advanced degrees other than medical. Robert Burns ably superviseed the studies and research of two men, Adrian Buyse and Thomas R. Forbes, who worked for their Ph.D's. in experimental embryology. Forbes went to the Johns Hopkins medical faculty and then to Yale, where he became a full professor of anatomy—a fair exchange for his teacher, Burns, who had taken his Ph.D. at Yale. We also had during my tenure five or six candidates, dental fellows and others, for the degree of master of science.[2] The academic career of one of these M.S. candidates is worth telling as an illustration of the remarkable flexibility of the University of Rochester as exemplified by the dean of the college, Arthur F. Gale, who also acted as dean of graduate studies in the 1930s.

William A. Ritchie began his career after high school as assistant at the Rochester Municipal Museum. Its director, Arthur Parker, encouraged him to seek professional training in Indian archaeology. Ritchie took his B.S. at the University of Rochester, but the master's degree was not available to him there, for want of a professor of his subject. Dean Gale kindly suggested that the department of anatomy in the medical faculty could with propriety take Ritchie for an M.S., anatomy being, as Gale said, the next thing to archaeology. I consulted my colleagues, Burns and Smith, both of whom were amateur collectors of Indian artifacts; they agreed, and we set up a course in archaeology, which simply meant that Ritchie came to our seminar room once a month during the academic year, to read to the three of us a chapter of a book that would constitute his M.S. thesis. It was a complete review of current knowledge

2. The original plans for the school included teaching dental students, but for reasons outlined in my biography of George Whipple, that plan proved to be impracticable, and instead the school provided postgraduate fellowships for dentists desiring to do research. Several dental fellows were attached to my department. See also W. T. McHugh, "Where's the dental school?" in *To each his farthest star: The University of Rochester medical center, 1925–1975* (Rochester, N.Y., 1975).

about Indian archaeology in the northeastern United States. This proving to be a truly educational process, at least for the three auditors, I certified Ritchie to Dean Gale as qualified for the oral examination. Gale named to the committee on Ritchie's candidacy Dexter Perkins, professor of American history, as chairman, Arthur Parker, and me. Because Perkins had a broken bone in his foot, we held the examination in his sitting room. Parker asked the first question: "What is the present state of Indian archaeology?" Ritchie replied learnedly for an hour; no other questions were asked. On the strength of his Rochester M.S. degree thus acquired, Ritchie was admitted to Columbia University for his Ph.D. He had had a long and productive career as curator of Indian archaeology in the great New York State Museum at Albany.

Between 1926 and 1940 nine scientists from other institutions came to Rochester on various fellowships to work for a year in our laboratory. Six of these were from foreign countries. Sidney A. Asdell was the first, in 1926, from Cambridge University on a Rockefeller Foundation grant, to study the reproductive cycle and the corpus luteum with me. After his year with us he returned to England, then came back to America to join the department of animal physiology at Cornell University, where he rose to a full professorship.

Seichi Saiki, assistant professor of gynecology at the University of Tokyo, followed in 1930. He worked on the ovary-pituitary relationship. Dr. Saiki was a friendly man of high character and intelligence. While he was with me, the crown princess of Japan, visiting the United States, fell ill in Buffalo, New York, and Saiki was summoned to see her professionally. Formal Japanese etiquette posed a dilemma for him. As I was his professional colleague and pro tem chief, protocol required him to inform me about his patient's illness; as physician to royalty he could reveal nothing. I absolved him from any duty to me. Saiki had a pleasant plan that I should go to Tokyo for a scientific address to the Japanese Gynecological Association, but World War II ended that idea. I never heard from him directly again but learned that he flourished in Tokyo University's school of medicine.

In 1930 also came Eduardo Bunster Montero of Santiago, Chile, an already prominent practitioner of gynecology, on a

Guggenheim Fellowship to broaden his knowledge of the physiology of reproduction. Friedrich Hoffmann of Düsseldorf, Germany, a Rockefeller fellow, worked with me on ovarian endocrinology in 1932. I lost track of him during World War II, but in 1979, to my great pleasure, I received a letter from him. As a professor of gynecology in Essen, West Germany, he was about to publish some recent research on the corpus luteum. Following a German scientific custom, he asked permission to dedicate the paper to me "as my teacher in endocrinology, for reason of your 90th birthday."

Graham Weddell from Cambridge, England, holding a fellowship of the Commonwealth Fund, spent the year 1937–38 with us, returning thereafter to England. After the war he settled at Oxford and ultimately became professor of anatomy there. He and I greatly enjoyed working together again at Oxford, which we did jointly with Dr. Wazir Pallie when I was Eastman Professor there in 1952–53. From Córdoba, Argentina, came in 1939 Doctora Inés de Allende, sent by the eminent physiologist Bernardo Houssay on a fellowship of the Argentine Society for the Advancement of Science. She and her handsome husband, a scholarly amateur, won many friends in Rochester. When I moved to Baltimore in 1940 Inés followed for another year and at the Carnegie embroyological laboratory began with Carl G. Hartman of my staff a study of the cyclic pattern of cellular change in the lining of the vagina of the rhesus monkey. After her return to Córdoba she applied in her gynecological practice the information gained in her research with us and wrote a book on the subject which I translated into English for publication in the United States. My three American visiting fellows were Jessie King, professor of physiology at Goucher College, Baltimore; Reginald Harris, director of the Long Island Biological Laboratory at Cold Spring Harbor, New York; and Samuel R. M. Reynolds, from Long Island Medical College, whose research with us is embodied in his magisterial book on the physiology of the uterus (1939). Later he joined me at the Carnegie Institution's laboratory in Baltimore. I shall have more to say of him in another chapter.

Human anatomy, the oldest branch of medical science, imposes upon its practitioners responsibilities for both the living and the dead. During my seventeen years in charge of an anatomical laboratory, I had four offers from people who wanted to sell us their own or someone else's body for future dissection. One of these was a destitute old woman whose needs were taken care of by the social service department of our hospital. Three young men in navy uniforms came to my office with a cheerfully stated proposal to sell me the right to dissect the youngest of the three when he should die, in return for an immediate cash payment. I told them that we did not buy bodies and pointed out that even if we had, I might not be able to collect the quid pro quo, especially in the case of a navy man, who might die anywhere in the world. They went away laughing. The third and strangest episode was a visit from a twenty-year-old girl who wanted me to buy the body of her younger sister who, she said, was dying of pneumonia. A telephone call to her home, after she left my office, was received with astonishment by her mother; the sister was in fact convalescent. I never learned what macabre idea the elder sister had in mind.

The fourth applicant was an elderly man, a gardener, sincere and intelligent, who said that he had been told by a doctor that he had heart disease and might die suddenly. He was not religious, he said, and wanted to dispose of his body without ceremony or expense to his family. He did not ask for money. I explained to him that his legal rights to his body would expire at death and that we could accept it only by permission of the nearest surviving relative. I drafted a letter stating his wishes, to be kept on his person. He thanked me, signed and pocketed the letter, and departed. Two months later he died suddenly at his work. His body was duly delivered to the medical school, with a message from his daughter asking me to assuage her mother's feelings by arranging a service. A Protestant minister kindly came to the laboratory. I turned our departmental seminar room into a chapel by removing a mounted skeleton and placed four chairs in front of the reading desk. My secretary sent out for some flowers. The corpse was wheeled in on our laboratory cart, covered with a clean white sheet. The minister read the service to a congregation of four—the wife and daughter, my secretary, and myself, and offered some consolatory words of his own. The two women were quite satisfied, and in due time the good man's body, treated with the respect for the dead that was always maintained in our dissecting rooms, was devoted to the education of future physicians.

The Rochester police asked us twice for expert advice on anatomical problems. The first was a pile of charred bones found in the ruins of a burned barn near the city. The police thought that these might be human; somebody had seen a stranger near the barn before the fire. They were not human; my guess was that they were the remains of a horse. My students were doing the histology of bone that afternoon. I put the specimens on the lecture table in the class laboratory and asked the students to file by and write on a slip of paper whether the bones were human or not. Everybody wrote "not human," which shows that first-year medical students are better anatomists than are policemen. One of the students, Benny Favata, with quiet assurance told me that they were the bones of an ox about a year old. This shows that a student sometimes may know more than a professor. Benny had studied veterinary medicine at Cornell before entering our medical school.

The other police case was a human leg somebody dragged out of Lake Ontario east of the steamboat landing where the Genesee River enters the lake. The police wanted to know what we could tell them about it, especially whether it had belonged to a man or woman. The leg had been severed from the body in a way that no surgeon or anatomist would have done and only a strong man with an axe could have managed. I thought that it had probably been severed by the propeller of one of the large steamboats that made the night run to Toronto. An x-ray picture showed the bones to be of adult age. The leg was intermediate in size between male and female. I made a tracing of the foot and showed it to an experienced shoe salesman, who said it could be a small male or large female foot. A bit of the pelvis was attached to the hip joint, but was too small to tell the sex. A telltale would be the width of the knee joint. The head nurse of our hospital's outpatient department was a woman of large frame. I explained the problem to her and she kindly let us x-ray her knee for comparison with our specimen. Her knee joint was narrower than that of the unidentified leg. I told the police that the leg was that of a man, and from the skin color and the length of the femur and tibia estimated that he was a young adult, brunet, about five feet five inches tall. Two weeks later the other leg, with male genitals attached, was found on the lake shore, well preserved by the icy water. No other part of the body ever turned up. The newspapers gave us a good rating for diagnosing the sex correctly, with the result that the Rochester Zoo asked me, soon after, to autopsy a dead lion and a seal. Later the zoo gave us a decrepit bear that it was about to put to death. Under terminal ether, with me as anesthetist, Wilbur Smith exposed and stimulated the "ursine lozenge," a configuration of the cerebral surface peculiar to bears that had wrongly been supposed to be an extension of the motor cortex.

When I first arrived in Rochester, George Whipple asked me to be chairman of the library committee, with Bayne-Jones and Clausen. When B.J. left for Yale, Karl Wilson succeeded him. The university librarian, Donald Gilchrist, had advised Whipple to commission James F. Ballard, director of the Boston Medical Library, to compile a list of books and journals most essential for the school's library. The list had been circulated to each professor for review and additions. Ballard had been buying books for us; it was a good time to start a library because in Europe World War I had forced the sale of many private libraries. By 1926 I could report to the chairman of the trustees' library committee that we had on the shelves about 1,100 journals comprising 30,000 volumes and about 3,000 individual books. My task was to lead the further development of the library and especially to gather works illustrating the history and literature of medicine. Henry L. Lemkau, a recent librarian of the school, has generously assessed my services during my seventeen years' chairmanship,[3] so I need not go into details here, but two incidents in which I was involved belong in my autobiography.

On a snowy November night in 1926 I was driving Dr. Mulligan home from a session of the Pundits. He took the occasion to say that he hoped the library committee was not neglecting the history of medicine. We should obtain, he said, all the great old medical books in English translation, so that he and other people not versed in Greek and Latin could read them. I had to explain, as gently as possible, that few of the Greek and Latin

3. Henry L. Lemkau, "Crossroads: The story of the medical library," in *To each his farthest star.*

classics had been translated into English. For example, there was no complete English version of Galen's works, nor a modern translation from the old French of the surgical works of Ambroise Paré, which (said I) I had heard him mention recently at one of his Sunday morning staff meetings at the Rochester General Hospital. There is, I said, an English translation of Paré's works printed in the seventeenth century, but it is rare. A copy might cost $150 or more, and at first we must spend our library budget on current books. Dr. Mulligan said nothing in reply, but just before Christmas President Rhees called me to say that he had received from Dr. Mulligan a check for $5,000, with instructions that it was to be used by Dr. Corner for rare books on surgery and anatomy. In each of the two following years he sent another check for $5,000. His terminal illness in 1929 ended his benefaction. In 1927 Mr. E. G. Miner rang me up, asking me to call at his house, bringing a suitcase. There I found him in bed with a bad cold. He said with a smile that he felt so miserable that his thoughts were on the uncertainties of life and he had decided to give us at once his collection of books and pamphlets on yellow fever. I brought away forty-one rare items but suggested to him that he continue collecting, expanding his interest to other epidemic diseases. The Miner collection now contains seven hundred volumes and pamphlets on yellow fever and cholera.

Medical history had been a hobby of mine since student days, as I have mentioned in chapter 4. In fact, at Berkeley when I was still in my twenties, the enthusiastic chairman of a medical society meeting introduced me as "the leading historian of medicine on the Pacific Coast"—a dubious statement because as far as I knew, nobody else on the coast was then doing serious work in the field. Now, at Rochester, I was expected to make my hobby a professional interest. President Rhees had said when he offered me the professorship of anatomy, that he would like me to develop the subject in the new school. I do not think that Dean Whipple would of his own accord have given me such an assignment. Great scientist as he was, his own research was in a field so new that it had no history, or so it seemed to him. He told me once that he had no need for books or journals more than fifteen years old. But his deeply admired teacher William H. Welch was a learned medical historian, and at Rochester not only the president of the university and an influential trustee (Mr. Miner) but also two of Whipple's most trusted advisers, Dr. Mulligan and Dr. Goler, were all strongly interested in medical history. With the dean's consent I took it upon myself, as soon as the school got under way, to organize a medical history club like that at Johns Hopkins. I simply announced a meeting, arranged a program, and took the chair. We operated without a constitution or membership list and had no elected officers. I had no great difficulty either in recruiting speakers or in attracting an audience. We were a self-centered suburban community, far from the movie houses and theaters. On a winter night the students found it pleasant to have dinner at the school and stay on for our eight o'clock meeting. Practically the whole school came, from the dean to the first-year students. Bayne-Jones and Wilson took a practical interest in helping me find speakers.

I tried to have at each of our five or six sessions each year a principal talk by an experienced speaker from our faculty or from the city physicians, among whom were several well-read men. We invited nonmedical people who knew about some marginal but relevant topic. Mr. William Bausch of the great optical firm of Bausch and Lomb told about his collaboration with Professor Charles Sedgwick Minot of Harvard Medical School in constructing the first automatic rotary minotome. Arthur Parker of the Rochester Municipal Museum, a member of the Seneca tribe of Indians, gave us a fascinating account of the ancient medicine of his people as he had experienced it when he was a youth on the reservation. Stanhope Bayne-Jones joined me one evening in a discussion of the mysterious "Genesee fever" that caused many deaths among pioneers in the valley early in the nineteenth century. I collected the historical data from old records and tombstones, and B.J. discussed in masterly fashion the symptoms and the clues to the identity of the illness. He never found time to write down his talk, which if put into print would have become the standard account of a puzzling disease.

I had somebody give a brief "curtain raiser" before the main discourse, and for this I tried hard to get some of the younger staff people, especially the residents, to take part. In the hierarchy of a medical school the residents hold a special place in the students' regard. Professors are a bit remote, even young professors like us. Having won their place in the world, they can afford to indulge their hobbies, but the residents are doing the daily practical work of the wards and outpatient clinics. If they show an interest in the history of the profession, the students are impressed. So now and then I managed to persuade a resident to give a ten-minute review of a new book or article on the history of his specialty or to discuss the historical background of an interesting case on the ward. In my own department I required from each student a term paper on a topic of his own choosing; in the list of suggested topics I always included two or three on medical history. During my seventeen years at Rochester five or six students produced papers on historical topics that were presented at the club meetings and with a little editorial help from me were accepted for publication in historical journals, the best of them by a talented young woman, Jean Captain, who built her term paper into a learned article on the history of the classification of the blood cells, published in 1940 in the *Bulletin of the History of Medicine.*

Such organizations as our medical history club usually have their ups and downs, depending upon the enterprise and hard work of a few enthusiasts or even of one leader. Our club flourished while I was there, then died down, but has been revived twice, once by a devoted medical student, and again by E. C. Atwater of the department of internal medicine. In honor of its founder, it is now called the George W. Corner Medical History Club.

I have said nothing as yet in this chapter about such part as I had in the general administration of the school. President Rhees and Dean Whipple adopted the Johns Hopkins plan of an advisory board made up of the dean, the director of the hospital, and the other department heads to direct the daily affairs of the school. The term "advisory" means advisory to the trustees. This is a democratic system from the standpoint of the department heads but an oligarchy from that of the junior staff. It works well as long as the individual heads consult their respective staffs and make them feel that they are well represented. I never observed any discontent with it on the part of my staff. The board met monthly in the dean's office, with Dr. Rhees presiding. There were few disagreements. An amusing situation developed during the first cold spell after the hospital opened. The clinical heads reported that their interns were complaining about the cold bare concrete floors of the staff house bedrooms. They wanted carpets. Dean Whipple, ever anxious to save the school's money for research and teaching, said that when he was a young man in New England, he got along very well without carpets on his bedroom floor. The debate continuing, Dr. Rhees put the question to a vote which came out nine to one for the carpets. Whipple took it without demur and had the floors covered.

At first, for two or three years, he kept a tight hand on our departmental budgets until he had accustomed us to his scale of expenditure. But he did not deny reasonable spending for needed purchases. William Bradford told me that during his first year on the faculty, when he was in Bayne-Jones's laboratory pending the opening of the hospital, B.J. asked him to make up a list of equipment for his room. Brad badly wanted a $150 electric centrifuge but thought that Whipple would not allow it. He did list a $50 desk chair like B.J.'s. When the list came back with the dean's comments, the chair was crossed off and a centrifuge added.

When I was working on the history of medicine at Salerno (my ventures into medical history will be described in a subsequent chapter), a copy of the *Opera* of Isaac Judaeus (1515) came on the market in Europe for $600. The book is very rare; I knew of only three copies in America, one at the Library of Congress, one at the Jewish Theological Seminary, and another in a private collection in Baltimore. I needed it for my historical study, so I asked the dean whether he would approve its purchase from the Mulligan fund, knowing that nobody else would possibly use it for years to come. "Of course," he said. "If you needed a microscope we'd buy it for you. If you are going to use this book as a research tool you must have it." So his firmness and tight hand were combined with generosity when he agreed with the need. As to teaching he was liberal. I used to tell him when I meant to try something radical, like not holding a final examination or letting a bright first-year medical student give a lecture in the anatomy course for pupil nurses instead of myself. No matter how unusual our whims, we taught as we pleased. I did not always agree with George Whipple. I was distressed when he and the president yielded to pressure from the clinical heads to abandon the strict full-time plan for the clinical professors, and when this important matter of policy came to a vote in the advisory board, I cast my lone nay against nine ayes. George Whipple smiled. He knew that I could be an impractical idealist.

We scientists of the medical faculty were not the only people doing front-line research in Rochester. The university's college faculty had in recent years recruited several able research men, and the city's technical industries, especially the Eastman Kodak Company, had on their research staffs physicists and chemists of distinction. With some of these we organized, at the instigation of Benjamin Willier, professor of zoology, a little group calling itself the X-Club. Our consorts, who met at the same hours for a literary evening, called themselves the X-Wives. The roster of our club as I knew it until my departure for Rochester in 1940 is worth recalling here. The initial members were Edward F. Adolph (physiology), George P. Berry (microbiology), E. K. Carver (chemistry, Kodak Research Laboratory), George W. Corner (anatomy), Elmer A. Cullen (zoology), Lee DuBridge (physics), Wallace O. Fenn (physiology), J. J. Gergen (chemistry), David R. Goddard (botany), B. Hoffman (physics), Brian O'Brien (optics), B. H. Willier (zoology), Vladimir Seidel (mathematics), Frederick Seitz (physics), Samuel E. Sheppard (physics, Kodak), and Victor Weisskopf (physics).

We thought of ourselves as the city's up and coming scientists, and so we were. Every one of us had a productive career, mostly as heads of university departments. This little group of twenty men included seven future members of the National Academy of Sciences, among them a president, a vice president, and a home secretary of the academy. Nine were chosen members of the American Philosophical Society. There was a future president of the Rockefeller University and a president of the California Institute of Technology, a dean of Harvard Medical School, and a director of Kodak Research Laboratory. At least six became presidents of the national associations of specialists in their respective fields. This remarkable (and short-lived) assemblage of scientific talent was bought together by the good judgment of President Rhees, his successor, Alan Valentine, and Dean Whipple of the medical faculty. We dined together several times each winter at the faculty club or the Rochester University Club to hear a paper by one of our members. After the 1950s, I am told, the X-Club allowed itself to grow to 100 members; its character changed, and ultimately it was discontinued. We, the original members, could not foresee how far any of us would go in the national and international scientific community, but we all knew the joy of successful research and the stimulus of intellectual companionship.

11

PROGESTERONE, LACTATION, AND THE CYCLE

In 1926 I began to plan an all-out attempt to find the hormone of the corpus luteum that Gustav Born of Breslau had predicted twenty-six years before. For this venture I felt that I was qualified by my thirteen years of hard thinking and intensive research on the ovarian cycles of the sow and the rhesus monkey. I possessed the requisite surgical and embryological skills, but what little biochemistry I knew would never suffice in the quest for a hormone. I found an excellent biochemist, Willard Myron Allen, to work side by side with me, but first I had to provide a physiological basis for the biochemical work.

Most discoveries of hormones, for example, adrenalin, insulin, and thyroxin, have resulted from somebody's observation of a physiological activity that is lost when a given organ or gland is impaired by disease or surgically removed. Insulin is a good example. If the pancreas is removed, the animal body can no longer metabolize sugar. Frederick Banting and Charles Best made an extract of the pancreas that restores the lost function.

There were clues of this kind pointing the way to look for a hormone of the corpus luteum. Ludwig Fraenkel, following up the conjecture of his former teacher, Gustav Born, that the function of the corpus luteum is to support pregnancy, had shown in 1910 that if he removed the corpora lutea of a rabbit doe shortly after she mated with a buck the embryos would not develop. What became of them he did not inquire. The French team of Bouin and Ancel in the same year provided part of the answer. When they removed the corpora lutea after mating a rabbit doe to a vasectomized (sterile) male, the lining of the uterus (endometrium) did not develop the progestational change (illustrated in Chapter 8, figure 3) which normally follows the appearance of the corpora lutea. The embryos of Fraenkel's rabbits must have died in utero because for lack of the corpus luteum hormone the uterus was not prepared to nourish them.

I began my investigation by repeating Fraenkel's experiments to see what actually happened to the embryos. I too used rabbits because of a useful peculiarity of that species. Rabbit does do not ovulate spontaneously on a cyclic schedule, as do most mammals, including our own species. In the ovaries of a rabbit half-ripe follicles are always present, but only after copulation will a crop of them mature and after ten hours shed their ova into the oviducts. Since rabbit does are almost always ready to accept the male, the experimenter can schedule tests at his convenience. I removed the corpora lutea eighteen hours after mating but did not wait two or three weeks, as Fraenkel did, to see whether or not the pregnancy continued. Instead I killed the does five days after excising the corpora lutea, when under ordinary circumstances the embryos would still be free in the uterus (they do not become attached until the eighth day). I found them there, but they were dead. They were not beautiful little blastocysts, semitransparent hollow spheres about 1.5 millimeters ($\frac{1}{16}$ inch) in diameter, as they should be at five days; they were wrinkled, opaque objects no bigger than a pinhead. Judging from their appearance they must have died on the fourth day after ovulation, soon after arriving in the inhospitable uterus, like the biblical seeds sown upon stony ground. If I left in place two or more corpora lutea the embryos survived. Thus I had confirmed the observations of Fraenkel and of Bouin and Ancel and had fully substantiated Born's hypothesis. I published these findings, with the necessary controls and tabulated data, in "Physiology of the Corpus Luteum, 1. The Effect of Very Early Ablation of the Corpus Luteum upon Embryos and Uterus" (1928).

Here, then, is a practical test for a hormone of the corpus luteum: mate your doe to a fertile male; eighteen hours later remove both ovaries (easier than digging out the corpora lutea separately), inject your extract daily for five days, kill the doe, prepare a cross section of the uterus, put it under your microscope. If the progestational change has occurred, you have a potent extract. This is the routine test. In a slightly more precise form it is called, in the scientific literature, the Corner and Allen test. If you want to make it deluxe, you may wash the tiny embryos out of the uterus and rejoice at the sight of them.

The stage was now set for the biochemist. I did not have to look far for him; Willard Allen, a very likable young man, was close at hand and ready to join me. That I chose a twenty-three-year-old first-year student for so important a venture may seem rash, but Bill had high qualifications, too. They will become evident as my story develops. Born on a farm at Macedon, New York, twenty miles from Rochester, he won his B.S. degree at nearby Hobart College at Geneva, New York, in June 1926, and in September of that year enrolled in the second class that entered our new school of medicine. At Hobart he was a star student, especially in chemistry. Once, on a written examination, he told me, he had earned a grade of 110 percent. The professor had included one question so difficult that he made it optional but promised a 10 percent bonus to any student who answered it correctly. Bill solved that hard one and also answered all the other questions with perfect accuracy, so the professor had to rate his paper 110 percent. At Rochester in 1926–27 Allen led his class in anatomy and biochemistry. I had at my disposal a fellowship for him if he would drop out of his class for a year to assist us in teaching microscopic anatomy and collaborate with me in research. As willing as I to take a long chance, he became the first student at Rochester to receive such a fellowship, and we began work together in October 1927.

Allen and I have each told in print the story of our collaboration, but I am telling it again here, to explain, for readers interested in a scientist's mental processes, my own precursory thinking that led to our successful collaboration, and to express my admiration of my companion in research. Philosophers of science have had much to say in recent years about serendipity, which *Webster's Dictionary* defines as "a gift for finding agreeable or useful things not sought for." An old adage says, however, that chance favors the prepared mind. In the discovery of progesterone serendipity played no part, nor did our well-prepared minds need the aid of chance. We carefully thought out in advance every step we took. I offer the following account to historians of science as a specimen of successful research based strictly on practical logic.

We bought fresh sows' ovaries for extraction in five-pound lots from the Rochester Packing Company. I picked out those bearing recent corpora lutea; one of us or a technician shelled out the corpora with a scalpel. From a week's or ten days' supply of ovaries we could harvest a 1,500-gram lot for extraction.

At first we were, so to speak, looking for a needle in a haystack. We did not know what solvent would extract our hormone from the gland tissue. Reasoning that most of the physiologically active substances in the animal body will dissolve either in water or in ethyl alcohol, we agreed that I should begin with an aqueous extract and Allen with an alcoholic. My aqueous extracts were for some reason toxic; I got only a few dead rabbits. That meant possibly a long effort to remove the toxicity. We therefore postponed such a tedious and uncertain task until we saw what Allen's alcoholic extract would do. Moreover, just at that time we got an unexpected hint.

A foreign scientist visiting my laboratory, to whom I explained our project, reminded me of an article published in 1915 by E. Hermann of Vienna, who had made alcoholic extracts of whole ovaries, of corpora lutea only, and of human placentas.[1] The effects he obtained we could confidently ascribe to the general ovarian hormone, estrogen, isolated by Edgar Allen and Edward Doisy in 1923, except that in one rabbit Hermann had produced the progestational proliferation of the uterine lining that was the telltale for our search. This was an instance of an unprepared mind not favored by chance. Hermann did not recognize that he had something special there, and anyway he did not specify the source of that particular batch of extract, whether from whole ovaries, corpora lutea or placenta. His picture, however, suggested to Allen and me that alcohol might work.

Bill set up an extraction column of Walter Bloor's design in which the vapor of boiling alcohol steamed up through a gauze bag filled with minced corpora lutea, was condensed on a water-cooled surface above, and dripped back through the bag. We ran

1. Edmund Herrmann, "Über eine wirksame Substanz in Eierstocke und in der Plazenta," *Monatshefte für Geburtshilfe und Gynäkologie* 41(1915): 1–48, figs. 11 and 12.

each batch through this procedure five times, one hour each, with fresh alcohol each time, pooled the extracts and distilled off the alcohol under reduced pressure. The residue was a few spoonfuls of a thick greasy semifluid material looking like a poor grade of cylinder oil. To get it into a hypodermic syringe and inject it we had to warm it up. A professor of anatomy from Germany whom I was showing through the medical school, looking into the room where we had our extractor and vacuum still, exclaimed, "Eine ganz besondere Anatomie!" ("A very peculiar anatomical laboratory!").

In our preliminary tests we used young unmated rabbits because they cost less than adults to buy and feed. These tests were mostly successful; the sought-for progestational state of the uterine lining developed. For an ultimate test we used mature rabbits, to see whether our crude extract would substitute for the mother's corpora lutea so fully as to preserve the embryos. Allen describes the results in his "Recollections of My Life with Progesterone." "There was much excitement," he says,

> in Corner's laboratory on that sunny afternoon when the time came to sacrifice the first adult rabbit which had received our crude extract. The rabbit had been mated with two fertile bucks 6 days before. About 18 hours after mating we had removed the ovaries taking care not to manipulate the tubes (oviducts). Rabbits ovulate 10 hours after mating so we presumed that fertilized ova in the 2, 3, or 4 cell stage were in the fallopian tubes when the ovaries were removed. The crude extract had been given subcutaneously each day for 5 days. We knew that normal blastocysts should be in the uterus if the extract contained the corpus luteum hormone. Corner excised the uterus, rather calmly it seemed to me, and injected salt solution into the uterus. There was a delay as the uterus distended. Then suddenly several transparent blastocysts popped out into the receiver. They were 1.5 mm in diameter, just the right size for 6-day rabbit embryos. Neither of us said very much but we both knew that much exciting work lay ahead of us.[2]

Following this success we carried two rabbits well past the stage of implantation and into the fetal stage, one of them to thirteen

2. Willard M. Allen, "Recollections of my life with progesterone," *Gynecological Investigations* 5 (1974).

days' gestation and one to seventeen days, twenty-one hours. These experiments had to be terminated because we ran out of extract. A photograph of one of these fetuses in situ in the uterus with its placenta, which I made to illustrate our scientific report, was accepted for a nationwide exhibition of artistic photographs, so that the little creature became an objet d'art as well as an object of science. The next year, with partially purified extracts we clinched the matter by carrying several rabbits through the whole term of pregnancy and the delivery of normal young.

As soon as reprints of our report of these experiments came from the printer, I gave myself the pleasure of sending autographed copies to Paul Bouin at Strasbourg and Ludwig Fraenkel at Breslau, each inscribed with a few words acknowledging our debt to their pioneer work, upon which we had founded ours. Bouin I had met in 1924, as narrated in chapter 9. Fraenkel I was to meet in 1941—at Montevideo. I found him a man of noble bearing and warm friendliness. Forced by the growing tide of German anti-Semitism to leave his home and university clinic at Breslau, he had settled in the Uruguayan capital, where his great experience made him a welcome addition to the medical faculty. Near him and his wife, happily, were his son-in-law Karl Slotta and another former student of his, Eric Fels, both of whom contributed in the mid-1930s to the growing knowledge of the structure and action of progesterone.

It had taken us about nine months to obtain a potent and usable crude extract—nine months not without delays and frustration. In the process of distilling off the alcohol, as the material became thicker and thicker it would often foam up in the flask and spill over into the condenser and be lost unless we instantly cut off the vacuum pump. For this reason somebody had to sit by the still for hours at a stretch. Such foaming can be avoided by adding a little butyl alcohol to the extract, but how could we know whether this would spoil the hormone? To find out took another rabbit, an operation with full aseptic precautions, and five days' time. Once or twice a defective distilling flask imploded, throwing hot muddy alcohol and broken glass over the electric heater. Once I went hurriedly up the animal house steps carrying a syringe full of the extract to inject into a rabbit, stumbled and fell and lost the world's entire current supply of our hormone.

The worst frustration came in the spring of 1929, when I had drafted our first reports. It occurred to me that I had never made a batch of the extract singlehanded; Allen had always led the chemical part of the work. We should not publish our findings, I thought, until we were sure that any competent laboratory worker could repeat them. We agreed that I was a sufficiently bad chemist to check the feasibility of our procedure. If I could make the extract alone, anybody could. Classes were over for the season, so I had time for the tedious job. We laid aside the typescript report, Allen left town for vacation, and I made a batch of crude extract alone. To my horror, my test on an immature rabbit was negative; the extract appeared to contain no hormone at all. I telegraphed to Allen to return to Rochester for a day and we gloomily canvassed the possible reasons for my failure. One of the most likely causes was that I had done the extraction and distillation in my sunlit private laboratory, whereas we had worked together in a room with northern exposure. Perhaps our hormone was sensitive to light. I had the windows blacked out and worked in total darkness; no luck, again a negative test. I tried one or two other hunches with similar results. When Allen returned from vacation, we made a batch together, I handling the material and the apparatus, Bill watching my every movement. He ran the test and found the extract potent. Later a young woman technician made a batch successfully.

The reason for my apparent failure was almost ridiculous. We were using, as already stated, rabbits eight to twelve weeks old. The uterus, we learned, will not respond to our hormone unless it is primed by the general ovarian hormone, estrogen. The ovaries do not produce enough estrogen to condition the uterus until the age of about ten weeks. When selecting rabbits for testing, I had tended to pick the younger and Allen the older ones. My solo preparations had actually been potent, but my rabbits had been too young to respond. Thereafter, to be certain of the test, to insure maximum action when measuring the potency of our extracts at successive stages of purification, and to work out a standard dose, we always used mature animals. The puzzle having been solved, we sent off to the *American Journal of Physiology* two papers announcing our discovery.

In daily conversations at our laboratory I had suggested to Allen that we name the new hormone "progestin" because it aids in maintaining pregnancy. The word is easy to spell and pronounce in many tongues, means something but not too much, and would not commit us to any theories that might prove untenable later. The name was first used in print by Allen in 1930, in a detailed paper on the preparation of the hormone. After the biochemists worked out the structural formula of the hormone, the name was by general agreement changed to "progesterone" to show that it contains a molecule of oxygen doubly bonded to a carbon molecule. My original name "progestin" survives as the general term for the class of related substances with similar activity.

After our announcement in 1929, fellow scientists elsewhere began immediately to follow up our work. In 1933 Frederick L. Hisaw and H. Fevold of the University of Wisconsin produced progestational (premenstrual) proliferation (see the latter part of this chapter) in monkeys, something I would have done myself if they had not accomplished it so promptly. In 1930 a well-known Austrian gynecologist, Hermann Knaus, prepared the first crude progesterone in Europe and showed that it makes the rabbit uterus insensitive to the stimulating action of pituitrin, a discovery useful in obstetrics.[3]

It was now Allen's task to purify the hormone. Our method of extraction had already eliminated the proteins and whatever carbohydrates might have existed in the tissue. Evidently the hormone was lurking amid the fats and fatlike extractives (lipids). Allen proceeded to eliminate these one by one, using selective solvents and other tricks well known to lipid chemists. For example, we could throw out the phospholipids by adding a large quantity of acetone to the alcoholic extract, which precipitated them. Of course, we could not know in advance which way the hormone would go—into the precipitate or into the supernatant liquid. Both fractions had to be tested on a rabbit—another five

3. Hermann Knaus, "Zur Frage der Standardization des Corpus luteum Extraktes," *Archiv für Experimentelle Pathologie und Pharmacologie* 141 (1930): 371–80.

days gone. Next came the neutral fats and fatty acids. Edward Doisy had easily rid his crude estrogen of neutral fats by turning them into soap with an alkali, but we had found that our hormone was destroyed by alkalis. Allen had to use a selective solvent.

When he had eliminated all the known lipids Allen went for advice to Walter Bloor, our professor of biochemistry, who was an expert on lipids and related substances. Bloor said that he had no helpful advice; Allen had done everything Bloor might have suggested. Allen was considering high-vacuum distillation, and we were figuring out the cost of the apparatus he proposed to construct. But just then we learned that Kenneth Hickman of Eastman Kodak's research laboratory had developed a high-vacuum still with which he was distilling oils of high boiling point—substances just like what Allen now had left of our extract. By permission of Dr. Kenneth Mees, director of research at Kodak Park, Bill and I took 200 milligrams of our precious oily residue to Hickman's laboratory and watched his elegant little still vaporize the oil and condense it into three successive batches of a few drops each of different boiling points. Back at our laboratory, tests on rabbits showed that one of the three fractional distillates contained almost all of the potency. Allen then built his own high-vacuum still, the cost of which was generously paid by Dr. Bloor from the funds of the biochemistry department (such was the brotherhood that prevailed in our school). With this equipment Allen sublimed a white waxy material and by fractional crystallization finally secured the pure hormone. On May 5, 1933, he came into my private laboratory holding a test tube containing a few cubic centimeters of some clear fluid in which floated a mass of fine white needlelike crystals. "This is it!" he said. "It's a steroid." "What's a steroid?" I asked. We were almost too happy to talk, but Bill referred me to James B. Conant's textbook of organic chemistry, which told me that steroids are a class of polycyclic substances resembling sterols—not very enlightening to me at the time. The estrogens are steroids, as is the later discovered testis hormone, androsterone, also Vitamin D.

Because Allen's supply was so small (he never had as much as half a thimbleful at any one time), the exact analysis of the hormone's chemical structure called for a microchemist. We enlisted the help of Oskar Wintersteiner, a young man at Columbia University, New York, who had the necessary microapparatus and experience. Allen sent Wintersteiner in all about 400 milligrams of impure but highly potent crystals with which in about a year he arrived at the empirical formula $C_{21} H_{13} O_2$. From this the two men independently deduced the structural formula. It is shown below for readers who understand the notation of organic chemistry.

Willard Allen was now no longer alone in the biochemical study of progesterone. I quote again his "Recollections":

> Corner and I realized, of course, that there would be competition in the race for the isolation of the hormone. At least four groups in addition to ourselves, entered the race—Slotta in Breslau, Butenandt and Westphal in Danzig, Hartmann and Wettstein in Switzerland, and Hisaw and Fevold in Madison, Wisc. The crystalline hormone was announced in the summer of 1934 almost simultaneously by Winterstein and Allen, Slotta, *et al.*, and by Hartmann and Wettstein. In a few months Butenandt and Schmidt had converted pregnanediol to progesterone and Fernholz had synthesized the hormone from stigmasterol. These endeavors established the structural formula in record time. What had started as progestin in Corner's laboratory in 1929 had now become an "international hormone" and by December 1934, an "international incident" was brewing. Wintersteiner received a letter from Slotta indicating that he (Slotta) and Butenandt had agreed that they would use luteo-sterone as a name for the hormone. This development did not appeal to us, as we had named the hormone progestin in 1930. On January 14, 1935 Corner dispatched a masterful letter to Slotta in which we suggested progesterone as a suitable name for the hormone. By giving up our name progestin, we hoped that Slotta would give up his luteo-sterone.[4]

4. Allen, "Recollections of my life with progesterone."

In 1935 Willard Allen was invited to attend a special international conference in London organized by the Health Division of the League of Nations in June of that year to consider standardization of estradrol, progesterone, and the even more recently discovered male hormone, androsterone. This was a distinguished group of sixteen or seventeen mostly young men under the chairmanship of Sir Henry Dale, one of the most respected English medical scientists. They included representatives of three of the four groups that had almost simultaneously discovered the exact chemical structure of progesterone, namely Butenandt, Slotta, and Allen, together with Doisy (estrone), Frederick C. Koch of Chicago (androsterone), E. C. (later Sir Charles) Dodds, and A. S. (later Sir Alan) Parkes, the latter two being widely experienced endocrinologists. The conference reached conclusions about progesterone that were acceptable to Allen and me. The name progesterone was recommended for use in the world's scientific literature. An international standard of progesterone was accepted, a stated amount of the pure hormone crystallized in the form of needles. The international unit was decreed to be the specific activity of one milligram of the international standard preparation—an amount practically identical with the unit Allen and I had adapted for our own computations.

The members of the conference, convened only four years before World War I, were talented and ambitious men of science, but they were also men of character, not inclined to petty disputes. They worked in harmony. Long-lasting friendships were formed there. But I believe that Willard Allen's calm Quaker persuasiveness helped to maintain the serenity of their deliberations. After the conference Adolf Butenandt, visiting the United States, came to Rochester to see me and stayed overnight at my home.

In 1935 Allen received a prize of $1,000 created by the Eli Lilly Company for the best biochemical research by an American under thirty years of age. He held his fellowship in my department for two years (1927–29), then resumed his medical studies, working on the chemistry of progesterone in what little time he had free in the afternoons and on weekends. After taking his M.D. in 1932 he had a one-year fellowship in pathology; next he was intern, assistant resident, and resident on the obstetrical-gynecological service of our Strong Memorial Hospital; and in 1940, at the age of thirty-six years, he was called to Washington University, St. Louis, as professor of obstetrics and gynecology. There he had a highly successful career. He is, at this writing in 1979, at the University of Maryland's school of medicine at Baltimore, in a postretirement position as assistant dean. Our friendship has continued unbroken for more than half a century. In his fascinating "Recollections of My Life with Progesterone" he tells of his important studies on progesterone after he and I both left Rochester in 1940.

At the time of our work together a number of biochemical discoveries made in American university departments were patented, usually with assignment of rights to the university in whose laboratories the work was done. We did not patent progesterone. A natural substance is not patentable; the method of extracting and purifying it may be patentable. The only step in the preparation of progesterone that was not in the public domain was the high-vacuum distillation, and that was Kodak's business. In any case opinion at the University of Rochester, led by Dean George Whipple (with whom I agreed), was that discoveries useful in medicine, supported by academic funds, should not be commercially restricted, even for the benefit of a university. One result of this high-minded policy was that drug manufacturers were not eager to put money into marketing a hormone without the protection of a patent, especially when the clinical uses were not entirely clear. When, however, they realized that a contraceptive pill could be made with progesterone or a derivative, several of them started a race to get into mass production. Progesterone is therefore now in big business. Fifty years after Allen showed me those first pure crystals, it is being made in kilogram lots to go into "the pill."

At first thought this seems a startling paradox. The reader will say: "You were looking for something that would support pregnancy, not prevent it. How can one hormone work both ways?" There is really no paradox there. One of the ways by which the corpus luteum protects the early embryo is by stopping the ovulation cycle so that another embryo will not come along to compete for space and nutriment in the uterus. Women do not ovulate during pregnancy. This was well known, and in

1918 Leo Loeb showed by experiments on guinea pigs that the corpus luteum is the blocking agent. I remember saying one day to Allen as we sat watching our extractors, that if we found what we were looking for and if it inhibited ovulation we would have a world-shaking boon—or a bane, depending upon how it was used.

When we had the pure hormone, I asked William Phillips, a medical student, to test its effect on the cycle of white rats, which become estrous every five days. He found that progesterone does indeed stop the estrous cycle, which implies (though it does not actually prove) that it prevents ovulation. This was as far as we carried that line of investigation. Allen was too busy with his chemical work, and I was occupied with physiological research on lactation and on the menstrual cycle of the rhesus monkey, now made possible by the use of progesterone. We simply did not have time to go farther in the matter of ovulation control. There were plenty of people elsewhere ready and anxious to take it on.

In April 1940, Allen and I were both summoned to the Federal Courthouse in New York City as expert witnesses in a lawsuit quaintly titled "United States of America versus six dozen boxes, more or less, each containing one dozen tubes of Lutein Tablets." These tablets were a relic of an earlier era of endocrinology when doctors were hopefully prescribing endocrine glands chopped raw or dried and powdered and pressed into tablets. Thyroid glands minced and served in sandwiches or powdered had worked in cases of hypothyroidism; maybe ovarian tissue would do some good for female complaints. It was in fact my former teacher at Johns Hopkins and my chief when I was an intern, Professor Howard A. Kelly, who had suggested to an honorable Baltimore drug house, Hynson, Westcott, and Dunning, that it make up corpus luteum tablets. It obligingly did so and found that they sold well; family doctors and gynecologists prescribed them and thought them helpful in various female complaints. Many other endocrine products of this empirical kind were on the market, some of them put out by much less respectable firms than Hynson, Westcott, and Dunning. The federal Food and Drug Administration, trying to abolish this dubious trade, made the mistake of picking out the Baltimore firm's Lutein Tablets for the initial attack rather than a more quackish product. To get the matter into a federal court they sent agents across state lines to seize the aforesaid six dozen boxes of tablets and charged that under the terms of the Pure Food and Drug Act of 1906 the tablets were "adulterated and misbranded." The drug company sued to get back the confiscated six dozen boxes. The government people, knowing of our work, asked Allen to assay the tablets. He found that they contained neither of the two known ovarian hormones, estrogen or progesterone. This was no surprise to us; Hynson, Westcott, and Dunning, to make the tablets palatable, had removed all the lipid content with a fat solvent.

The case came to trial before a celebrated judge, John M. Woolsey, widely known for the liberal judgment that forced the U.S. Customs to remove the ban on the importation of James Joyce's novel *Ulysses*. We were called by the government side. To my embarrassment the chief expert witness for the drug house was David Eli Macht of the Johns Hopkins medical faculty, who had been one of my teachers in the pharmacology course. Judge Woolsey evidently enjoyed presiding over this novel trial; full-faced, bald, with prominent forehead and heavy eyelids, he gave full attention to every detail of the testimony. At one time while I was testifying he asked me, Dr. Macht, and the chief attorneys on both sides to take paper and pencils and work out for his information an arithmetical problem concerning the relative dosage of estrogen and progesterone. I got off rather lightly on the stand; the government lawyers wanted me chiefly to provide the endocrinological background for their contentions. Allen had a much rougher time; he was cross-examined for many hours by the drug house's chief attorney, who tried every imaginable means to disparage his testimony. At the end of his ordeal Judge Woolsey commended him from the bench for conducting himself with consummate skill during one of the most exacting cross-examinations he (the judge) had ever witnessed. In his admirably clear ruling Judge Woolsey hinted broadly that he doubted the value of Lutein Tablets but pointed out that no one could say that they did not contain some unknown substance responsible for the vaguely defined good results the doctors had claimed to observe. So Hynson, Westcott, and Dunning got back the six dozen boxes of Lutein Tablets and was relieved of the charges of adulteration and misbranding; but the Food and Drug Administration won out in the long run by requiring manufacturers of gland products of unproved value to state on the label that the product contained no known biologically active substances. Such products, Lutein Tablets among them, have since disappeared from the market. Some of the ailments and malfunctions for which physicians had prescribed the ineffectual lutein tablets, for want of something better, are relieved by progesterone, but I postpone discussion of its clinical uses while mentioning two basic physiological aspects of progesterone which I or my immediate associates helped to elucidate.

I have mentioned the discovery by Hermann Knaus that crude progesterone acts upon the involuntary muscle tissue of the uterine wall, making it insensitive to the powerful stimulating action of pituitrin. This important finding was promptly confirmed in my Rochester laboratory by a young gynecologist, A. W. Makepeace. Samuel R. M. Reynolds, a physiologist then at Long Island Medical College, worked out an ingenious method of recording the spontaneous contractions of the uterus of the living rabbit. In collaboration with Willard Allen, who supplied the pure progesterone, Reynolds showed that the hormone greatly diminishes the spontaneous uterine contractions, an action doubtless evolved to keep the uterus quiescent when embryos are to be received and implanted. I returned to this subject in 1951 when I was the director of the Department of Embryology of the Carnegie Institution of Washington. Arpad Csapo, from Hungary via Sweden, came to our Baltimore laboratory bringing intimate knowledge of the chemistry and physiology of voluntary (skeletal) muscle. I taught Csapo what he needed to know about the reproductive cycle and the method for studying involuntary muscle in vitro. He and I carried out and published some preliminary experiments, and thereafter he went on to a long and productive career of research in the physiology of uterine muscle and its role in pregnancy and labor. The gist of all these researches is that progesterone reduces the transmission, throughout the uterine muscular tissue, of the impulses to contract. The clinical use of progesterone is partly based on this fundamental physiological action.

By 1937 Allen and I were able to announce with considerable satisfaction that we and our fellow workers had achieved with crystalline progesterone all five established effects of corpus luteum extracts upon the uterus, namely progestational proliferation of the endometrium, suppression of ovulation, inhibition of the action of pituitrin upon the myometrium, inhibition of uterine motility in vivo, and suppression of menstruation.

Two of our medical students, Abraham Teitelbaum and Louis Goldstein, at my suggestion added to this list another effect previously attributed to the corpus luteum which they could reproduce with crystalline progesterone. Leo Loeb had shown in 1910 by experiments on guinea pigs that when corpora lutea are present in the ovaries, any small injury to the uterine lining, such as a scratch with a needle, results in the appearance of a placentalike growth (deciduoma) at the site of injury. This the two students found could be effected in the absence of the ovaries by injecting a spayed guinea pig with progesterone.

Since the corpus luteum degenerates toward the end of pregnancy, we could surmise that the onset of labor is caused, or at least facilitated, by the cessation of progesterone action. As soon as we could easily isolate and partially purify progesterone sufficiently to assay the amount of it in sows' corpora lutea at various stages of pregnancy, I set Gimbo Kimura, a medical student, and another volunteer, William Cornwell, to work. They collected separate lots of ovaries from pregnant sows at successive stages of pregnancy and determined the amount of progesterone in each lot by the Corner and Allen test. The striking result was that corpora lutea from sows near term contain no measurable progesterone. This finding, of great importance for theorizing about the cause of onset of labor, was confirmed by other investigators more than twenty years later by direct chemical assay.

The production of milk by the mammary glands of human mothers and animals is induced by a hormone of the pituitary gland. For a few months in 1928–29 I thought that in the whole world only I and my immediate associates in Rochester knew that secret, but actually a couple of Frenchmen in Paul Bouin's laboratory at Nancy had already found it out and had published it before I had my report ready.[5] P. Stricker and E. Grueter did not tell how they happened to try the pituitary gland; I based my experiments on a simple logical process of adding and subtracting recently announced findings of two other workers. The general supposition had been that lactation is induced by the corpus luteum. In 1924 my friend and former chief at Berkeley, Herbert M. Evans, found that an aqueous extract of the anterior lobe of the pituitary gland causes persistence of corpora lutea of albino rats beyond their normal span in the cycle. Alan Parkes, then at University College, London, ingeniously used Evans's finding by mating rabbit does with a sterile (vasectomized) buck and then prolonging the life of the corpora lutea by injecting a pituitary extract. Their mammary glands underwent development as in pregnancy, a result that Parkes ascribed to the persisting corpora lutea.

At the time (1929) when Parkes published his findings, in my laboratory we were eagerly watching our rabbits to see whether our crude progesterone would affect the mammary glands. We found that the potent extract that had carried spayed does during the whole term of pregnancy, after which they lactated normally, did not cause lactation in a nonpregnant rabbit given the extract for twenty-eight days. This and similar experiments convinced us that lactation is not caused by the corpus luteum hormone. Obviously, therefore, Parkes's positive results must have been produced by the pituitary extract he had used to prolong the existence of the corpora lutea.

It is difficult for a research laboratory to collect sufficient amounts of pituitary glands for extraction. These small objects buried in the floor of the brain cavity are damnably hard to reach and dig out of the surrounding bone. So I asked the help of the large drug manufacturer, Parke, Davis, and Company of Detroit, who had a supply of been pituitaries from local abattoirs. They assigned a biochemist, E. P. Bugbee, to work with me. I set aside for study seven young mature virgin does that had been born in our colony and gave them each two cubic centimeters

5. P. Stricker and E. Grueter, "Action du lobe antérieure de l'hypophysis sur la montée laiteuse," *Comptes Rendus de la Société de Biologie* 99 (1928): 1978–80.

daily of an alkaline aqueous extract of the whole glands sent me by Bugbee. The daily dose represented about a half-gram of gland tissue. A few lines from my formal report ("The Hormonal Control of Lactation," *American Journal of Physiology*, volume 95, 1930) summarizes the story:

> The result of the injections in these seven rabbits was uniform and striking. On the fourth day or thereabouts, a single drop of milk could be expressed from the nipple. The next day there was usually more, and by the seventh many drops of milk could be obtained. At the beginning of the second week, thickening of the gland could usually be felt through the skin on rolling it between the fingers. By the tenth day the milk could usually be expressed in a stream, and the gland could be distinctly seen through the shaven skin as a dense white area spreading laterally over the abdominal wall. These changes seemed to reach their height about the fourteenth day, and thereafter there was in some of the experiments an apparent slight retrogression in the size of the glands and the amount of milk.
>
> At the time of autopsy, from the fifteenth to the eighteenth day, reflection of the skin demonstrated in all cases a general enlargement and thickening of the mammary glands, far greater than is ever seen in rabbits except during the last week of pregnancy. [Pp. 50–51]

Bugbee's efforts to isolate the active substance from his crude extracts ran into difficulties. The hormone seemed to be a protein or at least a polypeptide. At that time such substances were exceedingly difficult to isolate and identify. Much time was lost by a shortage of pituitary glands absurdly caused by a midwestern physician who claimed to have grown hair on bald heads by administration of pituitary extracts. If that hormone could be isolated, there was big money to be made, so serious scientists all over the nation had to wait months for pituitaries, until the baldness cure proved ineffective. Bugbee was not optimistic about his task, and I had plentiful other uses for rabbits and my time. We discontinued the research. It has in fact taken fifty years for top biochemists to straighten out the six or more hormones of the anterior pituitary lobe.

While writing my paper on lactation I came upon the brief article by Stricker and Grueter of 1928, which, of course, I mentioned. Thus in most subsequent reviews of work on lactation the two Lorrainers are quite properly given prior credit for the discovery they and I made independently. They buried their report in the *Comptes Rendus* of the Société de Biologie, in which for a hundred years French scientists have printed their preliminary reports, some of great import and some trivial. So far as I know, nobody in Europe followed it up by an attempt to isolate the hormone. My longer and more specific paper, however, stimulated my friend Oscar Riddle of the Carnegie Institution's laboratory at Cold Spring Harbor, Long Island, to try his experienced hand, which he did with some success. He called his partially purified extract "prolactin," a name now fully accepted. All subsequent work on the chemical problem, leading to the complete isolation of the hormone by the master biochemist Choh Hao Li of Berkeley, has been based on my paper and on Oscar Riddle's chemical report.

Our discovery of progesterone came at an opportune time in the course of my long-continuing effort to unravel the complexities of the primate menstrual cycle. During the whole exciting period of research from 1926 to 1935 I was also keeping up the observations and experiments on rhesus monkeys that I had begun in Baltimore in 1921. I could manage this along with teaching and the progesterone work because the daily chore of catching the monkeys and noting the occurrence of vaginal bleeding was carried on by my excellent caretaker of the monkey house, Fred Kesel, with notable reliability and devotion. Only at long intervals did an exploratory observation or autopsy take precedence over other duties.

My work with the sows, described in detail in chapter 8, had helped me understand the cycle in animals that undergo estrus. The object of my subsequent work with the monkeys was to learn about the stages of the cycle in a menstruating animal that might offer insight into the human reproductive pattern. The reader will recall that the sow undergoes a two- or three-day period of sexual urgency every three weeks. At that time, in summary, a crop of ovarian follicles matures; they discharge their ova and are replaced by corpora lutea; these persist for about two weeks and produce, by means of the hormone progesterone, a change in the lining of the uterus; the corpora lutea degenerate and the uterus returns to its resting condition.

We had begun to understand through the work of several European gynecologists that in women the ovarian follicle matures and ovulation occurs about the middle of the interval between two menstrual periods, without any outward sign like the estrus of domestic animals. Ovulation is followed by a corpus luteum phase and proliferation of the endometrium. When the two weeks' span of the corpus luteum ends, the proliferated endometrium does not simply subside; in women, apes, and the higher monkeys it breaks down and bleeds. Figure 4 illustrates diagrammatically this sequence of events, which may be compared with those of the sows' cycle (figure 2).

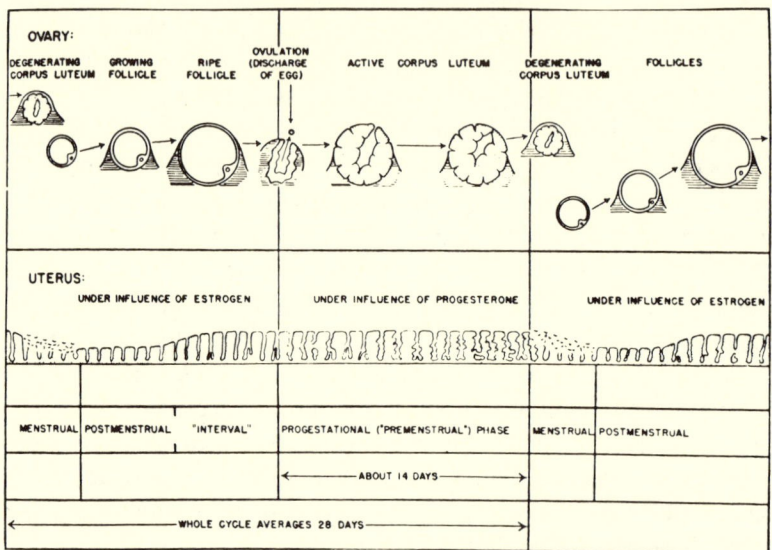

Figure 4. Diagram illustrating the sequence of events in the menstrual cycle of primates (apes, women). From G. W. Corner, The Hormones in Human Reproduction.

My studies of the monkey, begun in Baltimore, had revealed the same timing of ovulation and the corpus luteum phase that the gynecologists were seeing in the human cycle. In Rochester my first aim was to concentrate on the later phase of the cycle and to note the time of the breakdown of the corpus luteum in relation to the onset of menstruation. The observations were long and tedious, but by the generous actions of two friendly scientists who were carrying on similar research, Carl G. Hartman of the Carnegie embryological laboratory in Baltimore (who had succeeded to my monkey quarters there) and G. W. Bartelmez of the University of Chicago, I was able to compare their records and slides with mine and thus to prepare a comprehensive joint monograph ("Development, Organization, and Breakdown of the Corpus Luteum in the Rhesus Monkey"). This was not published until 1945, but by the time we had progesterone in pure enough form I had sufficient information from my monkeys to undertake experiments on the endocrine control of the menstrual cycle. This program of research was supported financially until the end of my stay in Rochester by grants to the University of Rochester by the Rockefeller Foundation and the John and Mary Markle Foundation.

The idea that menstruation is somehow brought about by the corpus luteum was not new. Ludwig Fraenkel, professor of gynecology at Breslau, had come very close to it in 1913; it was implied by the observations of the gynecologists Robert Schroeder at Kiel and Robert Meyer at Berlin and by the conclusions of Leo Loeb, pathologist at Washington University School of Medicine at St. Louis. I believe, however, that I was the first—certainly one of the first—to state it explicitly, which I did in a brief article in the *Journal of the American Medical Association*, November 26, 1927.

Fraenkel and the others mentioned here thought of the corpus luteum as acting positively to produce menstruation. My contribution was the idea that menstruation is brought about not by positive action of the corpus luteum but by its decadence. Some substance it produces, I said, presumably a hormone, first builds up the premenstrual (progestational) proliferation of the endometrium; when this substance is no longer available, the endometrium breaks down and bleeds.

This idea had occurred to me in London in 1923, well before I had any expectation of having an actual hormone for experimental test of the hypothesis. I wrote it down on a sheet of paper headed "X-deprivation theory of menstruation." This I filed away for future contemplation. In 1926 Edgar Allen of St. Louis (who, incidentally, had with Edward Doisy in that same year, 1923, isolated the general ovarian hormone estrogen) found that if he gave a mature female rhesus monkey daily injections of estrogen and then suddenly discontinued them, menstruation followed. He thought, therefore, that natural menstruation results from estrogen deprivation. But the situation is not as simple as that. In 1932 my former colleague at Berkeley, Philip E.

Smith, and a co-worker, Earl Engle, got ahead of me in putting progesterone (or rather a partially purified progestin) into the picture. They gave a monkey a continuous course of progestin. The expected bleeding did not occur until they discontinued the progestin.

By 1937 I was ready to report a series of careful quantitative experiments on monkeys. The progestin I used (Progynon) clearly suppressed menstruation in intact monkeys, and its discontinuance brought on bleeding. The next year a variation of the experiment gave an illuminating result. If I gave a spayed monkey a sufficient daily injection of estrogen for three or four weeks, no menstruation-like bleeding occurred. If I then added a daily dose of progesterone while keeping up the estrogen, and after two weeks discontinued the progesterone, bleeding occurred in spite of the continuing treatment with estrogen. Such a sequence of hormone action is obviously like that which occurs in the natural menstrual cycle in the intact female, whose ovaries produce estrogen more or less continuously, while the corpus luteum supplies progesterone for two weeks in each cycle. When the corpus luteum degenerates, bleeding occurs even though the supply of estrogen continues.

While I was running these experiments in 1935 and 1936, similar findings were being made in three other centers of research on the primate cycle that had sprung up following the discovery of estrogen in 1923 and progesterone in 1929. The workers were F. L. Hisaw at the University of Wisconsin, Smith and Engle at Columbia University, and Solly Zuckerman at Oxford. It dawned upon me that I could bring all their findings together with my own to form a working theory of the hormonal basis of the menstrual cycle, by introducing the idea that progesterone antagonizes the supportive action of estrogen upon the endometrium.

Let us assume that progesterone in some way or other has the property of suppressing the menstruation-preventing action of estrogen while itself holding off menstruation. Then in the normal cycle the uterus will not bleed during the first half ("follicular phase") because the ovaries are furnishing estrogen. It will not bleed during the second half of the cycle ("corpus luteum phase") because the corpus luteum is furnishing progesterone. The production of estrogen continues. By our assumption, however, the corpus luteum is suppressing the protective effect of estrogen; therefore when the corpus luteum undergoes retrogression, the animal is suddenly deprived of the action of both estrogen and progesterone, and the endometrium breaks down.

I first presented this modified hormone-deprivation theory at the annual meeting of the National Academy of Sciences in 1937 (*Science,* volume 85, pp. 437–38) and expounded it fully the next year in the *American Journal of Physiology* (volume 121, 1938, pp. 1–12). In that paper I was happy to mention that Solly Zuckerman had stated in the same year as I (1937) a conception of the antagonism of progesterone to estrogen, in the primate cycle, practically identical with mine. Solly and I, then as now cordial friends, had no reason to contend for priority in this matter. So far as I know, the basic hypothesis of an antagonistic effect of progesterone upon estrogen has never been disputed; in fact, a good deal of evidence has accumulated to support it, and the whole concept is now generally accepted.

The greatest practical application of progesterone and some of its chemical derivatives is as the principal ingredient in the birth-control pill. It is also prescribed by physicians for therapeutic uses based on its several physiologic actions—regulation of the menstrual cycle, reduction of premenstrual tension, relief of painful and excessive menstruation and postpartum uterine spasms, and the control or palliation of certain rather uncommon tumors arising from the endometrium. Progesterone has produced dramatic results in some cases of repeated spontaneous abortion. I know of two beautiful and intelligent young women who are the only offspring of a mother who first suffered four successive miscarriages. Treatment with progesterone in the fifth pregnancy was followed by the birth of a daughter; in the sixth the hormone was not used and another miscarriage ensued. In the seventh pregnancy progesterone was again used, with happy results. The father of these two girls—a physician-scientist and a friend of mine—is convinced that he owes his lovely daughters to the hormone.

A dozen years after Willard Allen and I announced our discovery of progesterone, I was in Buenos Aires for a few days and was invited to visit the maternity hospital of that city. Arriving with a local physician at the stated hour, I was welcomed by the director, Professor Alberto Peralta Ramos, who took us on a very impressive tour of inspection. The Buenos Aires Maternidad is probably the largest obstetrical hospital in the world and is certainly one of the most effective charities. Peralta Ramos was a man of distinguished bearing. He led us in state through the wards and laboratories of the immense institution and finally took us to a small room on the delivery floor. Here there was an ill patient, with nurses and a resident physician in attendance. I was not told what ailed her but guessed from what followed that it was a case of postpartum uterine spasms. Grouped around the bed were Don Alberto's chief of staff, the head nurse of the delivery floor, and some young doctors and nurses, about twenty of us in all. As we stood there in silence, Peralta Ramos gave a signal. The head nurse came forward with a filled hypodermic syringe; the chief of staff took it and administered its contents to the patient, whereupon the director turned to me and said, "Su hormona, Doctor"—"Your hormone, Doctor"—to which I could reply only with a grateful smile. Thinking it over later, I felt that Don Alberto had meant not merely to pay his guest a gracious compliment, but also to symbolize for his young people, by this little drama, the interdependence of the science and the practice of medicine. All our long hours at the microscope and the chemical bench, all his rich experience at the bedside and in the delivery room, had been focused upon one ailing woman, whose pain we were jointly able to relieve.

12

AT HOME AND ON THE ROAD

Rochester was a pleasant place for a young professor and his family. George Eastman once said, when calling upon his fellow citizens for their contributions to the Community Chest, that he wanted to help make Rochester the best place in the world in which to live and bring up children. Afraid, perhaps, that this might seem merely sentimental, coming from an elderly bachelor, he explained that superior living conditions would help him to attract and hold the thousands of skilled workers needed by Eastman Kodak Company. Since Betsy and I had children to bring up, we were grateful for all that Eastman and many other Rochesterians had done to make the city the healthy, orderly, and cultivated place it was. Col. Nathaniel Rochester had begun the good work by settling in 1818 at the lower falls of the Genesee, where the river races toward Lake Ontario. Beside the falls, source of power for industry, first a number of flour mills sprang up, then technical manufactories bringing well-trained mechanics and skilled administrators, engineers, and scientists. The Erie Canal and the New York Central Railroad gave the city easy communications east and west. Enlightened Baptists founded an excellent college in 1850, to which Eastman had given a school of music and a magnificent auditorium, the Eastman Theater.

The Corners, Betsy in particular, enjoyed the concerts of the Rochester Philharmonic Orchestra and the sociability that accompanied them, in the intervals of the programs when the intelligentsia of the city rose to promenade in a wide gallery just off the first balcony, to inspect each other's evening dress and spend twenty minutes in friendly chat. Betsy gladly joined the band of women who annually canvassed the city for subscriptions to the orchestra fund. There was also a theater to which the best New York road companies came, and an excellent local repertoire company played in another theater. Young George and I went two or three times a season to watch the Red Wings baseball team, a farm team of the St. Louis Cardinals, play in the International League. Two fine parks, Genesee Valley Park and Highland Park, were near enough to us for Sunday walks; a third, on the shore of Lake Ontario, was only seven miles away. Mendon Ponds Park, fifteen miles to the south, had picturesque tree-girt, pit-like tarns where ten thousand years ago an iceberg had settled down in the glacial till and melted away, leaving a deep secluded pond for frogs and salamanders. On the southern side of the city a long, wide reach of the Genesee River, beginning quite near the medical school, provides delightful canoeing amid the green lawns of Genesee Valley Park and on into the farmlands and villages of the countryside.

On our country drives we were usually accompanied, as the children entered their teens, by a new member of the household, a Scottish terrier named Jock. A canine aristocrat—his pedigree was registered with the American Kennel Club—Jock was a lovable companion to us all. Full of fun, he distributed his affection equally to each of us and also made himself agreeable to our friends if they were properly introduced. Of other human beings and large animals, such as horses and cows, he was suspicious. To all smaller species, from squirrels to St. Bernard dogs, Jock was a mortal enemy. He was the most belligerent creature I ever knew. The mere sight of a moving animal of any species would send him immediately into violent action.

Our children were growing up healthy, intelligent, interested in their studies, and generally in loving rapport with their parents. There were of course a few headaches and even transitory heartaches. The difficulty about adolescence is that its problems of adjustment within the family have to be solved by two parties, the child and the parents, both of whom have to learn the business as they go along. Both can make mistakes, but over the years our parental and filial affection stood the strain. Once when George was about seventeen and his sister fourteen they discussed, in my presence and without disrespect, my intellectual classification and declared me a Victorian, to them a term of gentle derogation. Fair enough; I admittedly liked Tennyson's poetry, still read Poe with pleasure, did not appreciate Auden, and could not always understand T. S. Eliot. In science and mechanics, however, my standing was not questioned in the family circle.

George and I tinkered with radio; we put together a crystal set and then a two-tube receiver that sometimes brought in short-wave broadcasts from London. One summer at Cold Spring Harbor, Long Island, I took time off and tediously ground a six-inch parabolic telescope mirror (from instructions in the *Scientific American*), silvered it, and fitted it into a tube a tinsmith made for me. We set it up on the roof of the medical school building. My young people enjoyed seeing the mountains of the moon, Saturn's rings, Jupiter's four major satellites, and some of the brighter double stars. My mirror was good enough to reveal clearly the ninth-magnitude companion of the Pole Star.

My colleague Wallace Fenn was as eager as I to interest young people in science. We both had heard, while in London, the superb scientific lectures for children staged at the Royal Institution (begun, I believe, by no less a scientist than Michael Faraday). At Wallace's suggestion we got the University of Rochester chapter of the scientific honor society of the Sigma Xi to put on a similar annual lecture. The public schools liked the idea, and we had audiences of several hundred, filling the new Strong Auditorium on the River Campus (no adult was admitted without a child). Wallace gave a beautifully clear lecture on muscle contraction, illustrated by actual experiments projected upon the screen. I staged a lecture on man's place in nature, describing the comparative structure of vertebrate animals, leading up to the similarity between man and the higher apes (without mentioning the word "evolution"; there were still anti-evolutionists about). After a series of lantern slides showing the similarity of form throughout the vertebrate phylum came the grand climax; at my signal the curtain behind me rose, revealing a black backdrop against which a spotlighted series of skeletons from fish to man was arranged as if in procession across the stage. The children were invited to come up and walk past the skeletons at close range.

In my day the parents of adolescent children were puzzled as to how to provide instruction about the physiology and morals of sex behavior. I was in a favorable position to solve the problem, for my own children at least. When Hester Ann was approaching puberty, her mother, remembering her own fright when, completely ignorant about the phenomenon, she first began to menstruate, asked me to provide the needed preliminary information for Hester Ann. So one Saturday I invited my intelligent young daughter to my laboratory and showed her, under the microscope, slides from my research on monkeys illustrating the menstrual cycle—the process of uterine bleeding and the accompanying changes in the ovaries. There was no embarrassment on either side; I might have been talking to one of the medical students. How much she may have heard already, from schoolmates' talk, I did not know; at any rate she got the facts from me without the taint of prurient curiosity or a vulgar terminology. I left it to her mother to add to my physical statement a woman's view of the dignity of sexual relations and childbearing.

For my son, I took another tack. By the age of fourteen he must have heard a lot of boys' talk, which according to my own experience was by no means accurate and was usually couched in vulgar terms. What was wanted was to place sexual physiology in an atmosphere not only of physical facts but also of human affection and responsibility. I typed a little homemade book describing the organs of sex and reproduction, with illustrations sketched by myself, adding a discussion of love and romance and of the common sexual deviations and maladies that a boy was likely to hear about. I gave it to George, asking for his suggestions before I sent it to a publisher. We had, in fact, no lengthy discussion about it; George said that he found it clear and instructive.

I gave copies to our psychiatrist at the medical school; to the Reverend Justin Nixon, the local minister I respected most; and to the superintendent of the Rochester public schools. All three men highly approved of the book. I had Nat Jacobs, our medical illustrator, make publishable drawings from my sketches, and I sent the manuscript to one of the best-known general publishers. It was politely declined by them and by five other commercial publishers. I next tried the Young Men's Christian Association, which had begun to be interested in sex instruction. They, too, returned the typescript with an appreciative note from a highly placed national staff executive saying that I was too permissive —I had discounted the alleged dangers of masturbation. This might disturb some parents, he said, especially Roman Catholics, with whom the YMCA was trying to develop closer relations. I tried once more by submitting the book to Paul Hoeber, a keen young man who had succeeded his father as a publisher of medical books in New York. He accepted it at once, provided that I would write a similar book for girls. He took both *Attaining Manhood* and *Attaining Womanhood* with him to Harper when he merged his firm with the New York publisher. The two books sold more than 100,000 copies, bringing me royalties of $1,000 or more annually for thirty years. They appeared later in a slightly bowdlerized English edition. As I write, they are going out of print in the United States, but in 1978 Harper sent me a check for my share of the fee for permission to a Spanish firm to issue a translation in Madrid.

A few pages back I mentioned Cold Spring Harbor, Long Island, where I had spent a summer in 1921. In that pleasant village on the north shore of the island near Oyster Bay, about thirty miles from New York City, we lived for six weeks each summer from 1929 to 1933. The pioneer geneticist Charles B. Davenport had for many years conducted there a summer school of biology alongside the Carnegie Institution's Department of Genetics, where I had studied his twin-bearing sheep in 1921. His son-in-law, Reginald Harris, an enterprising young biologist, had taken over the summer school and was modernizing it by introducing courses in general physiology, endocrinology, and other current subjects in addition to the old-line field work in natural history. Because in the 1930s many graduate students and college seniors were looking forward to research careers in these modern fields, Harris had foreseen a need for instruction in the methods of experimental study of mammals, particularly experimental surgery. He had found a biologist with surgical experience to conduct such a course, but in the summer of 1929 the man was not available, and Harris, probably at Davenport's suggestion, asked me to direct the course. This was an opportunity to give my family a vacation on salt water, near enough to New York to visit the museums and the zoo and see a play or two. Harris assigned us fairly comfortable rooms in one of the old whalers' houses on the laboratory grounds. I had a private study and space for my class. The students—ten or a dozen each summer—were mostly young Ph.D.'s or graduate students. One summer six of my eleven pupils were Ph.D.'s.

I was qualified by my surgical experience to teach them basic methods of anesthesia, asepsis, and hemotasis, the use of special instruments, and practical suturing. The work was done mostly on white rats; we used a few cats and rabbits but no dogs. The procedures, always done under full anesthesia, included simple extirpation of endocrine glands and other organs, tissue transplants, intestinal anastomosis, and similar steps in preparation for physiological study. I felt that such use of animals was justified by the training of young research biologists to do experimental work on mammals skillfully and with minimal discomfort to the animals. Among my students at Cold Spring Harbor were Robert Gaunt, who was for many years a research leader with the CIBA Pharmaceutical Company, and Lawrence E. Young, a college senior, who was sufficiently impressed by my talk about the medical school at Rochester that he decided to study medicine there. In good time he had a distinguished career as professor of internal medicine and is still, as emeritus professor, teaching medical students and young physicians. Other members of the class who went on to biological careers were Warren O. Nelson and Charles W. Lloyd.

For my family Cold Spring Harbor was a good base for summer recreation. The two children learned to swim there, and in our last summer on Long Island Hester Ann had her heart's desire, a rented sailing skiff in which she cruised the inner harbor round and round for hours. Those who know Cold Spring Harbor will agree that we were pretty good sailors when I mention that we sailed the little boat around from her home port in Huntington Harbor and navigated her into Cold Spring Harbor under sail through the narrow, twisting "gut" between the sandspit and the village shore. That summer George joined Dr. Sidney Kornhauser's field course in natural history, greatly enjoying the exploration of ponds, streams, the harbor, and Long Island Sound for living denizens of the waters.

Now and then we drove across the island to enjoy seabathing at Jones Beach, the immense, well-managed state-owned bathing resort on the south shore. In the long summer evenings and on Saturdays we explored in our Ford Zephyr the whole of Long Island from Coney Island to sea-washed and wind-swept Montauk Point.

Reginald Harris's enthusiastic direction of the summer school and that of his successor, Eric Ponder, brought a number of lecturers whose discourses and personal acquaintance I treasured. At the adjacent Carnegie genetics laboratory I renewed acquaintance with old friends—the botanist Albert Blakeslee, Carlton McDowell, Oscar Riddle, and Clarence C. Little (afterward president of the University of Maine). C. B. Davenport still lived on the grounds and liked to talk with me.

Back at Rochester, in the fall of 1933, I took on a new avocation for the benefit of my seventeen-year-old son and his classmate Harmon Strong. The Allendale School had up to that time not carried its pupils through the full college-preparatory curriculum. The boys, sons of well-to-do Rochesterians, went off for two years to eastern boarding schools such as Groton and Lawrenceville. Allendale's headmaster, Barclay Farr, was, however, planning to add the last two precollege years to his curriculum. George Corner IV and Harmon Strong, who both intended to enter the University of Rochester, would constitute the first class to stay at Allendale through the fifth and sixth forms. The university required for admission a course in science—physics, chemistry, or biology—but Allendale had no laboratory, and no master was prepared to teach one of these sciences. When Mr. Farr mentioned this to me, I volunteered to conduct a course in elementary biology for the two boys in my private laboratory on Saturday mornings, if the university would accept so informal a program. Dean Gale and the professor of zoology, Benjamin Willier, willingly agreed. I have pointed out elsewhere in this book that the University of Rochester was very liberal in such matters. The boys had the use of my research microscopes. I bought from the celebrated Rochester scientific supply house, Ward's Natural History Establishment, some necessary materials—a culture of living amebas, a couple of preserved grasshoppers, and bullfrogs for dissection. Curt Stern, the eminent geneticist of the arts and sciences faculty, kindly selected from his stock of Drosophila (fruit flies) two strains that could be crossbred to demonstrate the Mendelian ratio and supplied the necessary culture medium so that the boys could do the experiment themselves. George Berry, then our microbiologist, provided a bacterial culture that the boys could transfer and study under the microscope. My two bright pupils responded enthusiastically to this exceptional opportunity. All three of us enjoyed working together, and both Harmon and George passed the college entrance examination in biology with high marks.

This episode had an amusing sequel. Word of it not only circulated through the medical school and the college, but the other local private schools got wind of it, too. In the spring when our course was almost finished, my wife and I had a visit at our house from the headmistress of the Columbia School for girls, one of Rochester's grand dames, who wanted me to conduct, next year, a similar course for eight sixth-form girls. She offered, as compensation, free tuition for my daughter, who was at the rival Harley School. I confess that I would have enjoyed teaching the girls, but considering the probable effect upon our medical students of a bevy of eighteen-year-old subdebs in their midst, I had to decline the headmistress's request. I was aware also that my two mentors, Dean Whipple and Betsy Corner, would veto any such carryings on in my laboratory.

The American Association of Anatomists, one of the strongest and friendliest of the medical scientists' special societies, meets annually for three days at one or another of the nation's medical schools. Its members like to have a look at the new schools. By 1929 I felt my department was ready for inspection by my fellow anatomists. Our plain but well-equipped laboratory rooms were showing signs of effective use. My staff of eleven, assistant professors Burns and Smith, instructors C. M. Thomas and Anton Schneider, and illustrator. Jacobs, research fellow Willard Allen, secretary Cornelia Clark, technicians Bessie Bodine and Charlotte Button, and our indispensable all-round helper Fred Kesel were working together smoothly. On March 27, 1929, the anatomists arrived from all over the country, 125 strong, including the heads of departments in many of the major schools of medicine.

We were ready for them; there were buses to carry them from and to the Seneca Hotel; the laboratories had been swept and dusted; in the students' big histology laboratory rows of microscopes stood ready for the visitors to set up their demonstrations. The school's auditorium awaited the plenary sessions, and small classrooms were available for the special sections. The secretary of the association, my friend and former chief, Lewis Weed, had arranged an excellent program which Professor Charles R. Stockard, our president, conducted with characteristic verve.

On the afternoon of March 28 we took the visitors in buses to visit the Bausch and Lamb optical works, where they could see the extraordinary processes of making optical glass and grinding and polishing the microscope lenses on whose working so much anatomical teaching and research depend. After our visit to the glass furnaces, which are housed in a building down in the gorge of the Genesee River, far below the city level on which the main buildings stand, the buses started up the steep roadway. The last bus, overloaded, stalled halfway up, and the driver asked everybody to get out and push. We got it moving just as the last passenger was about to step off the bus. This was Oscar Batson from Philadelphia, the tallest and heaviest anatomist at the meeting, six feet five or six inches tall and broad and thick in proportion. He could have pushed as hard as any two of the rest of us, but instead, taking advantage of the situation, he rode along on the bus step, waving his ten-gallon hat and cheering as the thirty of us pushed and puffed, yelling to Oscar to get off and help us, until we were out of breath.

Everything else went well all three days, thanks to the enthusiastic efforts of my staff. The technicians and secretary told me later that they wished we could have the anatomists every year. Before the guests departed they voted a resolution offering "congratulations to the University of Rochester upon the signal progress and achievements in the conduct of the medical education and research which it has so brilliantly inaugurated."

One final episode of the meeting remains in memory, evidence of an elder scientist's enthusiasm for his research and kindness to an equally enthusiastic youngster. William Patten, professor of zoology at Dartmouth College, who presented a paper in the comparative anatomy section of the program, had in the demonstration hall a striking exhibit, a dozen slabs of stone in which were imbedded the skeletons of fossil reptiles. I wanted my son George, then thirteen years old, to see these stunning specimens and took him with me to the laboratory on the morning of the last session, when the exhibitors were packing up their slides, models, and other exhibits. Dr. Patten, alas, had just finished wrapping his slabs in old newspapers and had carefully packed them in a carton. Seeing the boy's disappointment he unpacked the whole lot and discussed them, though in simpler terms than if he had been teaching a graduate student. Of such is the kingdom of science.

Whether or not as a result of this successful meeting at Rochester, the association next year elected me secretary treasurer in succession to Lewis Weed. I served for eight years, 1930–38. At the end of my term we had 650 members. My duties were light except during a couple of months before the annual meetings, when I had to collect and edit the abstracts of a hundred or more papers to be presented and arrange them into a program. As secretary I recorded the minutes of the business sessions and conducted the association's correspondence. As treasurer I collected the dues, then two dollars per year, and paid the bills. My departmental secretary, Cornelia Clark, competently did much of the clerical work.

The secretaryship kept me pleasantly in touch with the anatomical world. It was not without its odd episodes. A member who had sent in, rather prematurely, an abstract announcing in positive terms a small discovery in his field, sent me just before we sent the program to press a telegram reading, "Please insert the word *not* in the last line of my abstract." Poor troubled young man, he had probably obtained travel money from his university to enable him to present his paper and therefore could not simply withdraw it.

Simon Henry Gage of Cornell University, an elderly widower, was a revered member of the association. A regular attendant at the meetings, he annually gave a paper, talking to us as if to a first-year biology class about the anatomy of lampreys or some other out-of-the-way subject. At last, at the age of eighty, he did not come to the meeting. At the formal dinner, word went around that he was ill. Somebody rose to move that a message of condolence be sent, and I left the dinner table to go to the telephone and dictate a telegram expressing our concern and hope that he would soon recover. The next morning's newspaper informed us that far from being ill, he had been getting married.

Among the members of our association was another elderly man, a minor teacher in a medical school—I'll call him Dr. X— whose research was of dubious quality and no great significance. He had attended the meeting every year and paid his dues and was entitled like the rest of us to the privilege of being heard when he presented his findings. While I was secretary he once sent in an abstract that was almost incoherent. I could only guess what he meant to say and could not tell whether it was correct. I am a softhearted man and a good hackwriter; I rewrote his abstract, making it seem intelligible, and printed it with the rest in the *Anatomical Record*. Nobody else was working in his field; the 100-word abstract would do no harm. I was not present when he delivered his paper, but on my way out to the hotel for a little rest before dinner I was stopped by a reporter for the town's morning newspaper, who said: "Please explain Dr. X's paper to me. It sounded important but I didn't quite understand it." I was tired and in a hurry. I said: "Nobody could understand it. It's all poppycock. Don't put that stuff in your paper." He thanked me for my frankness and went his way. Thinking over my rash outburst, I got no rest that afternoon and lost a lot of sleep that night. I imagined next morning's headline: "Secretary criticizes colleague, calls paper poppycock." But the reporter was a gentleman; he did not quote me or even refer to Dr. X. Since then I have never spoken to a reporter without weighing my words.

My former chief at Berkeley, the unpredictable Herbert Evans, was president of the association for two years while I was secretary, and Edgar Allen of St. Louis, codiscoverer of the ovarian estrogenic hormone, was vice president. The endocrinologists seem to have been riding high at that time. In the first year of his term Evans failed to arrive at the meeting, sending at the last minute a vague excuse. I suppose that one of his domestic or departmental crises had overtaken him.

Edgar Allen had to preside. His sturdy build, large head, and snow-white hair (he was an almost complete albino) made him a striking figure in the chair, but he was inexperienced in the association's affairs and I had to coach him occasionally. The experience of working together made us good friends for the rest of his lamentably short life.

During my last two years as secretary treasurer our president was Frederick T. Lewis of Harvard Medical School, a first-class embryologist and a kind man at heart but often gruff and disdainful. Once in conversation with me he spoke tartly about some policy at Harvard that he did not like. "I thought that was your dean's idea," said I. "Yes," said Lewis, "if our dean may be said to have an idea." Knowing his critical ways, I was deeply touched when in his farewell address as president he spoke warmly of my services as secretary treasurer and gave me a present. Referring to my interest in the history of anatomy, Dr. Lewis said that he wanted me to have something that was on earth while Galen lived and thereupon handed me a charming little piece of antique glass—a Roman lady's cosmetic jar, its once smooth surface etched by time in a beautiful pattern of iridescent color.

In 1936 I accepted appointment as managing editor of the *American Journal of Anatomy,* an unsalaried post. The other members of the editorial board were Wayne J. Atwell (Buffalo), Sam L. Clark (Vanderbilt University), Harold Cummins (Tulane), and George B. Wislocki (Harvard). We were responsible only for the scientific contents of the journal. The association had turned over the business of publishing it to the Wistar Institute of Anatomy and Biology in Philadelphia. I had to read thirty or forty manuscripts every year and send them to other members of the editorial board for a second judgment. I saw to the literary quality of the articles and the reproducibility of the illustrations and, in short, made sure that the articles were sound and ready for publication. At least one of the other editors read each manuscript submitted. The Wistar Institute took care of routine copy editing, proofreading, and printing. I performed this interesting task through 1940, until I became editor of the Carnegie Institution's *Contributions to Embryology.*

Another service to my chosen field of science was membership on a special committee of the American Association of

Anatomists to consider revision of the nomenclature of human gross anatomy, in the hope of securing international agreement on the 5,000 Latin terms designating the areas and parts of the human body. I was the junior member; our chairman was Clarence M. Jackson of the University of Minnesota; the other members were Robert Terry of Washington University, St. Louis; T. Wingate Todd of Western Reserve University; and S. W. Ransom of Northwestern University. All were sound anatomists and adequate Latinists. The problem called for an international effort in which I also participated a few years later. Its history and outcome will be told in chapter 15. Meanwhile our American group held several sessions at annual meetings of the association and produced an American revision, never published, that was very influential in the international conferences of the next decade.

My long and active association with the National Research Council's Committee for Research in Problems of Sex began through my friendship with Robert Yerkes. I will not discuss the group's origins here, since Sophie Aberle and I did so at length in *Twenty-Five Years of Sex Research* (1953). The Committee's ultimate goal was understanding of human sex behavior, but at first there was much to be done on the underlying physiology of the reproductive system, by anatomists, embryologists, physiologists, and biochemists.

When I joined the committee in 1934, while I was still at Rochester, the other members besides Dr. Yerkes were Walter Cannon, physiologist at Harvard; Karl Lashley, psychologist, and Clyde Kluckhohn, anthropologist, also at Harvard; Frank R. Lillie, zoologist, University of Chicago; C. N. H. Long, biochemist, Yale; Adolf Meyer, psychiatrist, Johns Hopkins; and Clark Wissler, American Museum of Natural History. The committee met annually in Washington at the National Academy of Sciences to consider applications for grants to aid research in a wide range of sciences bearing on sex biology and psychology. Money for these grants came from an annual appropriation by the Rockefeller Foundation to the National Research Council. The grants had a very great effect on the progress of American research. The list of published reports by the committee-backed investigators from 1922 to 1952 covers 106 pages in the history that Sophie Aberle and I wrote. The grantees include almost every one of the nation's investigators in the fields related to sex and reproduction, notably the endocrinology of the sex glands. Almost all the leading workers on the ovarian hormones, for example, received financial aid. Only a few investigators requested help on studies of human behavior.

In 1940, however, Alfred C. Kinsey of Indiana University asked us to look into a bold program on which he had already embarked, a program of recording human sex activity by direct interviews of people of all social classes. After long and intensive study of insect behavior, this devoted biologist, then thirty-seven years old, had turned to our own species to find out exactly how people expressed their sexual urges. Dr. Yerkes met Kinsey and was impressed by his skilled technique of interviewing. The committee made a small exploratory grant for 1941–42. In that year Yerkes and I visited Kinsey in Bloomington and discussed his program in great detail. He was a full professor, married with adolescent children. While carrying on his teaching duties in the zoology department, he worked every available hour, day and night, traveling anywhere that people would give him interviews. He was training a couple of young men in his method of interviewing. Dr. Yerkes and I submitted separately to his technique. I was astonished at his skill in eliciting the most intimate details of the subject's sexual history. Introducing his queries gradually, he managed to avoid embarrassment and to convey an assurance of complete confidentiality by recording the answers on special sheets printed with a grid on which he set down the information gained, by unintelligible signs, explaining that the code had never been written down and only his two colleagues, Wardell B. Pomeroy and Clyde E. Martin, could read it. His questions included subtle tricks to detect deliberate misinformation.

Dr. Yerkes naturally did not discuss his own interview with me but let me know that he was deeply impressed. Dr. Kinsey, as an exceptional sign of confidence in me, asked me to sit with him through an interview with another subject, pledging me to secrecy as to the man's identity so solemnly that I can still say no more than that he was a prisoner in a state penitentiary, convicted of a crime of violence. I was much interested to see how Kinsey's questioning of a person with experience so different from mine brought out intimate facts as readily as from me.

Kinsey knew and used effectively the sexual vocabulary of the streets—or, I should say, of the back alleys and dives of the city —and he could question anyone from a convict to a fellow scientist without lessening the respondent's self-respect.

Kinsey was the most intense scientist I ever knew. He worked all day and often half the night, traveling incessantly to conduct interviews with people of all classes. He talked of little but his research. His only diversion, as far as I could see, was listening to records of classical music. Oddly, because I am quite unmusical, it was through this hobby that I first won his confidence. He had met so much unfavorable criticism and so much resistance to his research program from prudish and timorous people that he trusted nobody on short acquaintance, even professional scientists like Yerkes and me. He never got over the feeling that Robert Yerkes was "sex-shy" and therefore not to be admitted to his full confidence, in spite of all that Yerkes had done to support his work.

I won his full trust by two incidents. On one of my visits he took me home to dinner, carrying with him from his office a flat package, evidently a phonograph disk. As soon as our hats and overcoats were off and I had been introduced to Mrs. Kinsey, Alfred unwrapped his new record and placed it on his phonograph. As the rich tones of a trumpet ensemble welled through the room, he turned with a quizzical smile to Mrs. Kinsey and me and challenged us to name the composer of the music. She ventured no reply. I had heard my son, like Kinsey a lover of classical music, playing records of trumpet pieces by Henry Purcell. Kinsey's record sounded like those, so I ventured the guess that we were hearing something of Purcell's. Kinsey beamed. "This isn't Purcell, but it's early Handel. He was influenced by Purcell. You have done very well, Dr. Corner!" From then on he talked with me with less restraint. I must be O.K. if I knew that much about eighteenth-century music.

The other episode was more to the point. In conversation about his work I cited some facts from a recent extremely explicit book on the sex practices of homosexuals. "What!" he exclaimed, "you have read that?" with a tone of surprise tinged with approval. I had thus proved to him that I was not sex-shy, and he could let down his defenses when talking with me. I could understand his caution and his scorn of prudery, but I think he sometimes hurt his own cause by his assumption that he alone was emancipated from the old taboos.

I was to be involved in the support of Kinsey's researches for some years to come, for in 1947 I succeeded Robert Yerkes as chairman of the Committee for Research in Problems of Sex. But that story belongs to another stage of my career. I shall return to it in chapter 15.

Busy as I was at Rochester with teaching and research, I found time for the history of medicine, which was now becoming a serious avocation. An amusing incident in the autumn of 1929 told me that I had begun to win professional recognition for my historical studies. On October 17 and 18 of that year the new Welch Library at Johns Hopkins Medical School was dedicated with due ceremony. Karl Sudhoff of Leipzig, the world's foremost medical historian, was brought over to deliver the principal address, and there was an afternoon of brief communications in which I was invited to participate. I chose to speak on surgery at Salerno in the twelfth century, a critical period in the development of European medicine. When my turn came to mount the platform and begin my talk, Dr. Harvey Cushing was in the chair, and in the front row center sat Dr. Welch and Professor Sudhoff in patriarchal dignity. As I spoke I saw that Sudhoff, the chief authority on Salernitan medicine, was listening attentively. I knew that he had read my book of 1927, *Anatomical Texts of the Earlier Middle Ages,* for he had published a critique of it, generally favoring my conclusions and explaining in a schoolmasterly way several passages in the texts that had puzzled me; but he had either not read the program or as I spoke had not associated me with my book, for when I left the platform, passing close to the two eminent gentlemen in the front row of seats, I saw Sudhoff turn to Welch and heard him ask, "Wer ist das?" Welch replied, "Corner, aus Rochester." "Corner!" shouted Sudhoff. "I vill shake hands mit heem." Rising to his feet he put out his hand to grasp mine. By that time I was almost back to my seat near the center of the hall and had to return to the center aisle and down to the front, where amid loud applause from the audience we shook hands like old friends.

In 1930 I had two calls to distinguished lectureships far from my home base. The first of these came from the Mayo Foundation at Rochester, Minnesota, which was organizing a series of lectures to be given on a circuit of midwestern medical centers. On my tour I had a repertory of two lectures. I based the first of these, "The Discovery of the Mammalian Ovum," on a translation of Karl Ernest von Baer's Latin monograph on his discovery of the ovum in 1827 which I had made in the hope of publishing it as a centennial tribute in 1927 (I did not finish it in time). This lecture, presented in November 1930 at Northwestern University Medical School, Chicago; at the universities of Wisconsin and Minnesota, the Mayo Foundation in Rochester, Minnesota, and the Des Moines, Iowa, Academy of Medicine, covered the whole story of the search for the ovum of mammals, from Aristotle's conjectures to von Baer. It was published in the *Quarterly of Phi Beta Pi* (a medical fraternity) and in a volume containing all the lectures of the series, *Mayo Foundation Lectures on the History of Medicine*, 1930.

The other lecture dealt with the rise of Western medicine at Salerno in the twelfth century. I talked about the practice of internal medicine by the Salernitan doctors as revealed by their surviving works. Delivered at the Universities of Iowa and Wisconsin and the Mayo Foundation, it appeared in *Annals of Medical History* and in the volume of collected lectures.

Early in 1936 I received from London an invitation from the Royal College of Surgeons to give its Vicary Lecture on December 10 of that year. This is an annual affair, established in the twentieth century to commemorate the first master of the Royal College, the surgeon Thomas Vicary (d. 1561). I chose to speak on Salernitan surgery in the twelfth century, and worked on the subject in every spare moment of that busy year. I read the *Bamberg Surgery*, the *Surgery of Master Roger*, and other early Salernitan texts that had been published by scholars from the original manuscripts and looked up pictures for my lantern slides. In the late spring when I was in New Haven for an anatomical meeting, I chanced to encounter my former teacher Dr. Harvey Cushing. When I told him I was getting ready to give a Vicary Lecture on surgery at Salerno, he mentioned that he had just acquired a Salernitan surgical manuscript attributed to Ricardus Anglicus. We chatted briefly, and I arranged to see the manuscript when I next visited New Haven. A week later at Rochester, a Railway Express van left at my house a small parcel containing *Cirurgia Magistri Ricardi Anglici*, a fine

Latin manuscript in a twelfth-century hand. The parcel was insured for one thousand dollars. In a little note that came with it, Dr. Cushing said simply that if the book was useful for my lecture, I must keep it as long as I needed it. *Master Ricardus* was indeed a find. I kept it for a month, transcribing the text for continued study, and published an analysis of it in the *Bulletin of the History of Medicine*, volume 5, 1936.

Nineteen hundred thirty-six was the year of King Edward VIII's abdication. In America in the latter days of November we were fairly well informed about the crisis, but censorship in Britain had kept the people ignorant of the king's intentions. When I arrived in London about December 3 after a smooth voyage, they still had no definite news. On the afternoon of December 10, as I walked from my hotel to the Royal College of Surgeons in Lincoln's Inn Fields, I heard the newsboys crying, "The King Abdicates," and wondered how much attention I was going to get to a lecture on events of 750 years ago. British decorum, I found, can withstand anything. Inside the college the assembling audience was calm. I did not hear the king mentioned, in the lobby nor in the council room where the council robed for the formal procession to the auditorium. With measured pace we marched, led by a portly beadle bearing a red velvet cushion on which lay the golden mace, symbol of the king's patronage of the college. A dozen councillors followed, and after them the president of the college, Sir Cuthbert Wallace, and I at his side. Formally introduced, I read my lecture to a fully attentive audience and was thanked by Sir Cuthbert Wallace and warmly applauded. At tea afterward the conversation was of the usual casual, friendly sort. Sir Charles Sherrington, who had been so coolly critical and admonitory when I called on him in 1923, came up to shake hands and say some kind words about the lecture. Stricken as these people must have been by their king's downfall, they were not going to let a foreign guest be troubled by their sorrow.

That evening I was guest of honor at a dinner at the Savage Club, arranged by my friend of Baltimore days Henry Woollard. The party included a dozen of the younger professors and lecturers in London hospital schools of medicine. Again nothing was said about the king, but I felt a tension that showed itself in forced hilarity. A toast to me was followed by a round of other toasts proposed by each diner in turn, and then a second round, getting rather maudlin toward the end. As ten o'clock approached, the steward of the club came to our table, reminded us that the king's farewell speech was about to go on the air, and invited the whole party to his rooms upstairs where he had a wireless set. There we sat in silence, listening with solemn attention to that strangely affecting address. When it came to an end with Edward Windsor's final words to his family and his brother, now George VI, no one could or would speak. We rose silently, nodded our thanks to the steward, filed out into the cold night and dispersed without a word from one to another.

Later in private conversation with Woollard and other friends, I took occasion to say that I knew an uncle of Mrs. Wallis Warfield Simpson, Henry Warfield, respected banker and country gentleman, and had often seen another uncle, Edwin Warfield, governor of Maryland. I meant by this to show that the lady was no upstart; her people were gentry. The reply was always the same: the British public would have accepted an American queen but not a divorcee on the throne of England.

During the latter half of my seventeen years in Rochester I had to consider several times the possibility of moving to another post elsewhere, including two definite calls to important and desirable professorships. The first of these incidents was, so far as I know, quite illusory, though Dr. Whipple claimed to have inside information about it. The senior chair of anatomy at Harvard became vacant in 1930 and a search began for a new professor. I was certainly on the list for consideration, for that summer Edward Churchill, professor of surgery at Harvard, sought me out at a reception I attended in Boston and engaged me in a long conversation evidently intended to size me up. Nothing came of this, and in 1931 George Wislocki, my former colleague at Johns Hopkins, was appointed to fill the vacancy. When at the end of the year our annual letters of reappointment came (there was no formal academic tenure at Rochester) I found that my salary had been increased by a thousand dollars. When I thanked the dean he said that this was done in appreciation of my declining the Harvard chair. "But it was never offered to me," I said. "You can't make me believe that," said Whipple. "I know for certain that it was offered to you." I accepted the raise and have wondered ever since which of us was dreaming. Had I, in that conversation with Churchill, inadvertently given him an impression that I would not accept the Harvard post?

At Christmastime in 1930 I was in Baltimore with my family, spending the holiday with my parents. On Christmas Eve, in a last minute visit to Remington's Bookstore on North Charles Street, I found Dr. William H. Welch there among the crowd of shoppers. After a friendly greeting he told me that he was about to retire from the post of his later years, the directorship of the institute for the history of medicine at Johns Hopkins, and said that if I would consider succeeding him, he would nominate me for the position. This was truly astonishing; coming from him it was practically an outright offer. I asked for a week to think it over, coming finally to the conclusion that I should not give up my anatomical and physiological research that was going so well.

The next year came an even greater surprise. J. Whitridge Williams, the eminent professor of obstetrics at Johns Hopkins, died in 1931. At Rochester we thought that his successor would surely be Karl Wilson, our professor of obstetrics and gynecology. At this juncture I had a visit one afternoon, in my office in the anatomical wing, from my colleagues John Morton, professor of surgery, and William McCann, professor of medicine, who had come to tell me that if Wilson went to Baltimore they would propose that I should take over the department of obstetrics and gynecology—a startling idea, considering that my practical experience consisted of witnessing five or six deliveries and a year's internship in gynecology. I could see that my two colleagues wanted the women's clinic to make greater progress in research than it had under Wilson, a highly experienced practitioner but not a very active investigator. They knew that I was a good experimental surgeon and thought that I could transfer my skill to human patients. That was probably true, but when I thought of my total lack of experience in clinical practice, I was staggered by the proposal. I believe, however, that I would have undertaken the venture if it had come about. But Johns Hopkins did not call Wilson, and I was spared what would have been a brain-racking decision.

In 1934 another will-o-the-wisp loomed up. Robert R. Bensley was about to retire from the headship of anatomy at the University of Chicago, where he had built up a strong department. He let me know that he wanted me to succeed him and would nominate me to the university authorities. This time I was not at all interested. Bensley had with him at the time two men, older than I, who aspired to the chair, one of them highly placed in influential Chicago society and both quite unlikely to accept an outsider as their chief happily. Furthermore, three of Bensley's immediate family held appointments in his laboratory—his daughter-in-law as an instructor, his son as departmental photographer, and his daughter as a technician. I thanked the kindly professor and asked to be excused.

In 1934 G. Carl Huber, of the University of Michigan, one of the most respected American anatomists and, like Bensley, head of a large department, retired, and I was officially assured of appointment to succeed him if I was interested. I took this seriously enough to visit Ann Arbor to meet the dean and inspect the anatomical laboratory. The salary offered me was exactly the same as that which I was receiving at Rochester, but the administrative duties were much heavier, and there were four times as many students. The older people in the department were not, in this case, a problem. They let me know that they would be content with me as their head. I could see no advantage in the move, for my family or for me. Ann Arbor, though an attractive city, had no superiority over Rochester, in culture or climate.

A call in 1937 to the directorship of the Wistar Institute of Anatomy and Biology in Philadelphia was at first thought more tempting. The institute owned a farm not far from the city, where if I wished I could expand my monkey colony. I would be able to develop a center for research in the physiology of reproduction, uninterrupted by having to teach medical students. The institute's laboratories and museum were just across the street from the University of Pennsylvania. I had friends on its medical faculty. The College of Physicians of Philadelphia, with one of the nation's greatest medical libraries, was only a mile away. My wife, a music lover, could hear as often as she liked one of the world's best symphony orchestras. The city was nearer than Rochester to the Baltimore home of my aging parents. But the situation was not as simple as it looked at first. Philadelphia would be a good place to live, as I have since found out by living there, but the Wistar Institute's affairs were confused. Milton J.

Greenman, the late director, had let the income from endowment largely go into activities other than research—a printing plant publishing several scientific journals for the general good, including the *American Journal of Anatomy* and the *Anatomical Record*, and an active business of breeding and selling white rats of superior quality for research. The farm was not scientifically productive. Greenman's assistant director, Edmund J. Farris, an enterprising and ambitious young man, had settled his family in the excellent residence on the farm. He said that he would be happy to work under me but hoped that I would not want him to give up the house—on which my wife had set her hopes for our use.

Relations between the Wistar Institute and its neighbor, the University of Pennsylvania, were nonexistent. Milton Greenman, fearing that the university would absorb or at least dominate his institute, had avoided all cooperation with its faculty. Eliot Clark, professor of anatomy in the university's medical school, was not told of the offer to me, his former pupil at Johns Hopkins, and was indignant that he had been given no opportunity to urge me to accept the directorship. Worst of all, nobody at the Wistar Institute, not even the president of its board, Dr. Alfred Stengel, could tell me the amount of its annual income. Greenman had so closely integrated the expenditures for printing the journals and for breeding rats with those for research that a team of accountants had not yet untangled them. The institute was apparently solvent, but no balance sheet was to be seen.

My colleagues at Rochester were happy that I declined the Philadelphia post. George Whipple gave me, on behalf of the trustees of the university, a handsome sterling silver platter engraved with the signatures of the whole board. He also increased my salary by $1,000, and to justify the increase added to my official title of professor of anatomy the further designation of curator of the medical library.

The real bombshell came in the early autumn of 1939 in the form of a letter from Vannevar Bush, president of the Carnegie Institution of Washington, offering me the directorship of the Department of Embryology in Baltimore, one of its seven research centers situated in various parts of the United States.

This opportunity was far more tempting than the calls to

Ann Arbor or Philadelphia. The Carnegie embryological laboratory was founded by Franklin Mall, to whom I owed my start in anatomical research. After Mall's untimely death George L. Streeter took over the directorship and faithfully carried on the founder's plans, making it the world's foremost center for research in primate embryology. Its laboratory was located in one of the buildings at the Johns Hopkins Medical School. I was being called back to my native city and my alma mater. Although by that time both my parents had died, Betsy's father still lived in Baltimore, as did my brother and my sister. Betsy was from the first anxious that we should make the move. Always ambitious for me, she thought that it would put me on a wider stage than that of the University of Rochester. She feared, I believe, that I was in danger of settling down for the rest of my life in the shelter of a comfortable professorship under the protection of our forceful dean. Moreover, she felt cramped by the social milieu of faculty wives in Rochester, which was dominated by a small group of conservative grandes dames.

I was torn almost in two by Bush's offer. I was proud of my share in the creation of the Rochester medical school, which was yearly gaining greater national prestige. My colleagues were agreeable and trustworthy. I did not want to give up teaching medical students, especially in my course on histology, which I secretly thought was the best in the country and getting better every year. My regard for George Whipple had grown into strong friendship. He made it plain that my departure would sadden him. In a poignant conversation he offered to resign the deanship in my favor if that would hold me in Rochester.

In my distress, putting off the decision as long as I decently could, I finally drafted two letters, one accepting the proffered post and the other declining it. They lay on my desk for a day. Unable to settle the matter by further thought, I at last picked up the letter of acceptance and, hurrying to the nearest letter box lest I should change my mind again, posted it to Vannevar Bush.

RESEARCH DIRECTOR

13

THE CARNEGIE
EMBRYOLOGICAL
LABORATORY

Before we moved to Baltimore, Betsy and I drove down and scouted the northern suburbs for a house to live in. We found a modest but comfortable brick cottage in the Maryland colonial style in Merryman Court, Roland Park, a few blocks from the house my parents had built in 1904. The house was one of six designed some thirty years before by the architectural firm of my cousin, G. Corner Fenhagen. They stood, backed by tall trees, around three sides of a green lawn opening onto Keswick Road, a mile northwest of the Homewood campus of Johns Hopkins University and four miles from the Johns Hopkins Hospital and Medical School, where the Carnegie laboratory was housed. As one ascended the gentle slope from University Parkway, the sidewalks of Keswick Road were lined by dogwood trees that burst in springtime into layered clouds of pink blossoms. Behind our house we had about a quarter-acre of lawn bordered by high privet hedges, along which at the north side was a wall of forsythia bushes ten feet high, the first shrubbery to flower in April. The former owner had left us a few fine rose bushes. Though I was not much of a gardener, I laid out a flower bed along the eastern hedge and grew there zinnias and marigolds, easy to care for and a source of flowers for the house all summer long. To our hedges and trees came the summer birds of passage, bold bluejays jawing at the squirrels, cardinals flitting from bough to bough, and timid wood thrushes with their sweetly musical song. The redheaded woodpeckers that in my boyhood used to rattle on our trees and rainspouts no longer came to Roland Park. Baltimore orioles were rare. Although they wore the Calvert colors, they preferred New England in hot weather. In the evenings we sat outdoors watching the fireflies rise one by one from the grass until there were hundreds in the air above us on their nuptial flight. Across the lawn and beyond the lane were the grounds and old stone building of St. Mary's School for orphan girls, whose young voices could be heard at evensong when the chapel windows were open.

In the court we had good neighbors. At No. 1 lived Mark Watson, military expert of the *Baltimore Sun*, a New Englander who had learned gracious Maryland ways, with his sociable wife and two young daughters. No. 2 was inhabited by three elderly people named Harwell. The two ladies said little but contributed pachysandra cuttings from their garden for us to plant as a carpet for the rhododendrons beside our front steps. Their brother said nothing at all. He was visible only at 5:00 P.M. daily, when he came out of their house, strolled down the back lane to a cocktail lounge on Cold Spring Lane, drank his daily martini, and returned to disappear into the house. A dozen years later the Harwells were succeeded at No. 2 by Dr. Walter Buck, a skilled internist attached to the Johns Hopkins Hospital, and his young family. At No. 3 lived the household of Walter Boggs, a busy lawyer; at No. 4 the Corners; at No. 5 another lawyer, Alan Sauerwein, a taciturn middle-aged gentleman with a talkative wife. No. 6 was the home of the large family of Clinton McSherry, a handsome stockbroker, and his charming matronly wife, Marian. Their name was sufficient to suggest to Baltimoreans the old Irish Catholic gentry of Maryland. Clinton McSherry claimed descent from Niall of the Nine Hostages. He was a gentleman to the manner born, descendant certainly of honorable and devout ancestors.

With such neighbors as these we lived in unbroken amity for all our sixteen years in Merryman Court. When the Watsons served Christmas eggnog we all crowded into their dining room to sip it. When Mrs. Sauerwein received each April a hamper of lovely daffodils from her brother, a grower in Virginia, she distributed the golden blooms to her neighbors. When the Boggses' eldest son, Paul, was killed in Germany near the end of World War II, we all grieved with them at the requiem mass that Mrs. McSherry arranged in St. Mary's chapel. When the McSherrys' daughter was married in the old Baltimore cathedral, the Corners were seated in a front pew and heard the officiating clergyman read a special letter of felicitation and blessing from the pope. When the Corners had a family party on Thanksgiving Day so big that Betsy had to roast two turkeys, Mrs. McSherry lent the use of her kitchen. The two ladies became good friends. I believe that Marian McSherry had hopes of converting Betsy to Catholicism, perhaps even of bringing me into the fold, but social restraint kept her efforts within bounds.

My brother, Harry (Henry Evans Corner), and my sister, Hester, who was married to a likable and capable young businessman, Robert Wagner, both lived, with their families, ten minutes' drive from us. Harry, three years younger than I, after taking an M.A. degree in history at Johns Hopkins went into the advertising business, in which, I think, he was only moderately interested. Betsy's father, now widowed, was living in East Baltimore. So we had kinsfolk, and our son and daughter had cousins nearby. George IV was halfway through medical school at Johns Hopkins when we returned to Baltimore in 1940, and Hester Ann was in college at Bryn Mawr.

Soon after our return I was asked to be a trustee of the Samuel Ready School for orphan and half-orphan girls, named for its founder, a mid-nineteenth-century bachelor merchant. My grandfather, the first George Corner, and my father, the second, had each been president of the board of trustees, a post to which I myself was elected a few years after joining the board. The school's handsome new building in the western suburbs was designed by my cousin, G. Corner Fenhagen. My maternal great-uncle, Dr. John T. King, Sr., was at one time physician to the school. I was glad to have a small part in a distinguished Baltimore philanthropic service to which so many of my relatives had contributed.

The budget allocated by the Carnegie Institution to its Department of Embryology was sufficient to support the work of five or six investigators. At that time the institution did not rate its scientists by the usual academic titles, but the rank of member of the institution implied standing equal to that of a full professor or at least associate professor. I had a vacancy to fill at once because Warren Lewis, senior member under my predecessor, George L. Streeter, resigned at the end of 1939 to join the Wistar Institute in Philadelphia. My senior colleague at Rochester, Robert K. Burns, Jr., accepted my invitation to join me in Baltimore. I felt guilty about taking from Rochester so excellent a teacher. He might well have succeeded me as head of the department of anatomy but told the dean that he did not wish to be considered for the post. A Virginian married to a Maryland woman, he was happy to move to Baltimore. Thus our long association in research was continued for many years. Burns's keen intellect, wide biological experience, and solid friendship meant much to me.

I had hoped that Carl Hartman, who had been with Streeter for years, would stay on with me. A stocky, squareheaded, unpolished midwesterner, sixty-one years old in 1940, who had spent many years in Texas before joining the Carnegie laboratory, he was an enthusiastic, unselfish fellow worker. He had taken part with George Streeter and Chester Heuser in a brilliant study of the embryonic development of the rhesus monkey. Basing his mating program on what I had learned about the rhesus cycle, to which he added much by his own observations, he provided the dated embryos that Heuser skillfully sectioned and Streeter analyzed and described. The result was one of the greatest achievements of American biology in its day, being the first complete description of the development of a primate from the one-cell stage through the whole embryonic period.

Hartman was the only member of the Carnegie staff who might have felt hurt because he was passed over for the directorship. He welcomed me cheerfully, saying that he would have been content with any director whose first name was George, thus humorously referring to Streeter and me and to George Wislocki of the Johns Hopkins department of anatomy, who had been regarded as a likely candidate for the post. Hartman left us in 1941 to head the large department of anatomy at the University of Illinois medical school in Chicago. He kept in constant touch with me and with G. W. Bartelmez at the University of Chicago, comparing information about the ovarian and uterine cycle of *Macaca rhesus* until in 1945 I published our joint findings in the Carnegie *Contributions to Embryology*.

Margaret Reed Lewis was only a nominal member of my department, having moved with her husband, Warren Lewis, to the Wistar Institute. The Carnegie Institution, however, continued to pay her salary and the expenses of her research on malignant cells in tissue culture. For several years I signed the vouchers for her purchases of rats and chemicals, until she reached the age of retirement.

With the consent of Lewis Weed at Johns Hopkins, I offered a post to Louis B. Flexner of his staff, a brilliant physiological anatomist who brought to us his characteristic enthusiasm and energy. Flexner is a nephew of the late Simon and Abraham Flexner, whose contributions to American medicine need no explanation here. As the only medically trained member of the senior staff other than myself, he was a helpful adviser on many administrative problems.

In 1941 I appointed to my staff Samuel R. M. Reynolds, a Philadelphian who was trained at Swarthmore College, took his Ph.D. in physiology at the University of Pennsylvania, and had been at the Long Island Medical College in Brooklyn—another good teacher stolen by Carnegie from a medical faculty to do full-time research along with Burns, Flexner, and me. Reynolds had made himself the leading expert of the time on the physiology of the uterus. Like Louis Flexner, he was taken away from me by the army, to do secret and at times dangerous work on survival methods for aviators downed at sea.

Chester Heuser fortunately was not called away. A Kansan by birth and a graduate of the University of Kansas, he took his Ph.D. in anatomy at Harvard with F. T. Lewis. He was a master at the delicate business of preparing embryos to be cut into thin serial sections and mounted on glass slides. When Arthur Hertig (of whom I shall have something to say shortly) brought us a two-cell human embryo, the first ever seen at that stage, so small that it could barely be seen with the unaided eye, Heuser ran it up through the usual series of stronger and stronger alcohols, then a clearing oil, and imbedded it in celloidin, keeping track of its orientation, so that when he cut it into sections 1/2,400 of an inch thick, the middle one of the twenty sections was cut squarely through the middle of the nucleus of each cell. Heuser handled and sectioned far more early human embryos then anyone else in the world. He knew much more human embryology than I and could put his knowledge at the disposal of his colleagues by word of mouth, but he had some kind of block about writing, so that his research work was nearly all published in collaboration with Streeter. When I undertook to provide an article on human embryology for the fourteenth edition of the *Encyclopaedia Britannica,* I hoped that Heuser would write the first draft, but he got nowhere. After I wrote the draft, he helped me revise it. To illustrate the article I had to get together a stock of suitable pictures from which he helped choose the best.

The men I have mentioned, Burns, Flexner, Reynolds, and Heuser, once we were all together after the war, constituted the permanent senior staff of my department, each of them a leader in his particular field and all of us happy to work side by side. I must mention also Elizabeth M. Ramsey, trained as a physician at Yale, who before I took over had been coming twice a week from her home in Washington to study the arrangement of blood vessels in the human and monkey placenta, a problem that had baffled anatomists for two hundred years and on which she was making herself the leading authority. It was my privilege to assist her project by injecting the blood vessels of several monkey placentas with india ink so that they could be followed in sections—a procedure requiring a trained team. Dr. Ramsey's distinguished studies were recognized in 1949 by her appointment to the senior staff as research associate.

In 1952 I seized an opportunity to bring to the laboratory one of the country's most experienced embryologists. George William Bartelmez had reached retirement age at the University of Chicago, where he had spent his entire career in the department of anatomy. A quiet, sensitive scholar-scientist, he had not in recent years been happy with his associates, although he had loyal research students. After R. R. Bensley's retirement he had been given a trial as chairman of the Chicago department which, I have been told, lasted only two weeks, after which Barty returned, with relief, to his microscope. He had long been a welcome visitor to our laboratory. In 1939 when I was beginning to get together the final account of the ovarian and uterine cycle of *Macaca rhesus,* about which he and I had often talked, I invited him to join me for a month in the summer to make an intensive comparison of our material on the cycle. Barty accepted, provided that I would find a cooler place to work than Baltimore. The head of the biological laboratory on Mt. Desert Island on the Maine seacoast kindly gave us the use of a room.

I took a cottage at Bar Harbor for my family, Barty came alone, and we sat down together for six hours every day, comparing sections of ovaries and uteri with enlightening results.

After the day's work he and my son George and I often climbed the miniature mountains of that island paradise. At such exercise Barty, slim, lean, and wiry, was superb, leaving George, Jr., and me behind at the rockiest places. As a youth in New York City he had been a gymnast in a Turnverein. He often dined with us, delighting us with his wide-ranging conversation, adorned with quotations in German, from Goethe. We were amused by his mild eccentricities, such as ordering lobsters for dinner every one of the thirty days he was on the island, never failing to dissect out the luscious meat from the smallest joints of the claws. Betsy and young George (Hester Ann was away at a camp somewhere) took kindly to Barty, and he and I became close friends.

At the Carnegie laboratory from 1949 until the end of my directorship in 1955, Bartelmez went on with his unending study of the peculiar spiral arteries of the lining of the primate uterus, gaining profound knowledge which, being a perfectionist, he never rounded up in the magisterial monograph he might have written. To all of us on the staff he was an unfailing source of information on the whole range of vertebrate embryology.

Others who joined the staff of researchers later in my directorship were Walter S. Wilde (1944–46), physiology; David Tyler (1947–50), general physiology; Bent Böving (1951–77), physiology; Arpad I. Csapo (1949–55), physiology and biochemistry; and David W. Bishop (1952–77), general physiology. Their researches, like all of our work, are summarized in "Reports of the Director of the Department of Embryology," in the *Year Books* of the Carnegie Institution of Washington, fifteen of which I wrote in the hot Baltimore summers of 1941–55.

Of course we always had with us younger people as visiting fellows, many of them from foreign countries, also guests from medical school faculties, advanced medical students, and transient scientists from all sorts of places. During the sixteen years of my administration thirty-five men and women were listed formally in the *Year Books* of the Carnegie Institution of Washington as fellows of the John Simon Guggenheim Foundation or the Rockefeller Foundation or one or another foreign organization in South America, Europe, and Asia. Most of them came to us already holding doctoral degrees in medicine or biology. The happy relations developing from their work with members of our senior staff were summarized by one of the most distinguished of them, Dr. Luis Vargas, now dean of the faculty of biological sciences at the Catholic University of Santiago, Chile, in a conversation in 1978 with Dr. James D. Ebert, president of the Carnegie Institution. The members of our staff, Dr. Vargas said, had furnished models that were to influence him for many years to come. He spoke highly of their devotion to basic research, of their capacity for intensive, independent study while sharing a wide range of interests, and of the warmth and understanding with which they received colleagues from foreign shores.

There were usually ten or a dozen people at lunch every day in our library. Under Streeter's administration this had become a traditional affair. Everyone brought his own lunch in a paper bag. Somebody made toast and coffee for the group. We all joined in an uninhibited conversation that might range from the day's weather to some abstruse topic like the segmentation of the embryonic brain. The *Encyclopaedia Britannica* and the unabridged *Webster's Dictionary* were at hand to settle differences of opinion or terminology. Dr. Streeter, who had taken a room next door in the anatomical laboratory, often came over to join us for lunch and was as likely to present a conundrum or a new limerick as a subtle discussion of ontogeny. Visiting scientists took home to their own institutions reports of fine-spun wisdom and sophisticated jokes at the Carnegie lunch table.

Supporting the scientists' work were, in addition to about a dozen secretarial, technical, and administrative workers, James F. Didusch, our illustrator, who had been a pupil of Max Broedel, the celebrated artist of the Johns Hopkins Medical School; Osborne O. Heard, the modeler, greatly skilled in the reconstruction of exact three-dimensional plaster models of embryos from serial sections; and Chester Reather, our photographer, who toward the end of my directorship was called to head the photographic department of the Johns Hopkins Hospital.

When Dr. Streeter's secretary and administrative assistant, Miss Rebecca Hepburn, who had been with the department since its organization, retired shortly after my arrival, Arthur Rever,

Hartman's assistant in the monkey quarters, applied for her post. Having foreseen the opportunity he had enterprisingly taken an evening course in accounting at the Baltimore YMCA. I could not dispense with his skill in caring for the monkeys and keeping up the daily record of the females' cycles, so I gave him both jobs, and he was my mainstay, both in the office and in the monkey quarters, becoming my trusted friend.

With the help of scientists and parascientists (to coin a modern-sounding word), I was now directing the activities of a center of intense advanced research famous for a quarter-century's study of the development of embryos. Yet neither I nor any of the research staff except Heuser was in the strict sense a descriptive morphological embryologist. Franklin Mall's chief aim in founding the Carnegie Institution's Department of Embryology was to advance the study of the form and structure of the human embryo and its constituent tissues. Most of the research done during his brief directorship and that of George Streeter had been of such a morphological kind. The program had been remarkably successful. Streeter and his associates carried the knowledge of early stages back into the second week of gestation, and it was to be expected that within a few years the human embryo would be known day by day from the first division of the fertilized ovum to the end of the embryonic period. The classical embryology of the human species was about to become, practically, a finished subject, just as the investigation of gross human anatomy had been finished about 125 years before.

Discerning readers of this book will therefore not be surprised to see that the staff of the department as I reorganized it in 1940–41 was oriented toward experimental rather than morphological embryology. My own one piece of descriptive embryology, the account of Embryo 5074, was an effort made because I had obtained that precious specimen. My appointee Robert Burns, one of the country's leading experimental embryologists, devoting himself to the development of the sexual and reproductive organs, had done much of his previous work on amphibian larvae and was going on to work with opossum embryos, accessible at an early stage in the brood pouch of the mother. Flexner was bringing modern physical methods to the study of placental transmission. Reynolds was planning intensive physiological investigation of the uterus. I considered that my prime duty as director was to foster the trend of the department's work toward the physiology of development.

By no means, however, did we neglect the unfinished program of morphological study. Indeed, the collection and study of human embryos was, when I took over, in the midst of a remarkable recrudescence. Two Bostonian physicians of great enterprise and devotion to science, John Rock, gynecologist in chief to the Free Hospital for Women, and Arthur T. Hertig, pathologist at the Peter Bent Brigham Hospital, had joined forces to watch for and preserve early human embryos obtained from the operating room. They brought their valuable finds to the Carnegie laboratory to be sectioned by our skilled technicians and reviewed by Streeter and Heuser. During my directorship this happy cooperation continued. Human embryos younger than about twenty days were almost unknown, so much so that there was doubt whether the structure of the earliest stages was like that of known mammals. With increasing experience and skill Hertig and Rock obtained embryos from practically every day of the first three weeks, completing that phase of Mall's ambitious program. This was an achievement worthy of the Nobel Prize.

One of the most exciting hours of my life was one I spent in Heuser's laboratory room when Hertig, just arrived from Boston with a specimen he did not dare to send by mail, took out of his vest pocket a little vial of alcohol, emptied it into a small glass dish, put the dish on the stage of a low-power microscope and showed us the two-cell human embryo I mentioned a few pages back. I had seen and handled many such segmenting eggs of the sow and the rabbit; this one was human, one of our own species, a veritable jewel of science, at a stage never seen before. Then followed an anxious week while we waited for Heuser to get the embryo imbedded and sectioned. He had to handle it with a pipette like a medicine dropper but with a finer tip. Once and only once in his career he had lost an early human embryo, in the barely visible morula stage, while transferring it from dish to dish. This time all went well, and the sections, in two rows on a slide, were sealed for good under a glass cover slip.

George Streeter, who continued his morphological research until the very day of his sudden death in 1948, made great use of the Hertig-Rock embryos and other early specimens in the collection when completing his descriptive catalogue, "Horizons in Human Embryology." This is a series of chapters published in the Carnegie *Contributions to Embryology*, in which Streeter planned to gather the data on all well-preserved and reliably described human embryos in the world's literature, from the fertilized ovum to the end of the embryonic period at about forty-five days' gestation age. A large number of the cited embryos, especially of the early stages, are in the Carnegie collection. Streeter set up twenty-five stages or "horizons" of about two days each. He began his descriptions and analyses at stage 11, about twenty-four days. He had reached and covered horizon 18 when he died in 1948. Heuser and I in 1955 added horizon 10 (four to twelve somites, length 1.5 to 3.6 millimeters.) In 1973 Dr. Ronan O'Rahilly, now at the University of California at Davis, finally catalogued and reviewed the remaining early horizons, 1 to 9.[1] During the directorship of my successor, James D. Ebert, when the transition to physiological and biochemical embryology was completed, the Carnegie collection was transferred to the University of California at Davis, where it is available for study.

My own time for research was limited by executive duties and by ever-increasing calls to give lectures, write reviews, and serve on committees, all of which seemed to be part of a mature scientist's duty. I kept the monkey colony going with Arthur Rever's skilled help, and continued to gather dated ovaries and uteri to fill gaps in my series of stages in the menstrual cycle of *Macaca rhesus.* Finally, in 1945, I was able to put together in final form, with illustrations and tables, the results of many years' work on the ovarian and uterine cycle, in a major report in *Contributions to Embryology* ("Development, Organization,

---

1. The interested reader might consult: George L. Streeter, "Developmental horizons in human embryos, age groups 11 to 13," Collected Papers from the Contributions to Embryology, in *Embryology Reprint*, vol. 2, *Carnegie Institution of Washington* (Washington, D.C., 1951); Chester H. Heuser and George W. Corner, "Developmental horizons in human embryos: Description of age group 10," in *Contributions to Embryology, Carnegie Institution of Washington*, no. 244 (Washington, D.C., 1957), pp. 29–39; and Ronan O'Rahilly, "Developmental stages in human embryos: Part A. Embryos of the first three weeks (stage 1 to 9)," *Carnegie Institution of Washington*, Publication 631 (Washington, D.C., 1973).

and Breakdown of the Corpus Luteum in the Rhesus Monkey"). For the conclusive account Carl Hartman and George W. Bartelmez put at my disposal their extensive collections of rhesus material. Bartelmez also lent me a good-sized lot of sectioned rhesus ovaries collected by Harry B. Van Dyke at the Peking Union Medical College. Carl and Barty were unwilling to be listed as joint authors, since the original project was mine and their acquisition of material had been incidental to somewhat different investigations, but I found a way to couple their names with mine on the title page.

Looking backward on those years I see now that with this article, published in my fifty-fifth year, I reached the culmination of my thirty years of observation and experiment on the female reproductive cycle. There were still odds and ends to be written up. One major unanswered question still haunted me, to which between 1945 and 1955 I devoted many fruitless hours. Various workers, including myself, had shown that in monkeys experimental deprivation of either estrogen or progesterone results in a period of menstruationlike bleeding. This finding had since been confirmed for women by other observers, and I had built upon it a theoretical explanation of the menstrual cycle. In lower mammals the end of the corpus luteum phase produces only a quiet reversion of the endometrium to the unproliferated state. Why the breakdown and bleeding in the higher primates?

I conjectured that in these species the sudden reduction in hormonal activity when the corpus luteum regresses removes a protective effect of estrogen and progesterone against some substance that causes the terminal arteries of the endometrium to contract and shut off its nutrition. I made many experiments by injecting vasopressor substances, chiefly adrenalin, into the uterine cavity of monkeys, with just enough hints of positive results to keep me at it for a couple of years, but not enough to accept as valid evidence. So my last experimental effort to understand the cycle was unsuccessful. The subsequent discovery of those peculiar vasopressors, the prostaglandins, suggests that a solution of the problem might come from that quarter. As I write this page in 1979, evidence in favor of this idea appears to be coming to light.

In my last years as director there came a resumption of experimental work on my part, a kind of Indian summer of research, occasioned by the arrival in 1949 of Arpad Istvan Csapo, a young Hungarian physician who had done first-class biochemical work on uterine muscle at Budapest under the guidance of the celebrated scientist Albert Szent-Gyorgyi. In 1948 he got out of Hungary with his young wife and found a temporary home at Uppsala in Sweden. My colleague Reynolds and I read a couple of Csapo's papers, which gave us our first understanding of the contractile mechanism of uterine muscle and suggested that we might learn still more if we could put together our information with that of Csapo. I telephoned to Professor Szent-Gyorgyi, who had come to the United States and settled at Woods Hole, to inquire about Csapo. Would he come to Baltimore to work with us if I could get him a fellowship? Szent-Gyorgyi spoke highly of Csapo. My letter to Uppsala offering the young man a fellowship must have passed, in the middle of the Atlantic, a letter he had written to me. He had read articles by Reynolds and me which gave him his first knowledge of the hormonal control of uterine muscle. He asked whether I might accept him to work with us for a while.

Csapo arrived in Baltimore in the autumn of 1949, a personable young man speaking very little English, but so quick-witted that we promptly understood each other. I showed him the simple method by which my Baltimore students in 1910–13 had discovered the basic facts and by which I later, with Willard Allen and A. W. Makepeace, had carried on the study with pure progesterone. Csapo and I began working together, at first with sows' uteri from the slaughterhouse, then with rabbit uteri. He taught me how to refine our experiments by using isometric contraction (physiologists will understand that). We discovered that uterine muscle if repeatedly stimulated displays a "staircase phenomenon" like that of heart muscle (cardiologists will understand that). We began to get a glimmer of the crucial fact that progesterone depresses the transmission of contractility along the uterine muscle (obstetricians will appreciate that). My role in this work was hardly more than to encourage Csapo, the brilliant experimenter. I was able to continue his fellowship for a couple of years and then in 1951 to make him a permanent member of the Department of Embryology. When I moved to New York in 1955 he went with me to the Rockefeller Institute and when I finished that assignment, my former student Willard

Allen, then professor of obstetrics and gynecology at Washington University, St. Louis, called Csapo to a full professorship in his department. At St. Louis he has had a fruitful career, winning wide recognition not only in our country but in Europe and South America.

During these years I also published some studies of early embryonic abnormalities and a thorough review of single-ovum twinning and other multiple births and of the incomplete twinning that results in double monsters, that is, "Siamese twins," based largely on specimens in the Carnegie collection of embryos and fetuses.

As director of the Department of Embryology of the Carnegie Institution I missed, a little, the variety of the acadmeic professorial career, the daily challenge of teaching medical students and the association with university colleagues in all fields of learning. The atmosphere of a research institute is more professional than that of the campus. Administrative problems are broader, less often involving personal quirks and qualms. One deals mostly with mature, settled scientists, less with enthusiastic youths. Life in my research department was of course not constantly smooth nor even quite impersonal. I was called upon from time to time, just as I was at Rochester, to listen to perplexities and woes of all ranks of my little company of half a hundred people who frequented our laboratory. Training as a physician stamps the M.D. as a qualified adviser in all sorts of human problems, even if like me he has long ago laid aside his stethoscope and never writes a prescription. Those who sought my sympathy and sometimes my advice in that period of my life are mostly still living. Their troubles, however long past, are not to be discussed here.

I was still, moreover, to some degree a teacher. There were always a few medical students about the laboratory, engaged in joint research with me or staff members. Visiting fellows needed guidance in varying degree. My colleagues Burns, Reynolds, and Flexner and I were each invited once or twice a year to lecture to the Johns Hopkins medical students on our respective specialties until Lewis Weed retired in 1949 and was replaced by a self-sufficient successor who wanted no dealings with the Carnegie staff. During World War II I lectured on the reproductive cycle to select classes of the Women's Auxiliary Army

Corps, a change from studying wax models to teaching model WAACS, as I remarked to my listeners. This small task for the army was my only national service in 1941–44 except the chairmanship of two committees on war-related problems, to be mentioned in the next chapter.

But if I was no longer primarily a teacher, I was a member of a proud and wide-ranging organization. Every year during the annual meeting of the trustees of the Carnegie Institution the directors of the seven research departments also met at the handsome headquarters building in Washington at Sixteenth and P streets, N.W., to discuss common problems and acquaint ourselves with each other's researches. During my time I thus spent a couple of days each year with my eminent colleagues Walter E. Adams and later Ira S. Bowen, astronomy, Pasadena and Mt. Wilson, California; Leason H. Adams and Philip H. Abelson, geophysics, Washington, D.C.; John A. Fleming and Merle A. Tuve, terrestrial magnetism, Washington, D.C.; Herman A. Spohr, C. Stacy French, plant biology, Stanford, California; Milislav Demerec, genetics, Cold Spring Harbor, New York; Alfred V. Kidder, historical research and archaeology, Cambridge, Massachusetts.

On one day of each annual meeting we directors were asked to join the trustees at lunch, where we heard the casual conversation of Herbert Hoover, General Omar Bradley, Charles Lindbergh, and the rest of that ultradistinguished board of statesmen, bankers, lawyers, and men of affairs. Each department set up an exhibit of its current work, attended after the formal dinner by everybody attached in any way to the institution. One year, on the morning before the exhibit, I had occasion to make a final rearrangement of my department's show. I was surprised to find that someone had already entered the silent exhibition hall. It was Colonel Lindbergh, intently studying a large map of the world's magnetic fields set up by the department of terrestrial magnetism. Twenty years after his famous flight across the Atlantic, Lindbergh seemed to be looking for more seas to conquer.

My everyday directorial transactions with the institution's administration were carried on largely with the executive officer —with Walter M. Gilbert from 1940 to 1947 and thereafter with Paul Scherer, both of them efficient, calm, and friendly men. Dr.

Bush found time for me whenever I needed top-level or special support for my department. A Yankee to the core, he was tersely outspoken, sometimes fiery, sometimes humorous, often mildly profane, always shrewd. He had the quickest mind I ever knew. Almost before I could finish telling about my problem, whether administrative or scientific, he would see what I was driving at and would come back at me with a basic question or a solution. He readily understood the work of our department and even during the war years knew pretty well what we were doing. At first I was bothered by his self-assurance and abrupt decisiveness, but in the sixteen years I worked under his presidency I developed affection and sympathy for him, for I detected, I thought, a paradoxical weakness in his temperament.

By the end of the war Bush was a leading figure in national and international scientific affairs, at the head of the U.S. Office of Scientific Research and Development, which, I suppose, was the largest enterprise of applied science ever directed by one man. His intellect and driving force were adequate for that enormous task. The flaw I saw in him, arising, I suppose, from some hidden insecurity, was an urgent need that people should recognize and defer to his authority. He once told me with glee about an occasion when on war service a major general demanded his seat on a crowded military airplane and how with calculated drama he produced his credentials including a special order from the secretary of war, completely squelching the general.

The one time when I unknowingly wounded his sense of high position was trivial but illuminating. Our expert modeler, Osborne Heard, ran into a mechanical difficulty which he mentioned to Dr. Bush during a presidential visit to the laboratory. Dr. Bush, an expert mechanic himself, later sent over from Washington some suggestions about the difficulty and then forgot the matter. In my annual report for the *Year Book* I mentioned that Mr. Heard, with the president's help, had solved the problem. To explain Dr. Bush's reaction to this when he read it in the proofs of the *Year Book*, I must say that some of the other directors of departments prepared their annual reports from statements contributed by individual workers. While I was at P Street one day on departmental business with Paul Scherer, Bush sent for me and angrily said that Heard was impertinent and insubordinate to associate his name with that of the president of the institution. "Doctor Bush," I said, "of course I shall omit that passage, since it annoys you, but I want you to know that Heard knows nothing about it. I write every word of my reports myself. I thought I was complimenting you by implying that our president was interested in our problem and democratic enough to share his experience with our head technician." Bush, still angry, glared at me and rasped out, "Well, I'll be damned." That was the end of the incident. I could balance it by a dozen stories of Bush's generosity to members of my staff and personal kindness to me.

During these years our two children had grown to adulthood. George took his B.A. degree at Rochester. Preceding us to Baltimore in 1938, he was graduated M.D. from Johns Hopkins in 1942 and won an internship in obstetrics at Johns Hopkins Hospital. In World War II he was in the Philippines as a captain in the army medical corps. He took his casualty clearing company ashore at Leyte on the second day of General McArthur's occupation of the islands and set up a casualty clearing station in Leyte Cathedral. Rejoining the Johns Hopkins staff after the war, he was resident obstetrician in 1951. Hester Ann entered Bryn Mawr College in 1938, majored in classics, and was graduated A.B. in 1942. She stayed on for an M.A. degree and then went to Yale for postgraduate study. Since George had in 1942 married Elizabeth Jenkins, a graduate of Kansas State University and of the school of dietetics at Johns Hopkins Hospital, both our young people were by 1941 living away from home.

Early in 1948, while Hester Ann was at Yale, I had a letter from Dr. Ann Roe, psychologist, wife of the paleontologist George Gaylord Simpson, asking me to participate as a subject in a study she was making of the personality of twenty biologists whom she designated as eminent, for comparison with as many physicists and mathematicians.[2] I consented to an interview and tests and an appointment was fixed for a day in April.

A couple of days before that date Hester Ann, who had completed all requirements for the Ph.D. degree except that her dissertation was not yet finished, wrote to say that she was slightly ill and was entering the Yale infirmary. She thought that

2. Ann Roe, "A pscyhological study of eminent biologists," *Psychological Monographs* 65 (1951): 1–68.

she might have monocytosis, a debilitating sickness that had recently been prevalent in New Haven.

In my office an hour before Dr. Roe's expected arrival, the telephone rang and a man's voice said: "Dr. Corner, I am an intern in the Yale infirmary. Your daughter is a patient here. We think you ought to know that her leucocyte count is two hundred thousand." Appalled, I could only query, "Leukemia?" "Yes," said he gently. "You may want to take her home. She is strong enough to travel." I said that her mother and I would come to New Haven the next day and asked that the Yale professor of medicine Francis Blake be requested to see Hester Ann. Then I hung up and sat there in a daze, wondering how I could break the news to my wife.

Dr. Roe was announced. I took her into my little private laboratory for the interview and tests, but first I told her that I might not be a satisfactory subject that day; only an hour earlier I had received by telephone the totally unexpected news that my daughter was fatally ill. Dr. Roe kindly offered to postpone the session. "As you please," I said. "But if you feel like going on with your work I shall willingly respond." Dr. Roe chose to stay and for three hours mercifully kept me answering questions and doing the tests—a verbal-mathematical-spatial test; the Rorschach test; and the thematic apperception test ("Look at this picture and tell me what you imagine the people are doing or thinking"). Ann Roe told me later that she observed nothing in my responses that revealed a distraught mind.

I do not know how I took the tests. Even now, three decades after that dreadful day, as I write about it my hand trembles, and the tears I did not shed then come to my eyes. Some people are bowled over by a sudden shock, some do not feel the full blow at once; they reel and rally, yet the hurt reverberates a long time. I think that for me never a day has passed since then without a pang of sorrow for the loss of my daughter. As I grow older I feel more and more what I have lost. To have her with me in my old age, a mature, experienced, understanding woman—what a blessing that would have been.

I shall not dwell on the distress of the next hours and days —breaking the news to Betsy, driving in almost total silence to New Haven (what was there to say?). Hester Ann was glad to leave the infirmary. She rested in her apartment while we packed her belongings and settled with her landlady. We set out for Baltimore in our new Ford Zephyr, which Hester Ann had not seen before. She was pleased with it and when we were in open country asked if she might drive for a while. She took the wheel with her usual skill but tired in a half-hour. At home that night the Johns Hopkins specialist on leukemia, Dr. James Conley, came to our home and took blood samples, calling the next day to confirm the diagnosis of acute myelogenous leukemia. He suggested a stay in the hospital to try one of the new experimental drugs which had shown some power to stay the disease. At our daily visits we saw her rapidly fail and pass into coma as the swarming leucocytes invaded her brain. Eleven days after that telephone call, as I walked into the ward where she lay, an intern came up to me to say that in the small hours of the morning she had ceased to breathe. I think she never knew that she was mortally ill.

Betsy, in the acute phase of her grief that lasted for days and weeks, wished that our daughter's ashes should be deposited in the place where she had spent her happiest hours as a scholar, the library of Bryn Mawr College. President Katharine McBride granted the necessary permission. One afternoon in May Betsy and I drove to Bryn Mawr. In the dusk of evening when the library was closed Dr. McBride came in person to open the building and let us into the grassy inner quadrangle, then with a sympathetic word left us there. While Betsy stood weeping at the side of the quadrangle I strewed the last remains of our daughter under the shrubbery she had often looked upon when she lifted her eyes from her books. Our friends and her classmates gathered a fund in her memory and presented it to Bryn Mawr College to create a memorial prize for distinction in literature.

14

ON A WIDER STAGE

My wife's thought that the directorship of the Carnegie Institution's Department of Embryology would put us on a wider stage was correct, but in fact the stage had begun to widen before I left Rochester. In April 1940 I was elected a member of both the National Academy of Sciences and the American Philosophical Society. Like most high honors that come to scientists, these two both entailed responsibilities. I took pleasure in attending the annual meetings of the National Academy, held in its noble building on Constitution Avenue, in Washington. Its program of brief reports in all fields of science kept its members informed of front-line progress and won me the acquaintance of many of the nation's leaders in research. Soon I was being assigned to small roles in the academy's business. I was for a while chairman of the section of anatomy and zoology, a post of some influence in the academy's intricate system for choosing new members. Later I was chairman of two committees of the academy's subsidiary, the National Research Council, namely the Committee for Research in Problems of Sex and a special committee to advise the army on the care of its medical records of World War II. From 1953 to 1957 I was vice president of the academy, but since Detlev Bronk was president, my duties were nominal. The only service in that capacity that I recall, besides attending council meetings, was at a time when it was inadvisable for official Americans to hobnob with Russians. Bronk asked me to represent the academy, instead of himself, at a reception and recital at the Russian embassy. Betsy and I went, shook hands with the ambassador, heard Rostropovich play a sonata, and partook of a sumptuous collation. Being less prominent than the Bronks, we escaped the notice of the newspapers and the Un-American Affairs Committee. The academy, founded in 1863, with President Lincoln's approval, to provide the government with scientific advice, became so heavily involved in such service during World War II that it acquired some of the aspects of big business, for which I was not adapted.

I felt much more at home in the American Philosophical Society in Philadelphia. Benjamin Franklin's aim in founding it, "to promote useful knowledge," has in the course of more than two centuries broadened to include all fields of learning, literary, social, and historical as well as scientific: its semiannual meetings bring together scientists and humanists to discuss each other's ideas and findings. Members bring their wives (or husbands) to join its social gatherings. The walls of its eighteenth-century building, Philosophical Hall, on Independence Square, are hung with protraits of the greatest of our predecessors, from Franklin and Jefferson to twentieth-century scholars and scientists. The Society's library, a modern building, reproduces in its facade the original home of the Library Company of Philadelphia. It holds on its shelves the whole array of eighteenth- and early nineteenth-century American science and vast manuscript material on twentieth-century physics and genetics. The Society devotes almost one-third of its income from endowment to modest grants for research in all fields of learning which have aided hundreds of scientists and scholars, often at critical stages of their careers.

I am proud of my membership in this venerable institution. Under nine different presidents of the Society I have been in turn a member of the council, a vice president (1953–57), executive officer (1960–77), and editor of the Society's publications.

While still at Rochester I had begun to be wanted at distant places as a visiting lecturer, especially on medical history. In chapter 12 I told of the Vicary Lecture in London. I gave several performances of my lecture on medicine in the poems of Chaucer that I had prepared at Carmel, California, in 1916 and kept in my files ready to be trotted out now and then. With a portable lantern and my wife as projectionist I gave it once to an audience of three at the bedside of my ailing mother, who wanted to see and hear what her firstborn son was like on the lecture platform.

I met my most charming audience at Keuka College, a small but elite institution for women on Cayuga Lake in western New York. At Vassar, then another college for women only, with less social formality I talked to a physiology class about the female reproductive cycle. I spent the night there, was put up in the college's principal guest room, slept in Matthew Vassar's four-poster bed, and breakfasted in the refectory, the only man among hundreds of women. As late as the 1930s after a hundred years of Anglo-Saxon reticence between ladies and gentlemen on the subject of sex and reproduction, it was still a delicate matter for a man to discuss such a topic before a female audience. Having been born in the Victorian era, I grew up under the conventional restrictions. As a first-year medical student in 1909 I was surprised when associate professor Florence Sabin, talking with me at the microscope, frankly mentioned the female genitals by name. I learned later from her and from my own women students that the taboo could be broken by straightforward serious discussion, no apologies, no embarrassing hesitation, above all no jokes.

As a lecturer I was never an easy impromptu speaker. I found quite early, when as a medical student I gave talks about the Grenfell Mission, that I could not memorize a lecture. I was sure to omit some significant passage. Therefore I developed the habit of speaking from copious notes and on important occasions reading from a complete draft. I tried to read clearly and with proper cadence and emphasis. Only when called upon, as I was three or four times, to present a candidate for an honorary degree, did I memorize my brief speech. On those occasions in the sumptuous Eastman Theater, with two thousand people before me and the president and trustees on the stage behind me, I was trembling with stage fright.

But let us return to my years in Baltimore, 1940–55, when my career as traveling lecturer took on greater momentum. My first important appearance abroad while director of the Carnegie embryological laboratory was at São Paulo, Brazil, in March 1944. With my wife I had been to Montevideo as an official U.S. delegate to an international congress of endocrinology. For the fifteen-minute paper I read in Spanish my friend Inés de Allende carefully coached me to say in that language, "next slide, please," "the picture is upside down," and similar directions to the projectionist. A few days later we crossed the Rio Plata to Buenos Aires. The great Argentine physiologist Bernardo Houssay arranged an afternoon of scientific talks by the North American delegation to the Montevideo congress. The session was held in a large auditorium of the University of Buenos Aires. While I was reading my paper, anxiously striving for correct pronunciation, a newspaper photographer tiptoed behind me with an old-fashioned flashpan of magnesium powder and set it off without warning. There was a loud puff and a blazing light startling me almost out of my wits. The audience roared with laughter. I ventured a humorous remark. I meant to say, "I'm scared of those bombers" (this was in wartime), "Tengo miedo de aquellos bombarderos," but instead of "bombarderos" I said "bomberos" (firemen). There was another laugh at my mistake, but one of our U.S. party who knew no Spanish saw only that I had been startled and had responded with what seemed to him a witty remark, since the audience had laughed and applauded.

We had traveled to Uruguay by sea with agreeable shipmates, Frederick Koch of the University of Chicago and his wife, Oscar Riddle of Cold Spring Harbor, and Hans Selye of Montreal. We returned the same way. Aboard the ship were some of the Brazilian delegates to the congress, including the professor of internal medicine at São Paulo. On deck the first day out he told me that the medical society of São Paulo would be meeting while our ship was docked for a couple of days at the port of Santos. Would I address the doctors for a half-hour? I replied that I knew no Portuguese. "That's all right," said he, "We all understand Spanish." "But I cannot do that without notes," I added. "Write it out in English," said he, "and the young men who are traveling with me will translate it into Spanish." So I scribbled away in my deck chair and next day the two young physicians picked up the draft. One of them understood English but did not write Spanish well. The other knew Spanish but no English. The translation proceeded by steps, English to Portuguese, Portuguese to Spanish. The morning after we arrived in São Paulo by the alarming road up the mountian, a messenger brought to our hotel a neatly typed Spanish version of my talk. I read it to a hundred Portuguese-speaking doctors that evening.

I had purposely inserted a little joke in the speech. They smiled at it; my Spanish was being understood.

I have been called on three times to deliver commencement addresses at medical schools. The first of these was at Rochester in 1944, when a wartime class was graduated in the fall. I was touched by the call from the school that I had left so reluctantly four years before. Reflecting that wartime medical graduates and their parents, relatives, and friends who would form my audience in the Henry Strong Auditorium would appreciate an expression of encouragement and hope, I took my theme from St. Paul's message to Timothy, "God hath not given us the spirit of fear, but of power, and of love, and of a strong mind," and applied it to the physician's social responsibilities in war and peace. The University of Rochester printed *The Gifts of the Good Physician* privately and sent copies to all its medical alumni serving in the armed forces.

At two other medical commencements in the 1940s—at the Woman's Medical College of Philadelphia (now the Medical College of Pennsylvania) and at the University of Tennessee in Memphis—I spoke on the physician's need to recognize the individual mental and emotional problems of each patient as well as the physical ailment. Similar in style, though not a commencement address, was my talk at a weekly "collection" (a Quaker term for a college assembly) at Swarthmore College in February 1954. Borrowing my title from Sir Thomas Browne, "A Glimpse of Incomprehensibles," I ventured to display my brand of scientific humanism (or, if you will, materialism) by pointing out the extreme complexity of the human brain. Our mental processes, I said, are dependent on physical structure and chemical reactions, but the mechanism is so intricate that its products of thought and feeling can reach the heights of intellect, imagination, and spirituality. This essay must be my best, if judged by its popularity among scholarly people. It was first printed in the *American Scholar* (the journal of the Phi Beta Kappa Society), then reprinted in pamphlet form by the Carnegie Institution, by the Smithsonian Institution in its annual report, and by Hunter College in New York, where I gave a repeat performance at an honors convocation. To my further gratification it was included in a college textbook, *Expression and Persuasion.*

I was twice appointed to lectureships at Ivy League universities. The invitation to give the Vanuxem Lectures at Princeton in 1942 conveyed the committee's wish that I should discuss the hormones of the reproductive system for the benefit of a general audience, assuming on the part of my hearers no familiarity with biology. This was, so far as I know, the first time that an American university devoted one of the great endowed lectureships to the subject of human reproduction. I am not sure how well I succeeded in making my complex subject comprehensible to people with no knowledge of biology. The resultant book, *The Hormones in Human Reproduction,* was widely recommended to graduate students for collateral reading and was translated into five foreign languages—Swedish, French, Italian, Spanish, and Portuguese. It went through two editions in English. Twenty years after its first appearance it was republished in paperback form and, I believe, is still in print.

The founder of the Terry Lectures at Yale specified that the successive lecturers should "aim to build the truths of philosophy and science into the structure of a broadened and purified religion," but the speakers were held to no dogma and were given complete freedom of speech. In my lectures, which appeared in book form under the title *Ourselves Unborn: An Embryologist's Essay on Man,* I set forth what embryology has to tell us about our evolutionary relations to other animals (the one very early chimpanzee embryo so far seen cannot be distinguished from a human embryo of the same age), about prenatal fate and foreordination and the generality and particularity of human structure. My central theme is summarized in the concluding words of the book—"We bear through all our days the marks of intimate kinship with the animal world, tempered by powers of the mind that bestow dignity and honor upon the life of the body." The volume containing these three lectures was more widely reviewed than any other of my fourteen books. I listed thirty-eight generally favorable reviews from the London *Times* and the *New Yorker* to the *Nebraska Journal of Religion.*

Attractive invitations to lecture kept coming every two or three years. In the autumn of 1946 the Commonwealth Fund offered me a month's visiting lectureship at the University of Louisville School of Medicine. The supporting invitation from the university with true Kentuckian hospitality included "all the

Bourbon whiskey you can drink and free tickets to the races at Keeneland track," two privileges of which Betsy and I availed ourselves with moderation.

A few years later I made the most extensive lecture tour of my career. In the 1950s the scientific honor society Sigma Xi offered every year a visiting scientist to lecture at colleges and universities in each of the four quarters of the nation. I was asked to take the southeastern states. Betsy and I were delighted by the opportunity to see something of the deep South. Twenty-one institutions asked to have me come. I chose as my topic the menstrual cycle of the rhesus monkey. Sigma Xi headquarters in New York City made all the arrangements and sent me off for a month with a carefully planned schedule, marked maps, and a membership in the Automobile Club in case of trouble on the road. We drove from Baltimore to the Mississippi Valley, as far south as Baton Rouge and New Orleans, then back through Alabama, northern Georgia, the Carolinas, and Virginia, with a luxurious stay for Thanksgiving at White Sulphur Springs. At each stop there was a warm welcome, comfortable lodging, a standard faculty club dinner, usually with fried chicken and ice cream, and a friendly audience of students and faculty. I had feared that to give the same lecture twenty-one times would be dreadfully monotonous, but there was something different about each stop and each audience that stimulated me to renew my effort. I could understand how actors can bear to repeat the same performance time after time.

For both of us the high spot of the tour was at the University of Georgia at Athens, where my medical classmate Linton Gerdine was the leading pediatrician. After the lecture he came in his Cadillac to take us to the pre-Civil War home he had inherited, where he, a bachelor, lived with a sister. To meet us Linton had invited four or five gentlemen of Athens—the retired president of the university, a professor, Linton's pastor, and a prominent lawyer. The house was furnished in colonial mahogany, the conversation was cultivated, the gentlemen deferent to the two ladies in courtly Southern style. My New England wife, who even yet had not quite gotten over her feeling that Massachusetts is the only seat of American culture, was deeply impressed with this glimpse of the best of the Old South.

Passing over various other appearances on academic platforms between 1940 and 1955, I shall mention only two more that had special connotations for me. In May 1950, I was honored by an invitation to deliver the fourth annual Addison Lecture at Guy's Hospital, London, where Thomas Addison (1793–1860) had made his reputation as a medical scientist by describing "Addison's disease," resulting from degeneration of the adrenal cortex, and as a teacher earned fame by his lectures. The founders of this modern lectureship, Dr. Harry Spon and Dr. Peter Bishop, challenged the annual speakers not only to convey information on the topics of their choice but also to trace the development of the ideas of modern endocrinology, and above all to give a picture of the medical investigator in action, with all the fascination of his problem and his hopes of useful discovery. That was just what I had always tried to do for my own students, and I am still at it in this book. At Guy's I talked about the development of our knowledge of the menstrual cycle, 1910–50, combining the story of my own research with that of other investigators, most of whom were personal acquaintances of mine and some of them treasured friends. Two of these, Alan Parkes and Solly Zuckerman, were there to hear me, as were Dr. Spon and Dr. Bishop, both pioneers in the clinical application of the ovarian hormones. The lecture was printed in *Lancet* in April 1951.

In May 1952, I was the twenty-first Huxley Lecturer at Charing Cross Hospital, where Thomas Henry Huxley took his degree of doctor of medicine in 1845. My lecture was "The Events of the Primate Ovarian Cycle." Recalling Huxley's brilliant book *Zoological Evidences as to Man's Place in Nature*, I tried to show that studies such as mine on primate reproduction supported what I took to be Huxley's message. I summarized my own personal mechanistic view of mankind in my concluding words: "Possessing a generalized body with a highly specialized brain, our species has grown into a realm beyond the merely animal, in which we not only undergo the cycles and fluctuations of animal life but also seek to understand and direct them, a realm where sex and reproduction are at their best bound up with reason, a sense of beauty, and human affection." The *British Medical Journal* published this discourse in August 1952.

During my years at the Carnegie embryological laboratory

my pen was constantly at work. I am almost shocked when I contemplate the number of my published writings. Besides the lectures I have listed and several others not mentioned, between 1940 and 1955 I published about thirty-five book reviews, four obituary articles, fifteen annual reports of my department for the Carnegie Institution's yearbooks and enough scientific and historical articles to make a total of ninety-seven items in my bibliography. None of these papers was lightly tossed off. They were all written with care for critical readers.

To a book composed in the earlier years of my Carnegie directorship I gave much time and thought. About the time when I was elected to membership in the American Philosophical Society, its library acquired at auction the manuscript of the autobiography and commonplace books of Dr. Benjamin Rush (1745–1813), the celebrated Philadelphia physician and signer of the Declaration of Independence. The librarian, Dr. William E. Lingelbach, knowing of my interest in the history of my profession, asked me to edit these valuable documents for publication. For this fascinating task I had the enthusiastic support of my family. My daughter transcribed a large part of the material and did much preliminary historical and biographical investigation. My wife, who had the talents and some of the training of a reference librarian, joined me in running down in the libraries of Baltimore, Philadelphia, New York, and Washington the hundreds of men and women mentioned by Rush. Members of the American Philosophical Society, especially Gilbert Chinard, learned and witty professor of French literature at Princeton, took an interest in my work and advised me helpfully.

When I had the task well under way, Dr. Lingelbach heard from a young historian then teaching at Franklin and Marshall College, Lyman H. Butterfield, who was ambitious to edit Rush's voluminous correspondence with important people of the Revolutionary and Federal periods and asked for the Society's encouragement. Dr. Lingelbach wanted to know whether this would interfere with my undertaking. I met Butterfield, liked him at once, and decided that he and I could help, not hinder, each other. He brought out the letters, superbly edited, and went on to a long career as editor of the papers of the Adams family of Boston. We did help each other and became firm friends. I shudder a little to think that I could have vetoed his project, though of course with his dedication and talents he would have won distinction in some other great historical task.

My *Autobiography of Benjamin Rush* was published for the American Philosophical Society by Princeton University Press in 1948. After it appeared, a Baltimore physician and well-known antiquarian, Dr. J. Hall Pleasants, called at our house one evening to show me a little manuscript book that he had found in a local attic when helping some members of the Shippen family dispose of the possessions of a deceased brother. Dr. Pleasants recognized that the book was a diary of Dr. William Shippen, Jr. (1736–1808), of Philadelphia, first professor of anatomy and midwifery in the University of Pennsylvania, written in 1759–60 when Shippen was studying medicine in London. It contained a lively, well-written account of the young man's studies and diversions. Dr. Pleasants suggested that I should edit it for publication, but I was busy with other matters. I proposed that Betsy should undertake it. The result was a charming little volume published in 1951 by the American Philosophical Society (of which Shippen was a member), *William Shippen, Jr., Pioneer in American Medical Education.* As with my book on Rush, our family helped produce it. Our son, at that time on the resident obstetrical staff of the Johns Hopkins Hospital, commented on that side of Shippen's work, and I translated from Latin his Edinburgh doctoral thesis.

Betsy became greatly interested in what young Shippen had to say about Dr. John Fothergill, a prominent Quaker physician in London who had befriended three American medical students, Shippen, John Morgan, and Benjamin Rush, who became founders of the University of Pennsylvania's medical school (the first in the American colonies). Dr. Fothergill played by correspondence a great role in colonial Quaker affairs and in encouraging medical education that was very little known to general historians. He cooperated, for instance, with Franklin in a last-minute effort to avert the American Revolution by appeals to Lord North and Lord Dartmouth of the king's cabinet (both of whom were Dr. Fothergill's patients). Reading some of Fothergill's correspondence at the Historical Society of Pennsylvania, Betsy found a treasure-trove of colonial history that ought to be made known to scholars.

One of the sharpest husband-and-wife disagreements Betsy and I ever had broke out when she told me that she wanted to collect and edit Dr. Fothergill's correspondence. I opposed the plan because I thought her temperamentally unsuited to a long, tedious effort of transcription and annotation. She had already published some delightful, sprightly short articles about Fothergill and his medical friends.[1] I told her that she ought to continue writing brief essays; in a few years she would have the makings of a fine collected volume. But no; if I could write books she could, too, and would, all by herself. She continued stubbornly collecting materials for the big job she had set her heart upon.

In the early 1950s we visited England almost every summer because of my committee work on anatomical nomenclature, which I shall mention in the next chapter. Betsy talked about Fothergill with Dorothea Singer, who was as much devoted to medical history as her husband. The upshot was that the historical section of the Royal Society of Medicine asked the two ladies to present a joint paper about Fothergill at one of its meetings held in May 1953 ("Dr. Fothergill, Peacemaker" was subsequently published in volume 98 of *Proceedings of the American Philosophical Society*, pp. 11–22). Dorothea furnished some facts for this paper. Betsy wrote all of it and read it at the meeting. Leaving the hall after the session, we were stopped by a good-looking fair-haired young Englishman who introduced himself as Christopher Booth, medical registrar (equivalent to resident physician in the United States) at Hammersmith Hospital. He said that he had attended Sedbergh School in Yorkshire, where Dr. Fothergill had been a pupil in 1724–28. He had begun to collect Fothergill's letters and would like to talk with Mrs. Corner about them at her convenience.

At our lodgings that evening Betsy asked me what she should do about this potential rival. I thought to myself that this was an answer to my worries about her project. Booth was young and could carry on if she faltered. He could gather materials and make contacts in England. His enthusiasm would keep

1. Betsy Copping Corner, "Dr. Ibis and the artists: A sidelight upon Hunter's atlas, *The Gravid Uterus," Journal of the History of Medicine and Allied Sciences* 1 (1951): 1–21; "Dr. Melchisidek Broadbrim and the playwright," *Journal of the History of Medicine and Allied Sciences* 7 (1952): 122–35.

hers from flagging. Why not, I said to her, make it a joint undertaking? We had Christopher to dinner; an alliance was formed and a warm long-lasting friendship began with both of us. One night a year or two later, as we walked along the street after dining at the Garrick Club, Christopher told me that some of his associates had warned him against putting too much time on medical history. He asked my advice. I could only tell him that my own interest in the history of our profession seemed to have done my career no harm; in fact I thought that it had helped to win me my professorial chair at Rochester. We watched his progress with high hopes and saw him reach the chair of internal medicine at the Royal Postgraduate School of Medicine, one of the most influential clinical professorships in Britain. Betsy did not live to know of his present post as director of the Medical Research Council's division of clinical research.

In the task she had set herself, Betsy did not falter. I had underrated her persistence. With Christopher's constant friendly help, she finished her draft of the introduction and notes on the letters just as the infirmity of age overtook her.

15

AT THE CONFERENCE TABLE

Of the making of books there is for me no end, and the same may be said of service on committees. In the last year of my Carnegie directorship I was a member of nineteen committees, boards, societies, and academies that required my attention to executive affairs, fifteen of them holding meetings once to five times a year outside Baltimore. Such work never bored me. I enjoyed travel to other cities and the fellowship of eminent people. I am not sure how much I contributed to the various institutions and enterprises that I served, of which I will mention only a few here. It seems to me that I was an observer and encourager and sometimes a helper rather than a leader.

My place on the Board of Scientific Directors of the Yale (later the Yerkes) Laboratories of Primate Biology came as a natural outgrowth of my acquaintance with Robert M. Yerkes, which began through correspondence in 1919 when he was planning to set up a chimpanzee colony at Orange Park, near Jacksonville, Florida, and I was exploring ways and means to study the reproductive cycle of the rhesus monkey. Dr. Yerkes offered me a place on his staff when he could organize it, but I did not have occasion to accept the offer. In 1939 he asked me to visit his colony to discuss the design of an operating room that he was planning to fit up. In 1942 he appointed me to the board of the laboratories, then attached to Yale University. The other members of the board under Yerkes's chairmanship were Derek Denny-Brown (physician, neurologist) and Frederick L. Hisaw (zoologist), both of Harvard; Francis Blake of

Yale (physician); William H. Taliaferro (pathologist) of the University of Chicago; Leonard Carmichael (psychologist) of Tufts University; and later Karl M. Lashley (psychologist) of Harvard.

We met annually, usually in March, at Orange Park. After touring the grounds, we assembled in the library to hear reports by staff members on their current researches and to deal with the operative business of the laboratories. In the warm evenings of the Florida springtime we sat sociably outdoors beside a tall stand of bamboo, enjoying the fragrance of the flowering shrubs that Mrs. Yerkes had planted about the buildings, talking over scientific matters or listening to William Taliaferro's gossip about university people or to Fred Hisaw's stories of his boyhood in the Ozarks, told with the accents of the Missouri hill country that years at Wisconsin and Harvard had not worn off.

When Dr. Yerkes retired from the directorship in 1947 he was succeeded by Karl Lashley; tall, lean, long-haired and high-browed, he looked like a nineteenth-century poet or musician (he played the cello in Jacksonville's semiprofessional symphony orchestra). His acute intellect assured the laboratories of continuing research leadership. Rather surprisingly, he was also a good administrator. Soon after his retirement in 1955, Yale relinquished the station to Emory University at Atlanta, Georgia, where the founder's name is perpetuated in the title "Yerkes Laboratories of Primate Biology." I was unhappy about the move and resigned from the board, an act which as far as I can see did not impair the institution's progress under Emory's auspices.

During the 1940s the work of the National Research Council's Committee for Research in the Problems of Sex continued actively. The majority of the committee felt that Alfred Kinsey's work was closer than that of any other grantee to the original aim of its founders, to study human sex behavior scientifically. The amount of money granted by the committee to Kinsey was quintupled in each of the two years following the original exploratory grant. For the year 1946–47 he received $35,000 annually, which was one-half of the committee's total budget.

The appearance in 1948 of the first major report from Kinsey's group, *Sexual Behavior in the Human Male,* published by the W. B. Saunders Company of Philadelphia, caused a nationwide stir. It elicited surprised but generally favorable comment but also brought a good deal of unfavorable criticism. This in large measure reflected the conventional reticence of the time about sexual matters, but there were scientific critics as well. Adolf Meyer of our committee, for instance, one of the nation's most experienced psychiatrists, had long taught the importance of dealing with the patient as an individual. He exhorted his students to question what he considered the overclassification of mental disease—labeling one patient as schizophrenic, the next manic depressive, and so forth—admirable advice, no doubt, for the practitioner of medicine. Kinsey's statistical tabulations of human conduct seemed to Dr. Meyer coldly impersonal. He never quite grasped, I thought, the fact that Kinsey was reporting the ways of a whole people, not the maladjusted few. Some thoughtful critics felt that Kinsey's informants included many people who did not share the usual reticence about personal conduct. His figures, they said, must be overweighted by the responses of oversexed people.

In line with these criticisms, a number of professional statisticians said that Kinsey's informants did not include a reliable sample of the population. Kinsey had done all he could to meet this difficulty by obtaining, as far as possible, information from groups, with a response from every member of the group. He would explain his study at a meeting, then interview separately each person present—all members, for instance, of a college fraternity chapter or all the inmates of a women's prison. This did not satisfy the critics, who demanded a sample selected by a completely random method, such as sticking a pin in a telephone directory and questioning everyone whose name was perforated—a totally impracticable method of getting information of an intimate kind. With astonishment I heard one prominent professor of statistics say that he would consider the testimony of three people chosen strictly at random more reliable than that of twenty-five chosen by Kinsey's method.

By this time I was chairman of the Committee for Research in Problems of Sex, Dr. Yerkes having retired in 1947. We now had on the committee Lowell J. Reed, a distinguished statistician, director of the Johns Hopkins University School of Hygiene and Public Health. Reed had himself been interviewed by Kinsey and approved both the interviewing procedure and the method of selecting interviewees, which he thought was as sound as could be achieved in practice.

I called a conference at Kinsey's institute in Bloomington, Indiana, including the members of our committee, Kinsey and his senior staff, and six statisticians, three who, we knew, were sympathetic to Kinsey's work and three unfavorable. We had a two-day battle across the conference table. Kinsey kept his temper admirably. At the end we all shook hands, but without an expression of agreement. In Kinsey's second book, on the sex behavior of women, he took care to explain and justify his statistical methods more acceptably than in the first book. This was almost thirty years ago. Since then other people, favored by lessening resistance to such work, have published studies of the same kind. Their findings in general agree with what Kinsey showed us about the wide range of human sex behavior.

It must be remembered that the Rockefeller Foundation was helping to pay for Kinsey's work through the National Research Council. Dr. Alan Gregg, head of the foundation's division of medical research, had enthusiastically approved our committee's growing encouragement of the Kinsey group. The trustees of the foundation included, as I learned via the grapevine, a few members who disapproved of Kinsey, but as long as the National Research Council and our committee stood between them and the public, the majority of the board voted the annual appropriations. When, however, in the early 1950s the Rockefeller Foundation became the object of suspicion by rabid anti-Communists of the McCarthy type, and a general investigation of its affairs by a congressional committee was threatened, the trustees and Dean Rusk, the president, feared that its indirect support of Kinsey's work might also attract unfavorable attention.

The atmosphere of the time was so full of suspicion and fear that instead of asking me directly to go to New York to talk to him, Rusk sent an emissary who with an air of profound concern divulged to me that Mr. Rusk would appreciate a letter from me asking for an appointment to see him. I obliged. This brought a cautiously worded invitation to the foundation's office for discussion of unspecified matters. At Mr. Rusk's office I found that he had called in one of his chief legal advisers. I was quizzed at length about our committee's business. When my replies had (as

I took it) established that I would show reliability and common sense if I were called upon to testify in Washington, the lawyer coached me thoroughly as to how I should reply to the congressional interrogation. Mr. Rusk, I felt, was deeply worried. I was almost disappointed when months passed by and I was never called to testify that the Committee for Research in Problems of Sex was by no means an un-American activity. The alarm unfortunately strengthened the hands of those trustees of the Rockefeller Foundation who opposed supporting Kinsey on the grounds of impropriety of his research. We were informed that the foundation's grant to the National Research Council would be continued with a provision that our committee would no longer grant funds to Kinsey's group. I was so upset about this that I proposed that we should dissolve our committee, but cooler heads among us pointed out that this would cut off support of the other noncontroversial grantees. As for Kinsey, the royalties from his two books were so large that he could get along without our committee's grants.

During my chairmanship some of the older members dropped out. Several new people, mostly of my choosing, took their places—my former co-worker Willard M. Allen of Washington University, St. Louis; Wallace O. Fenn and John Romano of the University of Rochester; James V. Neel of the University of Michigan; and Howard Taylor of Columbia University. Frank A. Beach, then of Yale, since of the University of California at Berkeley, succeeded me as chairman and kept the work going for several years. Research on the physiology and even the psychology of sex had become so well established in the universities that special support by the National Research Council was no longer imperatively needed. The Committee for Research in Problems of Sex was finally discontinued, after almost forty years of extremely useful service.

In chapter 12 I mentioned my membership, while at Rochester, on a committee of the American Association of Anatomists that was set up to revise the terminology of gross human anatomy. The names of the parts of the body in European languages had become very diverse. Our committee, as I have mentioned, put a good deal of time on the drafting of its own list of terms, which we hoped could be discussed at an international congress of anatomists, which finally met in Oxford in 1950, having been delayed by the war. Its president, Sir Wilfrid Le Gros Clark, set up a thirty-six-member international committee on nomenclature and a smaller working committee to which he named professors Pedro Ara (Buenos Aires), A. Beau (Nancy), Nello Beccari (Florence), G. W. Corner (Baltimore), Bo Ingelmark (Gothenburg), Thomas B. Johnston (London), and M. Woerdeman (Amsterdam). Teizo Ogawa of Tokyo joined us later. An invitation through diplomatic channels to the Russian Academy of Sciences to send a delegate was not even acknowledged. UNESCO made a grant for the committee's expenses. The CIBA Foundation of London (an agency of the great Basel drug firm) provided a comfortable meeting room and living quarters at its guest house in Portland Place. We met there for three or four days at a time in 1953, 1954, and 1955. At the first session I was unanimously elected chairman, and T. B. Johnston secretary.

I shall not go into the technical details of our task. The principal difficulty was that of agreeing on terms for the relative position of parts of the body—superior, inferior, medial, lateral, anterior, posterior—that would apply to four-footed and limbless animals as well as to the erect, two-legged human body, so that comparative anatomists and veterinarians could use the same names. Harmony prevailed; each of us knew enough Latin for the task, and we were all enthusiastically interested in reaching agreement. Our sessions were agreeable and successful.

At a meeting of the whole thirty-six-member International Committee on Anatomical Nomenclature held in Paris in July 1955, on the eve of the Sixth International Anatomical Congress, the list submitted by our working committee was unanimously approved, even by a Russian delegation that unexpectedly arrived, and it was then accepted by the congress. We agreed for diplomatic reasons to name the new list of more than 5,000 terms the *Paris nomina anatomica*, even though it had been worked out in London. Since that congress the anatomists of the world have possessed a workable Latin nomenclature to which they can relate the equivalent terms in their own languages, using the Latin for added clarity when they write for international use.

My trips to England on this project gave my wife and me many opportunities for travel. What with these trips, the Fifth Anatomical Congress at Oxford, in 1950, a year at Oxford as

Eastman Professor, to be described in the next chapter, and my installation as a foreign member of the Royal Society of London in 1955, Betsy and I, both fond of travel, managed to see a great deal of Britain and something of the Continent. I have driven a car in every county of England, half of the Scottish counties, and half of the Welsh. I have made twenty visits to England, fifteen of them with Betsy.

At the Fifth Anatomical Congress, Oxford University honored me and three other members with the degree of doctor of science, the others being Lord Addison, British statesman, who had been a professor of anatomy, L. S. B. Leakey, the famous paleontologist of Olduvai Gorge, and M. V. Woerdeman, professor of anatomy at Amsterdam. We were robed in the magnificent fifteenth-century divinity school and were led by a black-gowned beadle to the nearby Sheldonian Theatre, together with the vice chancellor and the public orator. To the audience of congress members the public orator read one by one in Latin his citations of our scientific merits, and the vice chancellor in the same tongue declared us to be honorary doctors of the university.

After the end of World War II the United States Army had on its hands an enormous mass of records of medical examinations of draftees, five million men and women. The surgeon general asked the National Academy of Sciences what to do with the records, in view of their possible value for research. They included, for example, millions of chest x-rays. President Bronk of the academy asked me to be chairman of a committee to look into the problem. We met four or five times in Washington. The army had no further use for the records, but it seemed a pity to discard these records of so large a sample of young Americans, possibly useful to scientists. The statistician pointed out that nobody could deal usefully with five million medical records. Somebody suggested retaining a random selection, say every tenth or hundredth or thousandth record, but nobody wanted them badly enough to pay the cost of pulling out the sample. The problem solved itself when the Veterans' Administration declared that for its purposes all the records must be kept as long as the last draftee of World War II is alive. We reported this to the surgeon general, and the committee was dissolved.

Before 1949 I had only a slight acquaintance with Henry

Allen Moe, chief administrator of the John Simon Guggenheim Memorial Foundation with the title of secretary (later president) and the director of its great program of grants in aid of scholarship, science, and the fine arts. A Minnesotan of Norwegian ancestry, Henry Moe was one of the early Rhodes Scholars. After taking a law degree at Brasenose College, Oxford, he returned to the United States and began to practice law in New York City. By some service rendered he attracted the notice of Sen. Simon Guggenheim, who asked him to draft a plan for the foundation the senator wished to set up in memory of his son. Moe's plan was so satisfactory that Mr. Guggenheim put him in charge of the foundation, which became a lifework for the young lawyer.

In 1949 Henry asked me to join his jury for Latin-American fellowships, I suppose because he knew that I could read Spanish. After a year's apprenticeship on that committee, in which I learned his simple but thorough system for getting information about the candidates, he promoted me to the committee of selection for the United States and Canada. The chairman of that committee was Louis B. Wright, director of the Folger Library of Shakespeareana in Washington, D.C. Others with whom I served were Willard F. Libby, chemist, at the University of Chicago and later at the University of California, Berkeley; Robert K. Merton, sociologist, Columbia University; Carl Sauer, geographer, Berkeley; Samuel E. Thorne, Harvard Law School; and E. B. Wilson, mathematician, Harvard, a polymath who had stored away in his brain a larger stock of useful information on many subjects than any other man I ever knew.

In the late winter of each year we received a huge bundle of applications for fellowships accompanied by letters of recommendation. Henry Moe had read and graded them all, classing them under each field of learning by a simple pattern of listing them, so that we could know how he rated them. This system made it possible for the committee, when we met in New York in March, to work through a thousand applications in three days. Very seldom did the committee disagree with Henry's judgment. When we did, he took it kindly. One of his staff sat with us to check the applicant's budgets and fix the amount of financial aid in each case.

This was a truly shipshape operation—an adjective that

Henry would appreciate because he had been a volunteer naval officer in World War I. While on active service a falling spar struck him, broke both legs and left a chronic bone infection that in those preantibiotic days never fully healed in spite of many operations. With quiet courage he bore his burden of lifelong pain. During my sixteen years of service on his committee I developed a deep affection for this wise and kindly man.

One of the joys, for me, of this experience was the association with my learned and friendly fellow members, whose wit and wisdom bubbled up when we dined together after the long days at the conference table. After the last session each year Henry, something of a gourmet and an expert judge of wines, set up a specially selected dinner at the Century Club. He always had a choice vintage for us as with relaxed minds we rejoiced in good food, good drink, and sparkling conversation with our benign and cultivated host. A year or two after Henry retired from the presidency of the John Simon Guggenheim Memorial Foundation his successor, Gordon Ray, gently retired me and one or two other members of the committee, but my association with Henry Moe remained intimate as we worked together in the American Philosophical Society. In all those years of our friendship I often went to him for advice on personal problems, never failing to receive prompt, sensible guidance and brotherly encouragement.

In nineteenth-century Baltimore, racism was not a crime. When the wealthy merchant Samuel Ready made his will, he specified that an orphanage he was endowing should be open only to girls of white Protestant families. His friend, my grandfather, the first George Washington Corner, was president of the Ready School's board of trustees. I remember being taken at the age of seven, by my dignified, white-haired grandfather and my jolly, plump grandmother, to a graduation ceremony at the school and being greeted by the lady principal, elderly Miss Rowe, as jolly as my grandmother and even plumper. My grandfather presided over the ceremony, my grandmother awarded a prize to the girl who had baked the best loaf of bread. Even at that age I was entranced by the sight of a hundred girls, some of my own age, others tall teenagers dressed in pretty clothes that they had made themselves. Miss Rowe, discarding the uniforms traditionally worn by orphan schoolchildren, had bolts of dress goods sent to the sewing room and let the girls choose the fabrics for themselves. To be a Ready girl was a distinction in Baltimore. They went out to get good jobs in banks and offices, or as schoolteachers, or to find (those who wanted them) good husbands.

My father succeeded my grandfather as president of the Ready board. My cousin, G. Corner Fenhagen, a leading architect, designed a handsome new school building in a western suburb when in my father's presidency the old school and grounds at Broadway and North Avenue were sold to Sears, Roebuck and Company. My great-uncle John T. King, Sr., was for a time physician to the school. Such was Baltimorean respect for family connections that in 1949, my father having died, I was elected to the board and soon after became in my turn president of the school. I held the post as long as I remained in Baltimore, appreciating the opportunity to serve in my small way a respected local philanthropy as so many of my family had done and as my brother and sister were doing more broadly for other institutions.

My colleagues of the board were all men of standing in the city—the head of the Baltimore Gas and Electric Company, the president of Goucher College, a prominent lawyer, a banker, a leading realtor. They hardly needed such guidance from the chair as I could provide, but I could help the principal in some matters of policy through my medical training. In the case, for example, of an unhappy sex-ridden adolescent I think I saved the girl from open disgrace by aiding the principal to steady a shocked grandmother. By the 1950s economic and social changes among the middle-class Protestants diminished the need for residential care of orphans and half-orphans. At the same time the school's income from endowment was seriously reduced. The expenses became dangerously close to income. With reluctance I proposed to the board that we should close the dormitory and classrooms, increase the endowment by selling the building and grounds, and use the income to provide scholarships in local private schools for girls. This solution was too radical for the board. Their answer was to open the school to paying day students from the surrounding well-to-do suburbs. As president of the board, I had to sound out the school's alumnae as to the feasibility of teaching paying day pupils in the same classes with the orphan boarders. I called a meeting of the alumnae and received a resounding judgment that the plan would work, and so it did. To help avoid invidious distinction between the two groups of pupils the alumnae advised me that all the girls should be dressed alike in an attractive uniform—an about-face from the time, a half-century before, when the school had shunned uniforms to protect the orphan girls' self-respect.

In 1978 further inflation of the currency made continued operation of a combined residential and day school impossible. The change of policy I had proposed twenty-five years earlier was instituted, with the result that Ready Scholarship girls attend local private schools. The building was sold to another, quite different philanthropic organization. I am left with the memory that three George Corners had the opportunity to help Baltimore girls start useful careers through the schooling and loving care of Miss Rowe and her successors. I suppose that if my son had remained in Baltimore, the trustees would have maintained tradition by making him a member of the board.

During the 1940s the Sunday afternoon concerts of the New York Philharmonic Orchestra were put on the air for millions of American radio listeners. At first the Columbia Broadcasting System filled out the intermissions of the concerts with talks by prominent music critics or musicologists. Toward the close of World War II, however, somebody—I suspect that it was Warren Weaver, director for the natural sciences of the Rockefeller Foundation—persuaded the financial sponsors of the orchestral broadcasts, the United States Rubber Company, that it would be a public service to devote the intermissions to the presentation of modern scientific work. Dr. Weaver, asked to organize such a program, invited me to join a formidable committee that he was assembling. Its scientist members, besides Weaver and me, were Frank B. Jewett, retired engineer, president of the National Academy of Sciences and former vice president for research of the American Telegraph and Telephone Company; Harlow Shapley, of Harvard College Observatory, one of the foremost American astronomers; and Wendell M. Stanley, biochemist, of the Rockefeller Institute for Medical Research (now Rockefeller University), Nobel Laureate in 1946. A nationally known newspaper editor and historian, Douglas S. Freeman of

Richmond, Virginia, represented the interests of the lay public.

At a preliminary meeting in Weaver's office we decided to put the scientists themselves on the air, to give the talks authority, dignity, and a personal touch. In the two years of our effort we recruited seventy-nine speakers whose names read like a roster of the nation's leading scientists: Henry Norris Russell ("Are the Planets Habitable?"); Isidor Rabi (on the nucleus of the atom); Linus Pauling (on the molecular structure of penicillin); Robert Cushman Murphy (on the penguins he had observed in Antarctica). Chariman Weaver chose me to give the concluding talk on April 13, 1947, at the end of the second and final season. Because I had learned from the preceding seventy-eight talks, my draft, "Light on the Blood Capillaries," passed the editors with practically no revision, but the speech coach had trouble getting me to speak slowly enough to make every syllable distinct.

As the moment approached, I was awed by the thought that for twelve minutes I was to be the voice of American science, heard by 13 million people. I told my unseen audience about the capillary blood vessels, those innumerable microscopic filtering tubes upon which depend all the functions of the body, even life itself. I told them how William Harvey discovered in the 1620s that the blood, flowing out through the arteries, gets back to the heart through the veins, but could only wonder how it passes through the tissues from one channel to the other. Marcello Malpighi, a few years later, with his little microscope first saw in the lung of a frog the network of capillary vessels joining the ends of the arteries to the beginning of the veins, and Anthony van Leeuwenhoek soon found capillaries in all the organs and tissues. Among the scientists now studying the capillaries, I said, there may be no such geniuses as Harvey and Leeuwenhoek, nor can we expect, in our day, such surprises as Malpighi's first sight of the capillaries. Planned experiment and accurate measurement are now the only way to discovery, but our understanding of nature becomes ever more complete through the persistent and laborious efforts of many workers. I finished my talk on time, thanks to my preceptor's signals. The series was a huge success. In 1947 Warren Weaver gathered all seventy-nine talks into a volume, *The Scientists Speak*, adding a thoughtful introduction of his own.

Toward the end of World War II Vannevar Bush, president of the Carnegie Institution, found that his immense wartime task as head of the Office of Scientific Research and Development, through which he had put the whole power of American science and engineering behind the Allied forces, was nearly finished. Wearied by exhausting work and burdened by the thought of all the destruction to which OSRD had patriotically contributed, he wanted to include among the last efforts of his vast enterprise some step toward healing the wounds of war. Under his direction engineers had developed missiles that could detect and trail those of the enemy in flight, and American physicists had augmented the powers of the magical British invention, radar. Might not the principles of such new devices be adapted to help sightless men find their way about, perhaps even to read? He asked me to undertake to head a Committee on Sensory Devices to look into the possibility of such help for veterans wholly or partially blinded. When I replied to this totally unexpected challenge that I was not an engineer but only an M.D., Bush responded with his tight-lipped, twisted Yankee grin. "Indeed you are not an engineer, and what's more, I don't think you are much of a doctor either, so you can see these problems with a fresh mind."

This was a command. Bush and I chose for my committee a group of distinguished experts: Henry A. Barton, director, American Institute of Physics; Anton J. Carlson, professor emeritus of physiology, University of Chicago; Wallace O. Fenn, professor of physiology, University of Rochester; Stacy R. Guild, Otological Research Laboratory, Johns Hopkins Hospital, Baltimore; Karl S. Lashley, psychologist, Yerkes Laboratories of Primate Biology, Orange Park, Florida.

I was promised a budget that seemed to me enormous, about as much as the cost of one combat airplane. We would of course need a well-staffed laboratory to work on our projects. It was OSRD's practice to contract with an established laboratory, academic or industrial, for such service to its committees. Bush suggested the Haskins Laboratories in New York City. This pleased me. I was acquainted with Caryl P. Haskins, a young man of keen, wide-ranging mind who was deputy director of the National Defense Research Committee, a division of OSRD under James B. Conant. Trained in both biology and physics, he had organized a nonprofit private research laboratory in New York City. His staff included several competent scientists— among them, Franklin S. Cooper, physicist, and Paul A. Zahl, a versatile all-around biologist. These men would be at our service. With them we began exploring some of the simpler projects that occurred to us.

We had gone that far when a tempest burst around my innocent head. The immense work of OSRD under Vannevar Bush's leadership had been organized in two major divisions headed by men of great ability and force. A. Newton Richards was vice president of the University of Pennsylvania and professor of pharmacology, and James B. Conant was president of Harvard University. Richards headed the biological and medical division; Conant presided over physics, chemistry, and engineering. Our little Committee on Sensory Devices was within the scope of both divisions, but Bush disregarded them. Either inadvertently or because the committee was a cherished project of his own, he made us directly responsible to himself. Newton Richards, as tense and war-weary as Bush, took offense out of all proportion to our importance. This was the only time in my sixteen years of association with Bush when I ever found him unequal to a crisis, large or small. When I went to him with Richards's bitter complaint I expected him to tell me to shut up and get on with the work. Instead he almost helplessly said, "Go see Jim Conant and ask him what to do."

I had never met Conant before. He sat at his desk with a dead-pan expression listening to my summary of the situation. He was of course as much entitled to be aggrieved as was Richards, but he showed no personal emotion. When I came to the end of my story Conant solved the difficulty with a few concise, crisp sentences. We were (as I remember after thirty-five years) to be listed as a joint committee of both divisions, reporting progress to both but subject to Bush's direct authority. By the time that I carried this Solomon-like judgment to Richards, he had cooled down enough to accept it. I can see now why Conant was so successful as postwar ambassador to West Germany.

We began our work without much idea of what we might really hope for. I conferred with Sir Ian Fraser, blind head of St. Dunstan's Hostel in London, and spent a day with Hector Chevigny, a highly intelligent blind writer in New York, to get their ideas. Our psychologist, Lashley, warned us that any attempt to imitate mechanically the human visual system, with its ability to receive and coordinate stimuli from the whole complex scene that confronts us when we look down the street or at a page of a book, would be enormously difficult.

I thought that we might well begin with something simple. Having heard that some blind people enjoy the sport of bowling on the ten-pin alley, I asked Franklin Cooper of the Haskins Laboratories to see what he could do to construct a direction finder to show a blind bowler the center line of the bowling alley. This Cooper did easily, with a source of light over the pins and a receiver on the bowler's head that gave a humming sound when he turned toward them. It was an effective toy but gave little progress toward what was most needed, namely an obstacle finder for the blind pedestrian. The Haskins Laboratories produced a device that would respond to a post or tree, a wall or another person in front of the wearer, but its practical use was limited. It did not give effective warning of curbs. Tried before the committee in the foyer of the National Academy of Sciences, it picked up an emblematic bronze plaque set in the floor as if it were a boulder in the user's way. In short, it was far less effective than a guide dog and added little to the unaided sensory powers of an experienced blind pedestrian.

For the aid of people with limited vision who can read if given sufficient magnification, Brian O'Brien of the University of Rochester designed a reading glass of previously unheard-of diameter, so large that it could take in a whole page of a book, superbly corrected for chromatic and spherical aberrations. Too expensive for general use and too large to carry about, it was highly praised by partially blind people who tried it out. Our most ingenious devices were constructed by Vladimir Zworykin of the Radio Corporation of America, one of the pioneer developers of the television tube. First, he made for us a modernized version of the Optophone, a reading device invented thirty years before that had not found practical use. A scanner not much larger than a fountain pen, held in the reader's hand and guided by a straightedge laid on the book or typed page, sent to an earphone worn by the reader three different tones as it passed over each letter. As it crossed a T, for example, the reader heard first the high tone from the crossbar at the top, then a brief mixture of all three tones as the scanning beam crossed the vertical stroke, then the high tone again. An L would give the mixed tones followed by the lowest tone. People with good discrimination of musical tones could read letter by letter with this device, after long practice, at the rate of a few words per minute.

From this attempt Zworykin went on to build a device that would pronounce the letters one by one. A rapidly revolving disk bearing the alphabet on its rim matched them to the letters of the text being scanned. When a perfect match occurred, a phonographic record was activated and pronounced the letter. However, reading letter by letter is distressingly slow and fatiguing. Experienced Braille readers can recognize several letters at a time, even short words, quite rapidly, and Braille contains many standard abbreviations. Zworykin's devices could not approach that. Furthermore the machine could match only one style of type and therefore could read only from specially prepared copy (I am told that a less limited machine is now being tested).

So our work, which came to an end when Dr. Bush disbanded OSRD soon after the war, yielded very little of practical utility. To save what little we learned and at least show future venturers into the field of sensory devices for the blind how difficult their task would be, I arranged that Paul Zahl of the Haskins Laboratories should edit a book reporting our efforts. He went much farther, assembling a volume on all phases of the problem of sensory training for the blind, by a broad group of experienced workers.[1] This, I think, was the most valuable product of the committee's work. The Veterans' Administration picked up some of our projects, but I have not heard of any noteworthy progress on obstacle finders or reading devices. When someone comes up with an instrument that will detect a step down at the curb, or warn of a boy on a bicycle coming toward a pedestrian, he will deserve a Nobel Prize.

Vannevar Bush saw to it that I received a presidential certificate of merit for service to the government through OSRD, but I felt no great sense of merit. For me personally the chief reward for my effort was the friendship of Caryl and Edna

1. Paul A. Zahl, ed., *Blindness: Modern approaches to the unseen environment* (Princeton, 1950).

Haskins, both of whom my wife liked and admired as much as I. As a trustee of the Carnegie Institution of Washington, a post to which he was elected in 1949, Dr. Haskins frequently visited the Department of Embryology, keeping himself well informed about our research and having always an encouraging word for each member of my staff. I was happy when Caryl succeeded Dr. Bush in 1956 as president of the Carnegie Institution of Washington, though my own retirement deprived me of the pleasure of serving under his presidency. His autobiography, if he will write one, should give an enlightening picture, from the inside, of Vannevar Bush and the Office of Scientific Research and Development.

While the Committee on Sensory Devices was still at work, I received a letter from Miss Helen Keller, the famous blind and deaf woman whose life story is a classic record of human achievement. She had learned of our program and wanted to know more about it. She and her companion, Miss Polly Thompson, came to my office in the Department of Embryology for an afternoon's talk. Miss Keller was then about sixty-five years old, of sturdy build and with a warm personality that overcame the barriers of her infirmity. She was unquestionably a great lady. We conversed without difficulty. The two women communicated by touch on each other's hands, Miss Thompson passing Miss Keller's words to me vocally. Occasionally Miss Keller spoke a few words in a guttural but understandable voice. Her response to my remarks as spelled out for her by Miss Thompson's fingers was so quick that she often interrupted Miss Thompson to make an apt reply before my words had been fully transmitted.

Miss Keller was especially interested in Zworykin's reading device. Of course she could not use it, being totally deaf, but she asked whether it would be possible to deliver the words somehow by touch. When I pointed out the intolerable slowness of reading letter by letter, she said that a transmission rate of twenty-five words per minute (expert Braille readers can double or triple that) would give her the satisfaction of reading typed correspondence without an intermediary. She hoped that we would keep that in mind.

During our conversation Miss Keller had shown considerable acquaintance with physical science, which of course she had acquired entirely through her companions, Anne Sullivan and

Polly Thompson. It occurred to me that she had never been able to sense directly the data of science, but our laboratory had many enlarged models of embryos which she could feel. I asked whether she would like to see a human embryo (one need not be embarrassed to speak to blind people about seeing; they use the word freely). She responded with delight. I brought to my desk a plaster model of an embryo of about twenty-five days' gestation age, about seven millimeters (¼ inch) long, enlarged to a length of thirty-five centimeters (about 15 inches). Miss Keller ran her hands rapidly over it, searching for the features she had heard about. "This is the head; these ridges in the neck must be the gill bars. Here's the arm—it's just a bud—and the beginning of a leg. It has a tail, just as they say." Then back to the head: "Where are the eyes?" I explained that the rudiments of the eyes were there, buried beneath the skin. The eyelids would not separate for some days. With something like awe, she exclaimed, "How long the little creature has to wait for light!"

Before departing, Miss Keller asked if I would permit her to see what I looked like. She passed her fingers gently over my features and told me that I had a kind face.

16

FELLOW OF BALLIOL

In the register of Balliol College, Oxford, for 1952–53, my name and title appear not far below the top of the list of the master, fellows, and students, reading simply "Corner, G. W., Fellow of Balliol." That I was also Eastman Visiting Professor in the University of Oxford was, from the Balliol standpoint, not highly relevant. As the *Blue Guide* to England declares, the university is "the inward and spiritual grace of which the colleges are the outward and visible form." From my own standpoint also, Balliol's brief designation had special significance. For a year I was to participate in the inner life of the ancient seat of learning as a member of one of its oldest and most prestigious colleges—to dine with the master and fellows at the high table, to share the companionship of the senior common room, to vote on Balliol's business in college meetings, to make Balliol my intellectual home for all three terms of that memorable year, to join the other Balliol dons, on festive occasions, in the time-honored toast "Floreat Domus." Therefore I proudly put my Balliol title at the head of this chapter.

In the spring of 1952 a letter from Frank Aydelotte, chairman of the U.S. committee on the Eastman professorship offering me the tenure of that Oxford chair for 1952–53, was a stunning surprise to my wife and me. We reacted in our respectively characteristic ways. Betsy, even more Anglophile than I, if that were possible, was entranced and wanted me to accept the appointment by return mail. Thrilled as I was, I had to think about it for a while. At the end of 1954 I would reach the age

331

of retirement from my Carnegie directorship. That would leave only one year after returning from Oxford in which to put things in order for my retirement. We had our house to consider; could we leave it empty for a year? Could I meet whatever requirements Oxford might have for me as visiting professor?

I went to Princeton to talk it over with Aydelotte. The chair offered me, I learned, had been endowed by George Eastman, the Kodak magnate. The American appointees were chosen by various Oxford University departments in turn; I had been named by the anatomy department, of which Wilfrid Le Gros Clark was head and Graham Weddell, who had been a visiting fellow with me in Rochester, was second in command. The professorship was attached to Balliol College. A residential flat was provided. I would be expected to reside in Oxford for at least two terms of the academic year, preferably all three, and to lecture six times in each of two terms. An office and research facilities would be available in the anatomy department.

I took the invitation to President Bush of the Carnegie Institution. He was pleased about it, so much so that he offered to ask the trustees to postpone my retirement for a year, giving me two years to prepare for the coming change in the department's affairs and my own. Other difficulties vanished as easily. My son and daughter-in-law would gladly move into our house for a year. Sam Reynolds would willingly serve as acting director of the Department of Embryology.

I relieved Betsy's anxiety lest I should stodgily decline the post by sending Aydelotte a grateful letter of acceptance. Forwarded to Oxford, this brought me from the university registrar a letter explaining that Mr. Eastman's deed of gift provided that the incumbent was to have all the rights and privileges of an Oxford professorship. The university required that a professor must hold a master's degree if he was to vote in convocation. The registrar had the pleasure to inform me that I had therefore been awarded the degree of master of arts by decree. His letter is the only evidence that I am an M.A.—Oxford does not issue diplomas—but I now had two Oxford advanced degrees without taking examinations or paying fees. This taught me something that I was to see over and over again in my year as Eastman Professor, namely that the English, who have so many ancient traditions and regulations, are very clever at getting around them when necessary.

Betsy and I sailed for Southampton late in September 1952, on the Cunard line's *Queen Mary.*

American visitors to Oxford who have stayed at the Randolph Hotel on Beaumont Street will remember Balliol College, just across St. Giles (Street) behind the Martyrs' Memorial, a large but not architecturally distinguished range of buildings mostly of Victorian design fronting southward on the Broad (Street). The college was founded in the year 1226. It was the college of John Wycliffe, John Evelyn, Cardinal Manning, Matthew Arnold, Algernon Swinburne, and a whole galaxy of nineteenth- and twentieth-century statesmen and soldiers including Lord Grey and Lord Curzon.

The flat provided for the Eastman Professor was several blocks from the college, on the second floor of a large house in Merton Street at the corner of Logic Lane, opposite the east end of Merton College. From its rear windows we looked down on the garden of University College. The house had been built about 1900 for a single occupant, the warden of Merton College, who had, we were told, fifteen servants. Our floor had two bedrooms, a sitting room with a fireplace, a modernized kitchen, and bathroom. The flat was high-ceilinged, roomy, and in winter very chilly. At bedtime from November to March, during that cold and stormy winter, Betsy and I used to fill up our chinaware "pigs," an English equivalent to rubber hot-water bags, place them under the bedclothes while we undressed before the sitting-room fire, then shivering in our nightclothes run to our beds as fast we could. Betsy made it a point not to complain to anyone that the flat was cold. When friends who knew the house asked whether we were comfortable in the Eastman flat, she always replied, "We are warmed by fires within."

Our comfort was also marred, at first, by a ridiculous situation at the Merton Street house. The first floor above the street, which had been the warden's ceremonial area, had a broad, heavily balustraded stairway leading to our floor. This first floor was now occupied by the university's department of Chinese language and literature, under the direction of a middle-aged professor with the un-English name of Homer Hassenpflug

Dubbs. He was, in fact, an American of Texas ancestry, born in China to missionary parents. His departmental library had overflowed his bookshelves and for some years Dubbs had been shelving the overflow on the stairsteps, permitting no one to pass up or down. The Eastman professor's family on the second floor, a nice old lady, a professor's widow, on the third, and their visitors, had to climb narrow, steep servants' stairs with no handrail, reached from Logic Lane by way of the coal bin and the dustbin (English for garbage can). Ada Notestein, when her husband was Eastman Professor, had been much annoyed by this indignity and being a determined woman had, according to gossip, carried her protest to the American ambassador in London without swaying the indomitable Dubbs. My immediate predecessor in the Eastman chair, Donald A. Stauffer, a relatively young bachelor, put up with the nuisance, but Betsy Corner was as much annoyed as Mrs. Notestein. Furthermore, one of Betsy's knees was making trouble, and we could not risk a fall on the back stairs. My appeal to Dubbs having no effect, I took the matter on medical grounds to the Regius Professor of Medicine, Dr. Arthur Gardner, who like Dubbs was a fellow of University College, and I also asked Arthur Goodhart, the American-born head of University College, to help if he could. This plan worked. Dubbs with fairly good grace called me to his office, gave me a key to the Merton Street entrance, and had a passageway cleared through the books. For use of the key Dubbs exacted a deposit of ten shillings and sixpence.

My wife was so determined not to be disagreeable in Oxford that she actually went out of her way to be nice to Dubbs. Hearing that his wife was seriously ill, she offered her sympathy, and later on, when the lady died, Betsy quite won Dubbs's heart by her condolence. I never reclaimed my deposit but gave the key to my successor, Willard Quine, and told him and Mrs. Quine to use it. I never heard what happened thereafter.

Betsy, who was gathering materials for her planned edition of Dr. John Fothergill's letters, found it difficult to work at the Bodleian Library because of the long stairway from the inner court to the reading room. The Bodley's librarian most kindly gave us a key to a lift hidden in the northeast corner of the courtyard, in which we found a typed list of old and crippled eminent Oxonians, to which Betsy's name had been added. Because of her lameness I had our car, the Ford Zephyr, out on the road every weekend and often on the long summer evenings. The car too was a source of some difficulty for me because it is hard to find garage space in the old part of the city.

This, however, concludes the list of our petty troubles. Relations with Balliol were always smooth and effective. The domestic bursar found us a retired "scout"—a manservant who looks after the students' rooms, sweeping and dusting, bringing up coal for the fireplaces, and carrying out the ashes. This admirable helper—his name escapes me; I'll call him Trotter—found butter and eggs for us in spite of the continuing postwar shortage; he enlightened me about college customs and told me when to wear my master's gown and when doctoral robes were required. He came every morning but Sunday, made a fire in the sitting room, and cooked breakfast and lunch for Betsy and me. He also had a discreet but helpful line of Oxford gossip. One day a friend brought a distinguished guest to tea, Lady Nuffield, wife of the millionaire automobile manufacturer who had been a generous benefactor to the Oxford medical school. A local woman, she had married Nuffield when he was proprietor of a small bicycle repair shop in an Oxford side street. Trotter served tea and cakes as primly and silently as any butler on the stage. When the guests had left I said, "Trotter, that was Lady Nuffield." "Yes," said he, "I recognized her. We went to school together."

I performed my statutory duty to Balliol by dining in hall at least twice a week. Betsy, aware that Oxford made few concessions to dons' wives, ate her lonely suppers with good grace, and spent the evening listening to BBC radio. We men gathered before dinner in the senior common room below the hall, put on our master's gowns, and filed up a narrow stairway to emerge on the platform of the hall. As we entered, the undergraduates, several hundred of them already seated, began a frightful din by banging the handles of their dinner knives on the oaken table tops. When the last fellow had taken his place at the high table, the banging ceased, the master (or if he was not dining in hall, the senior fellow present) said a Latin grace, and we began our dinner.

From reading English novels I had expected to hear much bright and witty talk at the high table. I had not counted on

Balliol's earnestness. If I happened to sit beside one of the science tutors (all five of them were fellows of the Royal Society) we talked science; if a literary tutor were next to me I tried to keep up with talk about books; if my neighbor was Thomas Balogh (now Lord Balogh), our political scientist, I was in for a quiz on American political or economic affairs, about which he knew more than I. I am not saying that the table talk was dull, but only that it was serious. I enjoyed occasional chats with men like Richard (now Sir Richard) Southern, a learned student of medieval church art and history (now president of St. John's College), or with Alexander Ogston, an able chemist, later president of Trinity College, who could mix humor with his science. When some friend at Magdalen College or Oriel invited me to dinner at high table I found the conversations more lively.

After dinner we returned to the senior common room for coffee. As the junior fellow by date of appointment, although at sixty-three I was actually one of the oldest, it was my traditional duty to serve the coffee. To the obvious discomfort of the two young men who were just ahead of me in seniority of appointment, I insisted upon my duty and right to pour coffee, but after a couple of evenings I resigned the task to them.

As was expected of me, I attended the stated meetings of the master and fellows of Balliol, held in the senior common room to discuss the business of the college. This was the feature of Oxford life that differed most widely from American ways. Under the chairmanship of the master, the fellows dealt with petty business as well as major questions of policy. We voted, for example, on a motion of the bursar to pay for a new roof on Farmer Jones's barn, he being the tenant of a farm belonging to the college. When the college gate needed painting, we voted on the color. The majority was for black, following an ancient custom, but Christopher Hill, a history tutor thought to hold Communist views, reminded us during the voting that the rest of us probably expected him to vote for red. Hill has since been master of the college without turning Balliol red. The college owns a number of Church of England livings, i.e., rights to appoint rectors of parishes. Had one of these posts fallen vacant while I was Eastman Professor I, a foreigner of no church affiliation, would have been legally entitled to vote on the choice of a rector.

We wore our master's gowns at dinner, as I have said, and when lecturing. In fact the gown was so much a symbol of rank and privilege that one carried it about town draped over his arm. It gave free entry to the precincts of any college and assured friendly service from college servants and tradespeople. One Sunday afternoon when Betsy and I went to evensong at Magdalen College, I carrying my gown, the beadle ushered me to a choir stall and took Betsy to a seat among the congregation. At Balliol one of the Sunday afternoon services was devoted to a memorial session for the well-loved professor of surgery, Sir Hugh Cairnes, who had died during the previous term. Our man Trotter advised me that for this special service I should wear a white linen surplice under my master's gown, so I bought one and wore it, feeling like a medieval clerk in holy orders. Betsy laughed at me so much that I never wore it again. Theoretically, I should have worn white neckbands with my gown when attending a university convocation, but that relic of the day when every Oxford don was a clergyman had lapsed to some degree. On important secular occasions I wore my scarlet and gray Sc.D. robe, as also at parties whenever the invitation bore the words "Mr. Vice-Chancellor will be present." I know no prettier sight than an Oxford garden party on a sunny afternoon with all the women in spring dresses and the men in scarlet robes.

The vice chancellor is the administrative head of the university, somewhat equivalent to the president of an American university, the chancellor being a peer of the realm or some other very distinguished person who presides only on great ceremonial occasions or when some matter of high policy is to be discussed. The vice chancellor when I was Eastman Professor was Sir Maurice Bowra, a well-fed bachelor, professor of Greek literature, and head of Wadham College. He was said to be the best conversationalist in Oxford. After a dinner at Oriel College given in our honor by Graham Weddell, at which Betsy was seated next to Bowra, I watched them across the table having a merry time over their glasses of Liebfraumilch. She confirmed the report as to his conversational prowess.

The department of human anatomy, which was to be my scientific base in Oxford, was housed in a rear wing of the University Museum in Parks Road. Its head, Professor Wilfrid Le Gros Clark, was a quietly friendly man sixty-one years old.

In his younger days he was for a few years in the colonial medical service in Borneo, then returned to London to be professor of anatomy successively at St. Bartholomew's Hospital, St. Thomas's Hospital, and Oxford. He had done front-line research on the anatomy of the nervous system and in physical anthropology, including profound study of the evolution of fossil man. He was one of the experts who in 1953 revealed the spurious character of the famous Piltdown skull. In 1955 he became Sir Wilfrid Le Gros Clark. Not as deeply interested in administering his department as in scientific investigation, Clark left everyday business largely to Graham Weddell, reader in anatomy, who had been with me in Rochester in 1935–1936 as a fellow of the Commonwealth Fund.

I was given a room in the laboratory close to the professor's office and equipped with a desk, a bookshelf, and a microscope. As a courtesy to my hosts and also from interest in their teaching methods, I asked for and was willingly granted the privilege of visiting the dissecting room and attending lectures. I need not add that I found the lectures excellent and the teaching thorough. Gross human anatomy was taught in England with a degree of detail that most American anatomists considered excessive.

At my first official call upon the vice chancellor I raised the question of the twelve lectures I was expected to give. I told Sir Maurice Bowra that although I was an experienced teacher of microscopic anatomy, a formal course of lectures on that subject could hardly add much to the teaching of Le Gros Clark and Weddell. My other special interests were too diverse for a systematic lecture course on any one subject. Sir Maurice relieved my worry by saying that the lecture requirement was to be interpreted liberally. I could make up my quota by talking on a miscellany of topics that interested me and the lectures need not be formally academic. I could even count toward the required dozen any talks that I might be asked to give at students' clubs. At Le Gros Clark's request I spoke to the first-year medical students on the mammalian and human reproductive cycle, the ovarian hormones, and the embryology of twins and other multiple births. I gave my often-repeated lecture on medicine in the poems of Chaucer to a small audience of teachers of literature and other humanists in the Old Ashmolean Museum. I spoke to a scientific group about the sex research of Alfred Kinsey; the discussion showed me that Oxford was then on the surface a prudish place. I narrated to another general audience the life and work of Dr. Benjamin Rush, wondering whether I could interest an Oxford audience in the trials and triumphs of an American colonial doctor, and I was relieved to note that the master of Balliol and Lady Keir, who sat in a front row, seemed to enjoy the discourse. In such ways I filled my statutory quota of lectures.

A couple of incidents associated with these talks stand out as illustrative of Oxford ways. When I first addressed the medical students I invited them to drop in at my office for a chat whenever they liked. Only a few responded; the students, a couple of years younger on the average than first-year American medical students, were timid about taking a professor's time. However, after my lecture on the reproductive cycle two women students appeared at my door with a question. I had mentioned the cyclic changes in the lining of the vagina, so distinct in the guinea pig and rat, which Charles Stockard and Herbert Evans had applied in fundamental researches on the physiology of reproduction. These two girls said that their biology teacher in a preparatory school had told their class that the alleged vaginal changes were nonexistent. I replied that if they could join me for a few minutes every day for a week I would demonstrate the validity of the rat's vaginal cycle. Weddell lent me a couple of female white rats and the three of us made daily vaginal scrapings and examined them under the microscope. Since the rat's cycle is only five days long, in less than a week the students were satisfied that the vaginal cycle really exists. Some of the anatomy staff people who heard of this demonstration expressed a degree of surprise that I could hardly understand. It seemed that in the first place such personal attention to students by a visiting professor was unusual, and in the second place it was even more unusual that students had openly questioned a professor's statement.

The other episode revealed only my ignorance. When I lectured on medicine in Chaucer's poems, in the Old Ashmolean building, next door to the Bodleian Library, I asked the Bodley's librarian to let me have on exhibition Caxton's first printing of the *Canterbury Tales*. This brought me a stiffly courteous reply that no book ever leaves the Bodleian. Even King Charles I was denied the privilege of taking out a book.

My privilege of working in the university's department of anatomy gave me the opportunity to answer a question that had long been on my mind. With my associates at Rochester and with Arpad Csapo in Baltimore I had studied the response of uterine muscle to the ovarian hormones. To what extent is the nervous system also involved in uterine motility? Almost nothing was known about the intrinsic innervation of the uterus. Graham Weddell, who had been studying the innervation of the skin, was familiar with the methods of investigating such neurological questions. I proposed to him that we should jointly undertake a study of the intrinsic nerves of the rabbit's uterus, upon which I and my earlier colleagues had worked. Weddell improved upon my proposal by recommending that we should enlist the help of Dr. Wazir Pallie, a visiting fellow from the University of Colombo in Ceylon (now Sri Lanka) who had been working on a neurological problem under Weddell's supervision.

To this project I brought little more than the basic question; Weddell brought his knowledge of modern methods of visualizing terminal nerve fibers, and Pallie contributed superb manual dexterity as well as a considerable knowledge of neurology. We obtained our best results by infusing rabbits' uteri, by way of the blood vessels, with methylene blue, an aniline dye that colors nerve fibers blue but not the surrounding tissues. Since the injections required teamwork and the observations had to be recorded at once, the three of us did the experiments together, a brotherly international team. In consultation with my co-workers, I wrote up our findings in a paper, "Nerve Terminations in the Myometrium of the Rabbit," which appeared in the *Anatomical Record*, April 1954. Pallie returned the next year to his native land but found conditions not favorable for research and moved to Canada, where he is professor of anatomy at McMaster University. In consideration of his skilled participation, Weddell and I put Pallie's name first on our paper.

The ceremonies of the university fascinated me. I had been through its impressive ritual of awarding honorary degrees in 1950 and therefore as an Oxford doctor of science received the following notice of a convocation at the Encaenia of June 24,

1953—a ceremony similar to commencement in an American university.

> Mr. Vice Chancellor invites Heads of Houses, Doctors of Divinity, Civil Law, Medicine, Music, Letters, and Science, the Proctors, the Public Orator, and the Registrar to partake of Lord Crewe's Benefaction to the University, meeting him in the Hall of Wadham College at 11:15 A.M. on Wednesday, 24 June. Thence they will go in procession to the Sheldonian Theatre, where will be spoken the Oration in Commemoration of the Benefactors to the University, by the Public Orator, according to the intention of the Right Honorable Nathaniel, Lord Crewe, Bishop of Durham.

Lord Crewe (1633–1721) had for love for Oxford bequeathed a fund for a Latin oration on Encaenia Day each year, to be preceded (presumably as bait to insure a large attendance) by fruit and wine for the high officers and all doctors (as of 1722; the D.Phil. being a modern degree, doctors of philosophy are not included). The endowment, like all such funds, has long since been depleted by inflation, and the vice chancellor has to pay for the party. It is held at his college, whichever that may be at any given time. Sir Maurice Bowra received us graciously at Wadham. The strawberries and champagne were excellent, the conversation friendly. Well refreshed, we marched two by two along Parks Road and Catte Street to the Sheldonian Theatre.

Charming touches of old customs marked the slightest occasions. On several Sundays I enjoyed seeing the university preacher of the day, a local or visiting divine, duly gowned, walking alone to St. Mary's, the university church, preceded by a beadle in black clerical robe with white neckbands and a gold-tipped staff, to show him the way. I believe that Englishmen, so often shy in personal encounters, find moral support in public gatherings by ritual behavior. At all the formal gatherings we attended, from a garden party to the grand procession at Queen Elizabeth's coronation, this national gift was evident. In April 1953, I was invited to a gathering of town and gown to celebrate William Shakespeare's birthday. I was directed to appear at the Oxford town hall, in academic dress (which for me meant the scarlet and dove gray Sc.D. gown with a mortarboard cap). There I found the mayor of the city, in his black robe with the gold chain of office round his neck, his lady, several professors of English and history, two American colonels from the U.S. air fields at that time still in operation in Oxfordshire, and a few other persons of less obvious status. We marched up Aldgate (Street) through the intersection at Carfax, and up Cornmarket (Street) through the midday crowd of shoppers, who politely left us a path, to an old inn where Shakespeare is said to have once stayed overnight. Upstairs in a dining room the tables were nicely set for luncheon. Waiters circulated among us asking whether we preferred hock or malmsey (Rhine wine or Madeira). The food was such as might have been served to Shakespeare in his day. After lunch we drank to the Queen and to the memory of William Shakespeare, and an elderly professor delivered a beautiful little speech on what Shakespeare meant to Oxford.

Although such instances as these of old traditions mingled with modern science and scholarship come readily to mind after a quarter of a century, it is more difficult to put into words the overall impression that Oxford made upon me as a guest of the university and of Balliol. The major response was immense affection and respect. Oxford has more power to tug at my heartstrings than any other city I know. How can any American of English descent look at the Martyrs' Memorial, or walk through Christ Church meadows, or see the chained books in Merton College library, or gaze at the portraits in any college hall without a surge of gratitude for the scholars who for seven hundred years have lived and labored there?

Yet along with reverence for Oxford's past (and its modern science and scholarship) went surprise at a streak of—what can I call it but boyish lightheartedness in Oxford's men and Oxford's customs. The first-year medical students, as I have mentioned, looked younger than Americans at the same stage. The undergraduates I met in two or three junior common rooms were younger still. I had to smile at the way in which discipline is maintained in Oxford's university area—the stodgy-looking "bulldogs"—ununiformed university policemen wearing bowler hats, under the command of the two proctors (who are junior professors), patrolling the narrow streets at night. The system works; Oxford seems an orderly place. One warm spring night, after dinner at Balliol, some of us went into the fellows' garden to chat in the fresh evening air. From an open upper window of neighboring Trinity College a young tutor looked down at us and shouted an insult at Balliol, whereupon the fellows and tutors I was talking with joined in a slanging match that went on for a quarter of an hour until they were all out of breath.

The problems of modern medical education at Oxford, I thought, had not yet been fully solved. Medicine has been taught there for centuries, by lectures and occasional dissections. In the late nineteenth and the twentieth century, laboratory teaching of physiology, biochemistry, pharmacology, microbiology, and pathology was developed under research-minded teachers. In 1952–53, however, the medical students were mostly enrolled in one or another of the old colleges, at least for a couple of years. They associated with undergraduates rather than the students of the latter years of the medical curriculum, who were based at the Radcliffe infirmary. Thus, unlike beginning American and Continental medical students, those in the preclinical years at Oxford did not profit by the companionship of men and women already immersed in the medical atmosphere. Such older students can influence and stimulate their juniors.

This segregation may promote the general culture of the young people who remain in the collegiate environment, but it deprives them of a sense of participation in medical affairs. This is true also, I thought, of those who teach in the preclinical laboratories, who are not as much a part of the medical faculty as are the members of the preclinical staffs of the London hospital schools. Pedagogically, it seems to me, there is an advantage in giving students of the preclinical sciences—anatomy, physiology, biochemistry, pharmacology, microbiology, and pathology —some idea of the way these subjects contribute to clinical knowledge. Whether the Oxford system at mid-century balanced this lack by producing physicians of greater general culture than Guy's or Bart's I had no way of knowing.

Oxford's long vacations between terms gave us opportunities for travel far afield. In the Christmas vacation of 1952 we went to Spain, traveling in our Ford Zephyr. English friends had recommended the little resort of Torre Molinos on the Mediterranean near Malaga for an inexpensive stay in the sunshine. I should perhaps not have undertaken just then so long a drive in unfamiliar country. Just before leaving England I had a quite severe virus infection in the upper respiratory tract which left me a bit weak and fatigable. We crossed the English Channel pleasantly enough by steamer from Dover to Boulogne and drove south by way of Rouen, Bordeaux, San Sebastian, Vitoria, and Burgos. After a visit to the somber Burgos cathedral, I had the most frightful nightmare of my life, the prelude to the last serious depression I have known. Next morning I pulled myself together and started for Madrid. Once there in a comfortable hotel I brightened up a little. We spent a half day at the Prado Gallery and another at the Royal Palace and made fascinating but fatiguing side trips to the Escorial and to Toledo. When the time came to resume the southward journey, however, I had scarcely enough courage to pack my suitcase and drive on. Betsy, alarmed, did what she could to help me and cheer me up, and I kept on to Granada, where we stopped at a *parador* (a kind of motel) next to the Alhambra.

We reached Malaga safely and at Torre Molinos found a comfortable inn, sunny weather, and a week of physical rest. Depression of the kind I had is always worse in the mornings. In the evenings as we sat on the hotel terrace looking over the blue Mediterranean to the distant Moroccan mountains, I began to find life almost tolerable again. Reports of snow in the Pyrenees, however, made me fearful about driving back to England. We drove to Gibraltar, put the car aboard a dingy old P. and O. liner bound home from Australia, and arrived at London feeling much better.

I was still depressed enough to see our physician in Oxford, who sent me to a psychiatrist. He put me on a carefully balanced regime of a barbiturate and amphetamine that enabled me to keep my lecturing engagements and continue the research with Weddell and Pallie. In the Easter vacation we drove to Cornwall and had a happy stay at St. Ives, resting at the Tregenna Castle Hotel, driving to Penzance and Land's End, and exploring the prehistoric sites in the neighborhood. I have never had a serious depression since.

Betsy and I had both, following advice, enrolled in the national health program for our year at Oxford. My doldrums and Betsy's inflamed knee joint were relieved by careful and sympathetic physicians. The only cost to us was a few shillings for registration. As far as we could see, socialized medicine was working. Doctors whom I asked about it varied from enthusiastic approval to resigned tolerance. I heard no outright opposition from physicians, though I met a few consultants who had enough private practice to permit them to avoid signing up for the national program.

Academic friends in Oxford, anxious that the Eastman Professor should get to know some of the university's famous men of learning, kindly arranged introductions for me. Two such meetings come to mind. C. S. Lewis was then lecturer in English, on his way to a professorship at Cambridge a year or two later. A mutual friend suggested to him that he should ask me to lunch at Magdalen College. I had read *The Screwtape Letters* (1942) and did not care for their smart-aleck style but thought it might be interesting to talk with a Christian apologist who seemed to be on good terms with the Devil. Lewis turned out to be so quiet and polite that I cannot even remember what he looked like. At our lunch in Magdalen's hall he directed the conversation so assiduously to me and my doings that I got no look whatever at his own thought. His autobiography had not yet appeared. I knew too little about him to turn the conversation toward his interests. The hour and a half I spent with him, though pleasant enough, was a failure for both of us.

Another friend told us that Sir William Craigie, the celebrated lexicographer, liked to have visitors at his lonely house at Christmas Common, Watlington, a few miles east of Oxford. Sir William, when we met him there, was eighty-five years old. We had read about an affectionate tribute to him a few months before at his college, Oriel. White-bearded, dignified, with sparkling eyes and a bright smile, he sat among his books and talked about his work. Having spent twenty-two years on the *Oxford English Dictionary* and ten years at Chicago on the *Dictionary of American English,* he was in 1953 nearing completion of his *Dictionary of the Older Scottish Tongue.* Our afternoon visit with Sir William and his woman secretary went by all too quickly, leaving us the memory of a great and friendly scholar.

Oxford has two chairs for American visiting professors. The Harmsworth Professorship of American History was held in 1952–1953 by Henry S. Commager of Amherst College. His wife and two younger children were with him at Oxford. The Commagers and the Corners made each others' acquaintance promptly after we arrived. They had us to Thanksgiving dinner in Henry's rooms at Queen's College, a gracious kindness because to travelers abroad the holidays of one's homeland always bring a sense of loneliness that was assuaged by the company of these sociable people and their merry children. While we were at Oxford we heard Henry lecture at Rhodes House on American political affairs. It was a lucid and authoritative discourse that made us proud of our fellow countryman.

The greatest event of the year in Great Britain, the coronation of Queen Elizabeth II, took place on June 2. Our Oxford friends took it for granted that Betsy and I would go to London to see the procession. I would have passed up that great occasion, for Betsy's arthritic knee was giving trouble. But she was eager to go, all the more so when Arthur Goodhart, who had some extra tickets for viewing stands, gave us two seats on the south side of the Mall opposite Waterloo Place. The orthopedist, patriotically anxious that we Americans should see British ceremonial at its grandest, made for Betsy a strong plaster splint fitting halfway around her leg, but it turned out to be unnecessary.

On June 1 we drove from Oxford to Earl's Court, garaged the car, and made camp at a lodging house. I laid in paper-bag lunches for the morrow. We had umbrellas and raincoats, for the weather prediction was rain. In case of emergency I took along Betsy's splint in a suitcase. On the second we reached our seats a couple of hours before the procession was due. A light, cold rain was falling, but the crowds were already assembling. Many young people had spent the night on the lawn of St. James's Park. A Guards regiment in full dress already lined both sides of the Mall, the men standing at attention with only brief breaks for rest. When the ceremony began in Westminster Abbey, we heard the trumpets and the organ through loudspeakers along the Mall. Finally came the solemn and sonorous words of the Archbishop of Canterbury, "This is your undoubted Queen." When at last the procession came through the Admiralty Arch and up the Mall, we saw with our own eyes what millions of people the world over saw on television, a military spectacle as great as any the world can present. The helmeted and plumed regiments of the Household Guards filled the entire Mall from the Admiralty Arch to Buckingham Palace with men marching to the exultant music of their bands. Betsy and I cheered the royal coach as heartily as the Britons around us, though we had only a dim view of Her Majesty in the dark interior of that ancient vehicle. Later in the procession, however, another royal lady, the plump Queen of Tonga, in full view in an open car, somehow maintained her dignity and, in spite of her rotundity, was cheered for her beaming smile.

When the spectacle was over and the crowds dispersed we walked across the park to St. Ermin's Hotel on Caxton Street, where we enjoyed a Coronation Day dinner of *Suprême de Volaille Reine Elizabeth, Artichaut Balmoral,* and *Pomme Windsor* (16 shillings each).

The ancient mercantile guilds of London nowadays combine sociability with service to the city in much the same way as do the Rotary Club and similar American organizations, though with far more dignity and ceremonial. Each of the guilds celebrated the coronation by a festive dinner. My scientific host at Oxford, Le Gros Clark, was at the time upper warden of the Worshipful Company of Salters. He arranged for Betsy and me to be invited to a dinner on July 7 and asked me to take part in the evening's proceedings by responding to the toast "Our Visitors" (i.e., the invited guests of the Salters' Company), a request to which I could hardly say no.

This was a quite formal full-dress affair. The Salters' Company had lost its own hall by bombing in World War II and therefore held its dinner in the hall of the Drapers' Company in Throgmorton Street, E.C. On arrival we were each given a souvenir program and a plan of the seating. Betsy was seated between Le Gros Clark and me, I was at her left, between her and the Viscountess Woolton, wife of Lord Woolton, who had helped to save Britain from starvation during World War II when he was minister of food, by applying the resources of nutritional science to the problem of feeding the people. I seized the opportunity to tell Lady Woolton how deeply American scientists admired her husband's wartime service.

After a good dinner with choice wines the formalities began. A professional toastmaster appeared, in a scarlet full-dress suit, as usual at large formal dinners. He called for silence. The master of the Salters' Company proposed the "loyal toast" to the

Queen. We drank to her health and then to that of the royal family and to "The Visitors." Then the scarlet-clad toastmaster declaimed, "My Lords, ladies, and gentlemen, pray silence for the Vice President of the United States National Academy of Sciences!" Thus called to my feet, I spoke briefly in praise of salt, the commodity that the company's founders had purveyed to Londoners—emphasizing what sodium chloride means to biologists as a substance essential to human warfare and to life itself. This seemed to please the Salters, and I took my seat amid decorous applause.

When Betsy and I read in the London *Times* that the Queen would have a garden party at Buckingham Palace on July 23, I wrote to the American Embassy asking to be recommended for invitations. In due course came engraved cards from the chamberlain telling us that Her Majesty had commanded him to ask us to her party. Arriving by taxi at the appointed hour of 4:00 P.M. we were led with other guests through long corridors to the rear of the palace and into the forty-acre garden. Many people were already there, standing about the spacious lawn. In the center of the garden was the royal enclosure, surrounded by a low fence, for the Queen and her special guests. Ordinary people like us remained outside but were courteously received by young courtiers in cutaway coats and striped trousers, who circulated about, greeting people and introducing them to one or another of the lesser royalty. We were introduced to the duke and duchess of Gloucester, the Queen's uncle and aunt. The duke, a portly old gentleman, had little to say. I felt a bit sorry for him, having to dress up and be agreeable to total strangers. I have seldom met a man with whom I felt I had so little in common. No doubt he felt the same about me. We exchanged polite remarks; but his alert-looking duchess and Betsy Corner took to each other, and carried on a bright five-minute conversation until one of the young equerries came up with other guests. We walked by the little lake in the garden, chatted with some acquaintances from Oxford, and had cake and sherry before taking our leave.

At home in America a few months later we were guests at the White House when President Eisenhower entertained the National Academy of Sciences, as is customary once in each presidency. The president's party was smaller and more democratic than the Queen's; he shook hands with everybody. I came away warmed by his friendly handshake and kindly greeting.

By midsummer of 1953 my obligations as Eastman Professor were fulfilled; my research with Graham Weddell and Wazir Pallie was ready to write up at home in Baltimore; and my successor to the Eastman chair, Willard V. Quine, and his wife were on their way to take over the flat in Merton Street. The last entry in our guest book is dated July 28. We took leave of Oxford —I was about to say, with regret, but that is not the word—with reluctance and with a touch of sadness, but a year abroad is a long time, and living away from home presents difficulties that no amount of kindness on the part of the natives can fully alleviate. Oxford had given us enough to think about for years to come. I had a feeling that in our year there by my assorted lectures and in the give and take of university and college life I had given less than I had received; but I was relieved later by hearing from Henry Allen Moe, who had a kind of pipeline for Oxford news, that my professorship was regarded in high quarters as successful.

For rest after the strain of saying farewells and of packing up, we retreated for a fortnight to a place of quiet comfort that Betsy had read about and wanted to see, Visby in Gotland, a medieval walled town off the coast of Sweden. We crossed to Gothenburg by steamer, traversed Sweden by the Göta Canal, a charming three days' trip at four miles per hour, had three or four days in Stockholm and went by night boat to Visby. After a delightful stay there we returned to London and sailed for New York aboard the French liner *Liberté*.

RETIRED BUT NOT RETIRING

17

HISTORIAN

Reaching Baltimore early in September 1953, I found that the Carnegie Institution's Department of Embryology had flourished during my absence. My first task was the recurrent one of writing the annual report for the *Year Book* of the Carnegie Institution of Washington. In the personnel section of the report I had the sad duty of recording the death in December 1952 of Lewis Hill Weed, my friend since our student days, my chief in 1915–19 when I was associate professor of anatomy at Johns Hopkins.

My executive duties at the Carnegie laboratory were not heavy in my last two years there. There were no major changes of the staff and no emergencies to prevent me from spending part of my time in scientific research. I wrote up the work in which I had taken part in Oxford with Weddell and Pallie. Bartelmez and I joined in a little monograph describing nine very early abnormal embryos of the rhesus monkey from the Carnegie colony. Published in the Carnegie *Contributions to Embryology*, volume 35, 1954, it is unique in the literature of primate embryology in that we could study, along with the embryos, the maternal ovaries and endometrium (lining of the uterus). The findings helped to lay to rest the old idea that embryonic pathology is always caused by uterine inflammation. In five of our cases the ovaries and endometrium were normal; the embryonic abnormality must have resulted from constitutional defects of the embryo itself. In the other cases the possibility existed that the abnormality of the embryo resulted from primary failure of the corpus luteum.

I also began a study which I never had time to complete, of the arrangement of the bundles of involuntary muscle in the walls of the uterus. I reported preliminary findings at a symposium at CIBA House, London, in the summer of 1954 (when I was there for a meeting of the International Committee on Anatomical Nomenclature).

Calls to address college and university assemblies kept coming, but time was slipping by, and I had to think about what I would do after retirement, which by grace of the Carnegie trustees was now set for June 1955. Having begun my academic career without significant savings, I had never been able to lay away enough money to live on after retirement, nor had the bequests of my parents and Betsy's added much to our resources. I had never in my life had to apply for a job, except for the post of doctor at Camp Kineo in the summer of 1914, and that was not job hunting; it was a lover's stratagem.

The job problem settled itself once more, thanks to Detlev W. Bronk, who in 1953 had become president of the Rockefeller Institute for Medical Research in New York City. For an hour between trains, over cups of coffee in the restaurant of Baltimore's Union Station, he told me that the Rockefeller Institute was approaching the fiftieth anniversary of its founding. The trustees wanted to publish a history of its origin and growth. He offered me, if I would undertake the task, a salary equal to that of the Carnegie directorship. An assistant and a secretary would be provided. We agreed that the task would take at least two years. Bronk, who seemed to thrive on travel and had homes on Mt. Desert Island and at Media, Pennsylvania, as well as Baltimore during both his presidency of Johns Hopkins University and his present position in New York, at first expected that I would remain at Baltimore, doing my writing at home in Roland Park with occasional trips to New York. When I told him that I would want to live in New York and work at the Rockefeller Institute, he willingly agreed and said that he would provide laboratory quarters for me and a colleague I might bring with me, and also offices for my historical assistant and the secretary.

This offer was too good to miss. I gave Bronk my tentative acceptance at once, subject to my wife's agreement, but I knew that Betsy would be delighted to live for a while in New York City, and anyway I preferred not to remain, after retiring, close to the place I was leaving. We put our household goods in storage and left for New York in the late summer of 1955. My colleagues at the Carnegie laboratory and friends of the Johns Hopkins medical faculty joined in a farewell dinner for us in the Great Hall of the Welch Library. The editors of the *American Journal of Anatomy,* urged by Sam Reynolds and others, set aside the first three numbers of volume 98, for 1956, as a Festschrift in my honor. Carl Hartman contributed an article, "The Scientific Achievements of George Washington Corner, M.D.," and Richard H. Shryock, professor of the history of medicine at Johns Hopkins, wrote "George W. Corner as Historian and Humanist." Other friends, including people who had been with me at Rochester and at Baltimore contributed articles based on their researches. It was indeed gratifying to find in the volume the work of such honored friends as George W. Bartelmez, Bent G. Boving, Robert K. Burns, Jr., Arpad I. Csapo, Louis and Josefa Flexner, Arthur T. Hertig, and Elizabeth M. Ramsey. Especially touching was it to find a fine paper also by George W. Corner, Jr., professor of obstetrics and gynecology, on dating the human corpus luteum, which remains to this day the standard source of information on that subject.

We found a pleasant furnished apartment on the twenty-first floor of the huge Manhattan House at 200 East Sixty-sixth Street, three blocks from the Rockefeller Institute. It had a balcony looking to the south over the mid-city skyscrapers, a magnificent sight, especially early on winter evenings when the towering office buildings were lighted up. At the Rockefeller Institute I was given a suite of rooms on the third floor of Theobald Smith Hall. It seemed a pleasing coincidence that I was to begin my postretirement years in a building named for the great microbiologist whose account of his research had stimulated me to study biology. My office was at the southeast corner of the building with a view of the ever-thronged Queensboro Bridge and the lower East River.

Between my office and the secretary's room was my small laboratory, where I set up my two microscopes which the Carnegie Institution had generously allowed me to retain on loan, one for dissecting under low magnification, and one for high-power work. The colleague I had brought from Baltimore, Arpad Csapo, had an office and a laboratory room large enough for his own experimental work and that of a research assistant or visiting fellow. At first I devoted half-days to work at the microscope, examining the arrangement of muscle bundles in the rabbit's uterus and looking for cyclic changes in the size of the individual muscle fibers, but these studies, too desultory to be called research, interested me less and less. I felt that I had carried my investigation of the ovarian and uterine cycle about as far as possible with the technical methods that I had learned how to use. Now it was the turn of the physiologists and biochemists like Csapo and others of his generation to carry on investigations of the reproductive cycle. Rather than continue a line of work that had had its day, I had better give full time to my new career of historian of science, in which, I hoped, I could do significant research and writing.

John Blake, my assistant, had preceded me to New York. During the summer months he had made at my request a study of the medical research institutions of Europe, including the Pasteur Institute of Paris and Robert Koch's institute in Berlin. He had also looked into the history of older research laboratories, such as those of the Italian cities dating from the Renaissance. His report ("Scientific Institutions since the Renaissance"), which was very helpful to me, was so excellent that it was published in 1957 in the *Proceedings of the American Philosophical Society*. John also made for me an invaluable card index of all the scientists and physicians on the Rockefeller Institute's staff since its foundation in 1901.

The sources for the history I was about to undertake were manifold—the records of the trustees and the board of scientific directors, the institute's publications, newspaper clippings, the correspondence of many key people. Much of this immense mass of material was in the institute's library and administrative offices and was put freely at my disposal. Dr. Bronk thoughtfully retained on the office staff an old lady, Miss Margaret Wuest, who knew where all the files were stored in the business office, in the basement of Founder's Hall, and in a dusty room on the top floor of the hospital. But since the institute was only fifty years old, much valuable information was stored in the memories of living people, some of whom recalled almost the earliest years. Eugene Opie, who had come to work with Simon Flexner in 1904, was available for talks with me, having returned to the institute after a professorial career elsewhere from 1910 to 1941. David Rockefeller arranged for me a telephone interview with his aging father, John D. Rockefeller, Jr., who was closely involved in the institute's first years.

My best informant was Peyton Rous, member of the institute, who joined the staff in 1909. He had retired in 1945 but was still at work in his laboratory. I had met him in Baltimore and of course knew of his brilliant research career. He was the first of the institute's senior men to welcome me and took deep interest in my task. We had much in common, although he was ten years older than I. Born a Virginian, Peyton grew up in Baltimore. We were both graduates of Johns Hopkins University, collegiate and medical, and we both had been interns in the Johns Hopkins Hospital. Peyton had known every one of the original workers at the institute. He had a novelist's eye and ear for personal characteristics and liked to talk about people. He gave me valuable information I could have gotten from no one else. He read critically each chapter of the history as I drafted it and, being an experienced editor and writer, never failed to point out an inappropriate word or a missing comma.

The one person who refused to help me to understand and write about his research (and in this case, also about his administrative career) was Herbert Spencer Gasser, director of the Rockefeller Institute from 1935 to 1953, winner of the Nobel Prize in 1944. When I was writing the history, he was continuing his research at the institute. We had known each other in our student days; he was a medical student at Johns Hopkins University in the second class after mine. At the institute our acquaintance had been resumed in a friendly though merely formal way. Since I have to report that he was deliberately unhelpful to me, and in one instance, at least, was cruelly insensitive to the feelings of some of the institute's staff, I must mention here a mitigating circumstance that I have never seen in print. Gasser was afflicted with an endocrine defect that is often accompanied by temperamental disturbance. He was eunuchoid, lacking the testicular hormone, as indicated by his boyish complexion, high-pitched voice, and long limbs. In his executive duties he was sometimes timid and irritable. When the institute's trustees made their momentous decision to close the Princeton laboratories of animal and plant pathology in 1947, it was Gasser's duty to inform the staff of the impending action, but (apparently for lack of courage) he failed to do so. Carl Ten Broeck, director of the Princeton division, told me that he first learned of the decision from a news story in the *New York Times*. I believe that Gasser was unwilling to discuss his administration with me or even to read what I might say of the Princeton closing and other personal difficulties he had had with the staff.

Another and to me more puzzling case of reluctance to review my narrative was that of Robert Loeb, son of the eminent physiologist Jacques Loeb. Bob Loeb, not connected with the Rockefeller Institute, was professor of internal medicine in the College of Physicians and Surgeons of Columbia University. A friendly acquaintance of mine for several years, his highly intelligent and mature personality gave no sign of inner tension or insecurity. When I asked him to read a chapter devoted to his father's work at the institute, he agreed to do so, but I waited for months to get the typescript back. When finally I urgently requested its return, it came back unopened, with a note from Bob saying that he had been unable to bring himself to read it or even to open the parcel. Peyton Rous gave me a clue to this strange reluctance; Jacques Loeb, he said, had been a severe parent. His son probably had memories he was afraid to revive. American-born sons of eminent European scientists apparently faced such difficulties: another man not connected with the institute, with a similar family history, was reluctant to have me tell all I knew of his distinguished father's career.

My interviews and combing of the files brought out many episodes of life in the great research institute, some of them bitter, some heart-warming. A mature scientist with years of profound research behind him sat beside my desk for an hour telling me, with trembling voice and clenched hands, of the frustration he had endured from the crabbed perfectionism of his famous chief, which had kept the younger man from publishing experiments on which he had expended many months of research. In contrast, I found in the files a note to Simon Flexner from a foreign-born member whose work had been going badly: "I did not think yesterday morning that my nerves would stand the strain much longer. I left you after our little interview cured and happy. This was happening right along repeatedly. . . . I value this growing—what shall I call it but affection—above all."

For me as historian of the Rockefeller Institute a major problem was to give a balanced account of the work and personalities of some of its most celebrated members. Many of them, for example, Peyton Rous and Oswald Avery, had done their great work within the institute's walls, without publicizable dramatics; on the other hand Hideyo Noguchi and Alexis Carrel had made themselves conspicuous by wide travel, had become legendary figures in their lifetimes, and had come to their deaths spectacularly, Noguchi under the cloud of his great mistake about the cause of yellow fever, Carrel under the more sinister shadow of alleged disloyalty to his native land. Both had been overidolized by the sensational press. For my accounts of their work at the Rockefeller Institute I sought informants who had known them well. Peyton Rous, with the gentle wisdom of advancing age and long personal acquaintance with these two men, helped me to see them clearly. Philip McMaster, member of the Institute, and Theodore Shedlovsky, associate member, afraid that I would accept the journalists' adulation of Carrel, made a point of getting me to sit down with them over a cocktail to hear them talk of his credulity—he was as superstitious, said Shedlovsky, as a French peasant. Their picture may have been exaggerated, but it helped me understand Alexis Carrel's *The Voyage to Lourdes*, the incredible tale of witnessing at Lourdes a miraculous, almost instantaneous cure of tuberculous peritonitis. After studying the records of Charles Lindbergh's collaboration with Carrel in the development of the Carrel-Lindbergh pump for organ culture, I wrote to Lindbergh, asking him to have lunch with me at the Century Club and talk about Carrel. Lindbergh, modest, friendly, and keen, admitted Carrel's credulity while giving me an affectionate account of his immense technical skill and personal charm. From Robert Soupault's biography (Paris, 1952), I learned to understand Carrel's visionary dream of a world at peace, dominated by science, that led to his docility during the German occupation of Paris in World War I.

When in 1925 Sinclair Lewis published his best-selling novel about medical research, *Arrowsmith*, he thanked Paul de Kruif, a former junior member of the Rockefeller Institute's staff, for help in portraying the characters in the story and in developing the philosophy of medical research on which the plot is based. De Kruif had done excellent research on bacterial mutations at the Rockefeller Institute; readers everywhere thought that some of the leading characters had been drawn, with de Kruif's help, from Rockefeller Institute people, including Jacques Loeb and Peyton Rous.

By the time when I was writing my history, de Kruif had become a best-selling author himself with his excellent popular book about the great bacteriologists, *The Microbe Hunters.* I asked to meet him, and the next time he was in New York he invited me to visit him at his hotel. I found him tense and restless. Although he looked well, he said he was suffering with various ailments and had a traveling medicine chest, packed with bottles full of pills and tablets, from which he took one or two during our conversation. Quite willing to talk about *Arrowsmith,* he began by denouncing Sinclair Lewis for promising to publish the novel under their joint authorship and then giving him in the book only a note of thanks for his help. How true this might be I could not tell. I know only that in the rest of our talk he deliberately lied to me about the characters in the novel.

He told me that with his help Lewis had drawn the benign, unworldly Gotlieb from his (de Kruif's) old teacher F. G. Novy and from Jacques Loeb, and Terry Wicker had come from John H. Northrup. This, I believe, was true, but other figures in the book, said de Kruif, were not based on individual Rockefeller Institute people. Tubbs, director of McGurk, and his suave, ambitious understudy Rippleton Holabird, for example, were pieced together by Sinclair Lewis from various traits of people de Kruif disliked. I put this into my *History of the Rockefeller Institute.* Only later, when my book was in proof, did I learn that de Kruif had filed away for future reference a list of the novel's dramatis personae matching names of Rockefeller Institute men to some of the most disagreeable people of the fictitious McGurk Institute. I will not help to perpetuate de Kruif's petty spite by citing the list here. Any historian seriously interested in it can track it down from a footnote in my book.

The two years that Bronk and I had thought the task might require went by all too rapidly. Bronk extended my stay to a third, a fourth, and finally a fifth year. Arpad Csapo was also kept on the staff, continuing his fundamental research on uterine physiology with a visiting fellow or two. Finally the typescript of my book was complete—text, footnotes, lists of personnel, appendixes, illustrations, all the apparatus of a formal institutional history, enlivened (I hoped) with many biographical sketches and anecdotes from comical to tragic, that would make the fifty-year narrative readable. Late in June 1960, I bundled up the typed pages, left the book at Dr. Bronk's office, and did not see it or hear from it again for two years.

At last, in 1962 the director of the Rockefeller Institute Press, William Bayless, let me know that the typescript was in his hands, cleared for copy editing. Bronk had deleted three or four pages but had otherwise expressed his satisfaction with my work; in fact, he supplied a glowing foreword that ended with high praise of its author, "a historian who is uniquely qualified to tell the story of this remarkable institution."

The passage that he had omitted implied that scientists could manage a research institution without the guidance of lay trustees. But Bronk was at that very time planning to transform the institute into a university with all the usual appurtenances —professorial titles and cap-and-gown commencements, Latin diplomas, a university press, and a board of trustees of the standard type. The history of the earlier days must not hint that it could get along without trustees. He made no other changes in the manuscript whatsoever, and the Rockefeller University Press published the book in 1964. At the 1976 commencement of the Rockefeller University I received from Bronk's successor, Frederick Seitz, the honorary degree of doctor of science.

My wife and I enjoyed being in New York and the opportunities we had to use the public library and that of the New York Academy of Medicine, to visit the Metropolitan Museum of Art, the American Museum of Natural History, and the Cloisters. On many Sunday mornings we drove to the Cathedral of St. John the Divine. Betsy loved the ritual and the music, and I, too, when I heard the choir's magnificent chanting of the Nicene Creed resounding through the immense spaces of the mighty church, could forget the fourth-century theology and let the worshipful serenity of the chant envelop my brain.

Often at these Sunday morning services the preacher was the dean of the cathedral, James Pike, who was even then getting attention for his outspoken views on social questions. I was rather surprised when he was called to be bishop of San Francisco but hearing him from his New York pulpit would not have detected the radical mysticism that drove him out of his California bishopric and to his death in the bleak desert of Judea.

I liked to drive whenever I could along the waterfront of downtown Manhattan. In those days many large transatlantic liners could be seen lying at their berths on the West Side. Now and then we put our car on the harbor ferry to Staten Island, drove to its southern end and picnicked on the shore to watch S.S. *France* or *Mauretania* or *United States* coming proudly in from Europe.

In the long summer evenings we liked to drive up the Hudson to dine at an inn beside a quiet lake somewhere in Westchester or Putnam County. These outings, and our interesting tasks, Betsy gathering materials for her notes on the Fothergill letters, I pushing ahead on the history of the Rockefeller Institute, kept us busy and contented. I look back upon those five years in New York as a kind of Indian summer of our marriage.

In August 1956 Betsy and I, after a visit to England that was becoming an annual routine in those years, went to Rome for a fortnight for a sightseeing stay. There I learned from a newspaper article that earlier in the year workmen driving piles for the foundation of a new apartment house on the Via Latina had broken into a previously unknown catacomb, the burial place of a Christian community of the fourth century A.D. It contained remarkable funerary paintings, one of which represented a physician presiding over a demonstration before a class of doctors or students. The subject of the demonstration was the body of a man with an abdominal incision or wound.

I would have liked to see the painting, but the catacomb had been closed to visitors pending arrangements for its protection. The tombs and paintings were under the care of Father Antonio Ferrua, S.J., secretary of the Pontifical Commission on Sacred Archaeology, with whom I succeeded in arranging a conference. Father Ferrua, a learned scholar, came to our hotel with a large portfolio of photographs. After seeing them and hearing Father Ferrua's description of the coloring and costumes, I concluded that the painting depicts a physician with his pupils; the scene is not a dissection, as some have supposed, but a demonstration of an abdominal wound. Father Ferrua told me that the subject's eyes are painted as living, not glazed by death. Although this fascinating discovery does not call upon us to revise the well-established view that human dissection was not practiced before the fourteenth century A.D., the picture is certainly the oldest known representation of a doctor with his pupils. I reported my conclusions (with which Father Ferrua agreed) in a brief paper read before the American Philosophical Society at its autumn meeting of 1956 (*Proceedings of the American Philosophical Society*, volume 161, 1957).

In mid-June of 1959 we made a brief trip to England, chiefly to give Betsy a chance to confer with Christopher Booth on the Fothergill letters. Then on July 11 we embarked on a 12,000-ton freight-passenger ship of the Blue Star line, destined for Buenos Aires by way of Lisbon, Teneriffe, and Recife—a delightfully restful voyage. At Buenos Aires I attended a scientific confer-ence and after that we traveled by night train to Córdoba to visit Inés de Allende for a few days; thence by air to Mendoza and over the Andes to Santiago, Chile, a rough, almost intimidating flight over the most forbidding mountains I ever saw. At San-tiago we visited Eduardo Bunster Montero, who had spent a year with me at Rochester. Flying northward we stayed a few days in Lima, Peru, and from there went by airplane to Cuzco and Machu Picchu. This was another horrendous, literally breath-taking flight, for the plane, which was not pressurized, crossed the Andes to Cuzco at an altitude of 12,000 feet. At Machu Picchu, which is lower than Cuzco, though rugged be-yond any other place I have ever visited, I was able to breathe easily.

When we returned to New York, the American Association of Anatomists asked me to be president of an international con-gress of anatomists that was to be convened for the first time in America in 1960. New York had been designated the seat. Because the congress was to coincide with the annual meeting of the American association, we had a congress committee headed by me and the association's president, Stanley Bennett of the University of Washington at Seattle.

After years of preparation the congress was held April 10 to 14, 1960, at the Statler Hilton (formerly Pennsylvania Hotel) on Seventh Avenue at Thirty-fourth Street. (Most of the out-of-town scientists stayed there, but a Russian delegation of eight or ten members was not allowed by its Soviet government leader to stay at the same hotel with the rest of the anatomists.) I opened the scientific part of the meeting with a presidential address on the history of anatomical research in America, and Stanley Bennett followed with a review of the current state of American anatomy. Then for three days we had the usual series of brief research reports on various subdivisions of anatomical study, several sessions going on simultaneously.

One afternoon we took the delegates for a circuit around Manhattan Island on one of the sight-seeing steamboats. We had an evening concert arranged at my request by a local musicologist with a sense of humor, at which a good ensemble of singers and instrumentalists performed music more or less relevant to anatomy from "These bones shall rise again" and "Ja, dies ist meine Nase" to a romantic love song in which a fair maiden's heart was favorably mentioned, followed by classical music of none too obvious relevance to anatomy, to let our foreign guests know that Americans really can play serious music. The Seventh International Anatomical Congress was, I think, a success scientifically and socially.

With the anatomical congress over and my history of the Rockefeller Institute needing only some final touches before it went to Dr. Bronk, I could give full attention to the coming events of that momentous year of 1960. First on my mind was the question of what to do next. I would still need a job, because my financial resources were not sufficient for the two of us in total retirement.

Again a job came looking for me. My friend Henry Allen Moe, president of the John Simon Guggenheim Memorial Foundation, had in April 1959 been elected president of the American Philosophical Society. The Society's executive officer, the eminent botanist William J. Robbins, wished to resign his post in the autumn of 1960, and Henry Moe offered it to me. This was a position of responsibility and dignity for which, I felt, my experience and tastes fitted me. My wife was reluctant to leave New York, but the Rockefeller Institute had no further need of me, and Philadelphia offered amenities—music, art, and literature— rivaling those of New York. I gladly accepted Henry Moe's offer. In Philadelphia Betsy found a comfortable-looking apartment on the nineteenth floor of the Savoy on beautiful Rittenhouse Square. It would be available in September.

We booked a flight to London on July 8, for a stay of three weeks crowded with notable events. First, on July 13, was the dedication by Queen Elizabeth II of a new building near Regent's Park for the Royal College of Obstetricians and Gynecologists, of which in 1955 I had been elected an honorary fellow. The dedication was conducted in full ceremonial style. I wore my Johns Hopkins gown of black silk with facings and sleeve bars of green velvet for the degree of M.D., and the hood of an honorary degree from the University of Chicago, lined with maroon silk and edged with broad bands of yellow velvet indicating the degree of doctor of science. After about thirty foreign fellows, dressed in the varied robes of their universities, came row after row of the British members of the college, wearing its blue robes. While we were all standing at our seats, trumpets sounded, and in came the Queen in a lovely pink dress and Sir John Peel in his presidential blue gown faced and barred with gold.

When the affair ended a man came up to me and introduced himself as the artist who had been commissioned to paint the dedication scene. He wanted to thank me, he said, for my help. "I have been in the rear balcony making sketches," he said. "I was worried about my color scheme. As I would paint the scene from the rear looking towards the stage, the whole front of the hall would be a dull mass of men in blue robes with their backs to me, with more blue on the stage. I arranged for the Queen to wear pink, but there would still be the unbroken ranks of men in blue. Then you marched in with that maroon hood with wide yellow borders and put a dash of bright color just where I needed it." I asked him how one gets a queen to dress to suit an artist. That was done, he said, through one of the ladies in waiting. Some years later I went to the college to see the painting. Sure enough, at the left front near the stage, I saw a tiny image of the back of my head and shoulders, making a splash of yellow and maroon amid the ranks of blue.

In another gathering of medical men and women, the next week, I had a more active part to play. A classmate of mine in the Johns Hopkins Medical School, Thomas M. Rivers, had retired from directorship of the hospital of the Rockefeller Institute, joining the National Foundation for Infantile Paralysis as vice president for medical affairs. After the introduction of a vaccine for poliomyelitis the foundation became the National Foundation, and turned its attention to the widespread and baffling topic of congenital malformations. Tom Rivers, wishing to publicize the new objective and stimulate research in the field, set his heart on a great international scientific conference to be held in London. Knowing that I had given a good deal of attention to congenital malformations and prenatal mortality, he did me the honor of asking me to deliver the theme address at the beginning of his conference. I was deeply touched by this appeal of my old friend. For him the conference was to be the climax of his career; for me it would be one of the memorable occasions of my later years.

Church House, London, stands at the heart of Westminster next to Westminster Abbey. In its impressive auditorium, designed for the conduct of weighty church business of the Anglican communion, the National Foundation on July 18–22, 1960, gathered 500 delegates from twenty-one countries, mostly physicians and scientists, to discuss one of the most distressing and most complex problems of modern medicine. The seriousness of my theme and the churchly setting called for words more poignant than science alone could provide. I took them in part from Holy Writ. "We have been brought together from many lands," I said,

> to discuss a problem of grave human concern and high scientific importance. That we are meeting not in a laboratory or an academic auditorium, but at Church House, in the very precincts of Westminster Abbey, is altogether appropriate. From that venerable shrine for a thousand years without cease prayers have been ascending to God to reveal truth, to relieve suffering and to solace the afflicted. In our laboratories and clinics we too seek the truth and strive to aid the maimed and the deformed. Like Jeremiah at Ramah we have heard the voice of Rachel weeping for her children. From this hall as from the Abbey's altars there rise to high heaven an aspiration and a resolve that our labors shall help to lift the burden of congenital abnormality from the race of man.

Then I briefly reviewed ancient knowledge of congenital defects and explained the older theories of their causes, from that of Ambroise Paré to that of my teacher Franklin Mall. I spoke of the repeated efforts to explain all damage during intrauterine life by inadequacy of the uterine environment, then told how in the twentieth century, genetic theory had ascribed embryonic defects to faults of the germ plasm in the ovum and the spermatozoon. I mentioned on the other hand the experiments of modern biologists working with birds' eggs and the ova of aquatic animals, who produced anomalies—spina bifida, cyclopia, anecephaly, by subjecting fertilized ova to mechanical injury, changes of temperature, or chemical toxins. I spoke of disastrous immune reactions such as that which causes erythroblastosis (which is now yielding to scientific medicine). I described the complexities of early embryonic growth and mentioned what hints we have as to how these processes may go wrong. I discussed our uncertainty about the possible role of the mother's psyche upon the intrauterine development of her offspring. The sum of my discourse was that congenital malformations have many causes, both genetic and environmental; to prevent them will require a multiple attack in many fields of science.

To my distinguished audience I had said nothing that they did not already know, but they were deeply attentive during the fifty minutes of my address. Tom Rivers was happy because he thought I had given his conference a good start. James Ebert, my successor at the Carnegie embryological laboratory, wrote a few months later that "This address will stand, not merely as a theme address, setting the stage for the Conference, but as a veritable scientific charter, a plan of attack for a new generation of students of congenital malformations." The address, "Congenital Malformations: The Problem and the Task," was published by the National Foundation in a small illustrated pamphlet shortly after the conference.

A few days later I was present at another, even grander ceremony. The Royal Society of London, the most venerable academy of science in English-speaking lands, celebrated June 18–26, 1960, the 300th anniversary of its founding in the time of King Charles II. This was a great affair, opened by a plenary session in the Royal Albert Hall, again with the Queen present to make an address, and with all the fellows of the Royal Society in academic robes. I was seated, robed in my scarlet Oxford

Sc.D. gown, with other foreign members in the middle of the immense hall; Betsy was in a gallery reserved for the families of the fellows and foreign members. On the following days there were scientific sessions and a formal dinner, and a *conversazione* of which I recall only a pleasant talk with Werner Heisenberg, author of the "uncertainty principle."

One afternoon during the commemoration Queen Elizabeth the Queen Mother held a reception at her residence, St. James's Palace, for the wives of the fellows and foreign members. When Betsy Corner rejoined me after the party she had a story to tell. Having arrived at the palace rather early, she said, she was one of a group of guests who were chatting together in a lobby near the entrance to the large chamber where the reception was to take place. The Queen Mother appeared, accompanied by a lady-in-waiting and leading a pair of her famous Welsh corgis. The lady guests hastily lined up in two ranks between which their royal hostess and her companions walked toward the reception chamber. As they passed Betsy she forgot that commoners do not speak to royalty unless spoken to first. She impulsively exclaimed, "What lovely dogs," whereupon the Queen Mother stopped, smilingly said "I see that you love dogs, too," and drew in the leashes so that Betsy could see the corgis more closely. They exchanged another remark or two before the Queen Mother remembered her duty and walked on. This little episode drew amazed comment, not untinged with jealousy, from some of the other American ladies and made Betsy the center of attention. As a little girl she had wanted to be a queen; now she had at least talked with one.

On July 27 we drove to Scotland for a stay at the quiet little town of Callander in Perthshire, whose Roman Camp Hotel we knew and liked. After the great affairs in London it was pleasant to sit and rest in the hotel's garden beside the little river Teith. Betsy had much on her mind her work on Fothergill's letters and wanted to gather information about his wayward brother Alexander. On our way back to London I drove to Wensleydale in Yorkshire, where we stayed a few days at the village of Bainbridge, visiting archives nearby.

Then, as we had planned, we took Swan's Hellenic cruise, led by experienced scholars. That year the chartered ship, a small passenger liner of American build now registered in Turkey, sailed from Savona in northern Italy, an overnight trip by railway from London. The ship took us first to Syracuse in Sicily, to see an ancient Greek amphitheater and the Fountain of Arethusa. Thence we went to Olympia in Greece, where noble, well-scoured temples stand on grassy lawns, bright ruins in a green park. We went ashore at Heraklion in Crete, for the Minoan palace at Knossos, then to Rhodes for a touch of the Middle Ages, and to the Hippocratic island of Cos. We landed at three dusty little Turkish ports and rode by bus to three sites of great renown—Troy, surprisingly small for the amount of history and legend that has come from its lonely mound on the Anatolian plain; Pergamum, a healing shrine well preserved; Ephesus, a whole city fallen to the ground. Our ship passed without stopping through the Dardanelles and the Bosporus into the Black Sea and on to Varna in Bulgaria. Returning, we spent three days at Constantinople. At Delos, shrine of Apollo, photographing the ruins, I fell ten feet into a dry cistern of the Roman period, breaking one of my nineteenth-century American toes, so that at Athens a couple of days later I had to limp about the Parthenon and at Corinth could not make it to the top of the acropolis.

The lecturers who accompanied the tour were first-class. John Chadwick was with us, who with Michael Ventris deciphered the Minoan A script. In one of his shipboard lectures he told us how it was done. Lord David Cecil, in spite of his exalted ancestry and his own considerable learning, was a modest fellow traveler. A rumor I had heard about him, that the English he spoke was so hoity-toity Oxfordian that nobody could understand him, was a libel. The few words he exchanged with me, as even shy Englishmen will do without an introduction, on shipboard, were quite intelligible. A lecture he gave us in Athens, on the Greek tragedies, in the ancient theater of Herodias Atticus on the south slope of the Acropolis, was superbly clear and illuminative. An elderly Anglican canon, to whom we listened in the amphitheater at Ephesus, read from the Acts of the Apostles (19:22–41) with moving eloquence the story of the uproar against St. Paul in that very place where we sat listening.

After a breezy homeward passage from Patras to Savona we reached London September 10. Betsy remained there for almost a month to consult with Christopher Booth and to work with the Fothergill papers preserved at Friends' House Library, London. In the meantime, on September 14, I left by airplane for New York and proceeded to our new home in Philadelphia.

18

EXECUTIVE OFFICER

The American Philosophical Society, Held at Philadelphia for Promoting Useful Knowledge, our oldest learned society, has occupied since 1789 a dignified building on Independence Square in the simplest Federal style. The Society carries on its stated function in four ways. It brings together twice a year some of the nation's most knowledgeable people and their spouses, who also know a thing or two, to share their knowledge by formal lectures and (without undue insistence upon usefulness) by amiable conversation. It publishes two periodicals—the *Transactions* and the *Proceedings of the American Philosophical Society*—and a half-dozen scholarly monographs in book form each year. It makes grants for research in all fields of learning. Just off Independence Square, across Fifth Street from Philosophical Hall, stands the Society's library, which contains a vast treasure of American scientific history in books and manuscripts gathered and cherished for more than two hundred years.

Since 1932 the Society has been able to augment the traditional amenities of its meetings, bring out its publications, build up its library, and install the program of grants, through a bequest from a wealthy member, R. A. F. Penrose, who left half his fortune to the Society. This money and other funds donated and bequeathed since the late eighteenth century have been carefully invested by a wise committee of financially experienced members. Its total endowment now exceeds $20 million and brings in an income of more than $1 million annually.

Until the Penrose bequest came in, the Society's daily affairs could be managed by the president, a secretary and assistant secretary, and the librarian, but the broadened program beginning in 1936 called for a salaried executive officer. This post, which I was now to hold for seventeen years, was first held as a part-time post by Edwin G. Conklin, professor of biology at Princeton University, then by Luther P. Eisenhart, mathematician, also of Princeton. William J. Robbins, director of the New York Botanical Garden, held it for a couple of years, commuting from his base in the Bronx once or twice a week. Henry Allen Moe, elected president of the Society in 1957, decreed that the executive officer must live in Philadelphia and give full time to the work. This meant, as Henry Moe and I agreed, full time in the same sense that a university professorship is a full-time job. I was to have time for scholarly writing and occasional lecturing. Besides carrying on the daily business of my office, with responsibility for preparing the annual budget and controlling expenditures, I was also to be editor of the Society's publications, chairman of the committee on meetings, and of the committee on research, which directs the grant program, and member of the committee on the hall and several other special committees. The library was under my care only to the extent that its annual budget came to my desk for discussion and approval before going to the council. The management of its daily affairs was in the hands of a highly competent librarian, Richard H. Shryock, who had been professor of American history at the University of Pennsylvania and later director of the Welch Institute of Medical History at the Johns Hopkins Medical School. In 1965 Dr. Shryock was succeeded as librarian by Whitfield J. Bell, Jr., associate librarian, with whom I have worked as happily as with his predecessor. Julia Noonan, titled assistant secretary and later associate secretary (there being an officer of the Society historically called secretary who had only perfunctory duties), was in charge of my office. She has served the Society under thirteen presidents and has assisted and to a large extent gently guided four successive executive officers in their daily work.

This part of my life is too recent to be narrated in the reminiscent mood of earlier chapters. Of the four presidents under whom I have served I can write with some detachment only about Henry Allen Moe (1959–70). He was, from the executive officer's standpoint, almost an ideal president. He had long executive experience as president of the Guggenheim Foundation, knew almost every important scholar and scientist in the country, and was literate and wise, with a lawyer's self-confidence. He had a broad outlook, knew England about as well as his own country, and was deeply concerned about the individual men and women whose careers had been affected by their Guggenheim Fellowships.

I said, a few lines above, that Henry Moe was almost an ideal president. In some few ways he fell a bit short of perfection. In the chair at meetings he spoke with such a low voice that he could hardly be heard. At the council table he was patient and diplomatic except when the council or a committee could not arrive at a decision on some debated point. Then he would assume a firm judicial manner and declared, as if from the Supreme Court bench, "I will rule thus and so." Such arbitrary decisions cut short many a fruitless discussion. Henry's mildly autocratic style had grown on him, I think, because in the daily administration of the Guggenheim Foundation he was the only decision maker.

In spite of occasional rumblings in our Society, successive nominating committees kept Dr. Moe in the presidency for ten years; then, with a keen sense of timing, he declined to accept renomination. I greatly missed his wise and thoughtful leadership, for he had always encouraged me in my executive duties. In particular, he supported me in the chief innovation I made in the Society's activities, an annual musical evening at the autumn general meeting. In 1968 we elected to membership Ralph Kirkpatrick, the distinguished harpsichordist, chosen by the Society for his scholarly biography of Domenico Scarlatti rather than for his superb performances of classical music. Henry Moe, assuming his dictatorial manner, told Ralph that he must acknowledge his membership by giving us a recital. His performance, in the beautiful reading room of our library, so delighted the members that I proposed that we have a recital or concert at each autumn meeting. Henry Moe affirmed the plan and saw to it that I was allotted an adequate sum for the purpose. Although I have no musical talent whatever, my wife had taught me to appreciate good music. Somehow I managed to find talented performers, a soloist or quartet, or a chamber orchestra. That my critical wife, as well as Henry Moe, approved them made me feel that I was something of an impresario.

Dr. Moe's successor in the presidency was Leonard Carmichael, former president of Tufts University and later secretary of the Smithsonian Institution. In his earlier days he had done pathfinding research in developmental psychology. As our president for three years he especially enjoyed carrying on the Society's traditions, for example, the eighteenth-century formula of admitting a new member, which he recited in well-practiced tones. I have heard him criticized by a fellow scientist who thought him overcautious in executive action, but I think that he was conservative rather than timid.

Dr. Carmichael was followed by Julian P. Boyd, historian and editor of the complete papers of Thomas Jefferson. Imaginative and impulsive, he guided the Society through the bicentennial of the Declaration of Independence in 1976, keeping us out of some overambitious plans. I am grateful for one of his impulses, which was that the Society should have a portrait of me among those of men who have served it in various ways. Julian gathered subscriptions from a hundred members to a fund that paid for a bronze bust by the American sculptor Joy Buba that stands on a pedestal below Albert Murray's painting of Leonard Carmichael in the Members' Room of Philosophical Hall.

Julian Boyd was succeeded as president in 1976 by Jonathan E. Rhoads, Philadelphia's leading surgeon, professor emeritus in the University of Pennsylvania. It is difficult for me to write about Jonathan; the days of our association in the Society's work, in which he has been very generous to me, are too recent. I have also been his deeply grateful patient in a surgical operation. Fortunately that occasion required only a modest display of his surgical skill, but he also gave rare kindness and sympathy in a time of uncertainty.

My editorship of learned works differs from that of a literary editor because the material to be judged and prepared for press is mostly beyond the intellectual range of the editor, who must depend on specialist advisers. The manuscripts are submitted by their authors, not solicited by the publisher like most magazine articles and many novels. When a new manuscript comes in I make a tentative judgment as to its suitability for submission to the committee on publications. Then, unless it is clearly unsuitable, I send it to somebody I think competent to judge it expertly—either a member of the Society or some other recognized scholar or scientist to whom we will pay a modest honorarium. To find the right reviewer is one of my most important editorial duties and sometimes is a difficult task. Since we publish, generally speaking, only the results of research, the author of a submitted manuscript may himself be the only expert in his field. I try to find readers of broad interests at least generally acquainted with the relevant field of research.

Most of our authors, being scholars or scientists, write good English and understand the technical details of preparing their work for the press. Now and then, however, we get an article or a book manuscript based on competent research but poorly arranged or written in English below our high standard of clarity and literary style. We generally return such manuscripts to the author, asking him or her to get a friendly teacher of English or other experienced writer to go over the work word by word. A few times, when all else has failed, I have myself rewritten a manuscript in a field far beyond the range of my expert knowledge. The committee on publications has chided me for such use of my time, but I rather enjoy doing this work; it is as entertaining as a crossword puzzle and more useful. The authors I have helped in this way have mostly been grateful.

In my work as executive officer I have also served as chairman of the committee on research, which means, practically speaking, the direction, with the committee's advice, of the Society's program of grants in aid of research. This task I am still carrying on, along with the editorial work, in my ninth decade, although I am no longer executive officer. The committee awards about three hundred grants every year, averaging $1,000 each, to aid individual scholars and scientists with specific research projects in all fields of learning. As chairman I read all the applications, noting the applicant's qualifications and the nature of the project as far as I can comprehend it. I look at the requested budget and the list of the applicant's research publications and then assign each application to some one member of the committee with special knowledge in its field.

My post as executive officer gave me diverting glimpses of

prominent people, not only our eminent members, but also public figures, including three presidents of the United States. Some of these incidents were occasioned by the Society's roll book. At the beginning of each session any newly elected member present for the first time is called up to the front and requested to sign this book, in which a line has been reserved with his name engrossed in elegant gothic letters. The secretary then introduces him by name and title to the president, who formally declares him a member, shakes hands with him, and gives him his diploma of membership.

Sometimes we elect a new member who does not come promptly to a meeting to be enrolled, for example the late Kurt Gödel, the world's best known logician of his time but a frail reclusive scholar. In such cases we get a member who knows the reluctant neophyte to persuade him to come at least once. When Gödel came he said that because of poor digestion he could not join us at the buffet luncheon, so Miss Noonan had to give him shelter in her office and feed him on crackers and milk.

Among others who did not come to sign the book were some artists and literary people who were timid about hobnobbing with scientists and scholars. Perhaps we should follow the example of European academies, which have distinctive costumes or insignia. There is nothing like a uniform to support the ego. We should not need the pomp of the French academies—military tail coats, epaulettes, cocked hats, and swords. For Americans academic gowns would be sufficient, or even a broad ribbon across one's shirt front would brace up the shy new members.

Another eminent person who did not attend a meeting was Herbert Hoover, elected to membership in 1918, long before he was elected president of the United States. Hoover was so busy with national affairs from 1918 on that we could not inveigle him as we did Gödel and the artists, but at last in the early 1960s he came to Philadelphia to make a patriotic speech on Independence Square, next to Philosophical Hall. With his permission, obtained through his personal staff, Miss Noonan and I carried the roll book to Independence Hall and interrupted the former president's walk to the outdoor platform. Courteous as ever, he signed the book, shook hands, and went on. Miss Noonan and I stayed to hear him. I got a glimpse of the notes for the speech.

He must have had some defect of vision, for the notes were typed in letters half an inch high.

During my time as executive officer two incumbent presidents of the United States who were not members of the Society brought the quiet routine of Philosophical Hall to a stop when they visited Philadelphia. Richard Nixon came to Independence Square on October 20, 1972, to sign the bill H.R. 14370, the revenue-sharing bill, for which he and his advisers had earnestly striven—an achievement for which he should be kindly remembered. The occasion was considered so important that he chose to sign the bill at the nation's historic shrine. The White House staff wanted to have a place available before and after the address in case the president should wish to rest or confer with someone. They chose my office in Philosophical Hall and sent the Secret Service men and Philadelphia police to make the usual inspection and set up precautions for the presidential visit. I vacated my office that day but stood by with Miss Noonan in case we were needed.

The president did not come to the hall, but we had another, more entertaining visitor, Daniel Patrick Moynihan, elected a member of the Society in 1968. Nixon had specially invited him to the signing of the bill because he had been deeply concerned in drafting it. Arriving in Philadelphia early, Moynihan came to Philosophical Hall to await the president's arrival. Having no one else to talk to, he sat down with Miss Noonan and me and turned on his Irish charm in a long, amusing chat. He saw to it that Miss Noonan and I were each given one of the souvenir pens that were distributed to witnesses of the signing.

My office was again requisitioned for presidential use on September 5, 1974, when Gerald Ford came to address a governors' conference in celebration of the 200th anniversary of the First Continental Congress. This time the official preparations tied us up for a couple of days. Federal, state, and city policemen inspected every room in the hall. A Secret Service man looked in all the drawers of my desk to make sure there were no firearms hidden there. A "hot line" telephone to the White House was installed on my desk alongside my own telephone. An armed policeman was posted at an upstairs window watching the president's route to Independence Hall. Our building was crowded for hours with civilian and army police and White House staff. Telephone messages from the airport kept us posted as to the presidential party's arrival. The Society's president not being on hand, a staff man directed me to stand just outside the front door to welcome Mr. Ford. At last the motorcycle squad came up Fifth Street followed by several cars from one of which the president alighted with his immediate companions, shook hands as I bade him welcome, and was escorted to my office, leaving his entourage to add to the crowd of officials in our little lobby —military men, including at least one major general, policemen, politicians plus a reporter or two. There was further bustle when the governor of Pennsylvania, Milton Shapp, arrived by appointment for a conference with the president. Miss Noonan and I sat in the lobby feeling quite useless, but duty kept us there. At last Mr. Ford and Governor Shapp finished their conference and departed by the rear door toward Independence Hall, followed by their retinues. The hall lapsed into its accustomed calm and its memories of the days when our president, Thomas Jefferson, was also president of the United States.

My wife would have preferred to live in the suburbs of Philadelphia after our five-year taste of city life in New York, but she did not insist on her preference. Her choice of the apartment on Rittenhouse Square made it easy for me to get to and from Philosophical Hall on Independence Square. In our car, until I thought best to quit driving, we spent many weekend afternoons in fair weather, driving over the pleasant countryside west of Philadelphia or along the upper Delaware River above the city, usually dining at one of the picturesque riverside inns and getting home by bedtime. There were longer drives, which Betsy always enjoyed, to visit our son's family, first in Baltimore, then after 1963 to Sayre, Pennsylvania, where George, Jr., was a staff member of the Robert Packer Hospital and Guthrie Clinic. In winter when driving was not pleasant, the city offered all the entertainment and social life we cared for. The meetings of the American Philosophical Society, three days in April, two in November, brought to Philadelphia many of our friends of the academic world. Betsy took a season ticket for the Philadelphia Orchestra's Thursday afternoon concert, and it became our regular custom to meet after the concert for dinner at the Bellevue Stratford Hotel. Friends put me up for membership in the Franklin Inn Club, where I often lunched and whose Friday evening monthly dinners of members and their ladies made us acquainted with many local artists, writers, librarians, and some highly literate newspaper men.

Our writing projects and my scientific associations often took us out of Philadelphia. At the request of the alumni of the University of Rochester's School of Medicine and Dentistry, I undertook, soon after we moved to Philadelphia, to write a biography of my former chief and lifelong friend George Hoyt Whipple. I had to go to San Francisco to consult the files of the Hooper Foundation, which he had organized and directed (1914–24). We enjoyed crossing the continent again by rail and seeing Berkeley, where we had begun our married life. We returned by the northern route to visit Betsy's nephew Bernard Copping III at Bozeman, where he was treasurer of Montana State College.

In the autumn of 1962 my wife received a tentative invitation to a meeting in London of the Osler Society, a group of people interested in historical and literary aspects of medical practice. Christopher Booth wrote that the Osler Society was planning a session at Hammersmith Hospital on October 18, the 250th anniversary of Dr. Fothergill's birth. Dr. Booth, at that time professor of internal medicine in the Royal Postgraduate Medical School, had (I believe) suggested the topic, and Betsy was asked to address the meeting. She wanted me to accompany her, but October is a busy month at the American Philosophical Society, and moreover I thought that it was good for her to be on her own, since she had been so determined to write a book of her own. I saw her off for England aboard the S.S. *France;* Booth met her at Victoria Station in London. She stayed at the Mt. Royal Hotel, Marble Arch, which we both knew well.

At the meeting of the Osler Society, held at Hammersmith Hospital, Christopher spoke of John Fothergill as a physician. Betsy talked about his services to the American colonies, and Cuthbert Dukes, a distinguished urologist and medical historian, discussed Fothergill's role in the medical societies of London. The meeting, I was told, was a great success; Betsy's talk was enthusiastically received, and she came home with pleasant memories of kind English friends.

In 1964 the British Society for Endocrinology invited me to be Dale Lecturer at their annual meeting of that year in London. In my lecture I sketched the early history of the ovarian hormones and the conclusive isolation of estrone by Edgar Allen and Edward Doisey in 1923. To my great pleasure Sir Henry Dale was present and also Alan (now Sir Alan) Parkes, who had received the Dale Medal the year before, with his wife and co-worker Ruth Deanesley and several others who had contributed to our knowledge of the ovarian hormones. Sometimes I take the Dale Medal from my desk drawer to look at the portrait of Sir Henry and to recall the other men who were Dale medalists before me—Charles Best, Bernardo Houssay, Sir Charles Dodds, Adolf Butenandt, Philip Smith, and Alan Parkes. I have known them all, those friendly, high-minded scientists of five nations. My name engraved on the reverse of my medal will tell my grandsons that the old professor lived in the golden age of modern endocrinology and had his own part in it.

During these years things had gone well with us and life was interesting, but beginning in 1961 or thereabouts Betsy began to alarm me by occasional spells of depression and insta-bility. She had always been touchy, sensitive to fancied slights, and occasionally depressive, but more often cheerful, especially when we were traveling and when her seemingly interminable research for the book of Fothergill letters was going well. Her episodes of irritability had always for me been outweighed by her normal affection for me and by my delight in her intelligence and always impeccable taste in literature and the arts. Now, however, at the age of seventy-two or seventy-three, these moody episodes began to be more serious. As Christmas of 1963 approached, she surprised me and our son by deciding for no stated reason that she did not want to spend Christmas with the family. I took her, instead, on a Caribbean cruise that went very happily.

In the following summer a great event for us found her in excellent mood. This was my designation by the British Society for Endocrinology to be president of an international congress to be held in London (August 17–21, 1974), an honor which I ascribe to my endocrinologist friends—Sir Alan Parkes, then of Cambridge, Sir Charles Dodds of Middlesex Hospital Medical

School, and Emmanuel Amoroso of the Royal Veterinary College. For a restful vacation before the congress we sailed for England aboard the S.S. *France* on June 11 and went to North Wales for a fortnight at the fascinating resort of Portmerion in Merionethshire and later at St. Ives, Cornwall. At the opening session of the congress in the Royal Albert Hall on August 17 I gave the presidential address. I recall waiting behind the scenes for Amoroso, chairman of the local committee, to lead me onto the stage; I remember the large audience before me in the immense auditorium, but I cannot recall a word of my address.

That evening was given over to receptions for the members of the congress, British and foreign. There were so many people attending (1,200, I was told) that the local committee organized no fewer than five receptions in famous meeting places. It was my duty as president and Betsy's as first lady of the congress, to greet all the members. Emmanuel Amoroso hired a Rolls Royce with a uniformed driver to transport us and himself to each of the receptions. Amoroso, an enthusiastic and quite imposing coloured man from Jamaica, held the chair of anatomy at the Royal Veterinary College. He and I were in full evening dress (white tie and tails), and Betsy looked grand in a modish light blue dress. We drove first to the Royal College of Physicians at Regent's Park, where Sir Charles Dodds, P.R.C.P., and his fellow officers in their robes of office awaited us to form a receiving line.

Betsy nearly disgraced herself by giggling at a sight that only she and I could fully appreciate. Dodds, the distinguished biochemist, was short and a bit stout. In his heavy black robe reaching to the floor and glittering with gold embroidery, holding a gold-tipped black staff too tall for him, he looked rather comical in spite of his high office. Betsy and I both recalled a painting in the British Museum that had amused us, by Zoffany (1769), showing the actor Samuel Foote in a comedy taking off the Royal College of Physicians. In the picture Foote as president wears a medical wig and carries a sword instead of a staff, but otherwise it is a perfect caricature of Sir Charles Dodds as we saw him that night. Betsy stifled her amusement and was quite ladylike in her curtsy to Dodds.

After we had received the guests and had had a sip of sherry, Amoroso carried us off to the Royal Society of Medicine in Wimpole Street, Apothecaries' Hall in Blackfriars Lane, the Royal College of Surgeons in Lincoln's Inn Fields, and grandest of all, Lancaster House off Pall Mall, a ducal palace now used by the government for official functions. Amoroso, Betsy, and I ascended the broad marble staircase and held court at its head. This reception was reserved for the VIPs of the congress. Betsy was poised and charming; I had never seen her in better social form. This is a memory I have cherished during the sad years that were to follow.

19

EDITOR AND BIOGRAPHER

December 28, 1965, was the fiftieth anniversary of our marriage. Betsy and I decided to celebrate it with a golden wedding dinner —but where? Our son and his family were living in northern Pennsylvania at Sayre. Our closest friends were scattered, in Baltimore, Rochester, Philadelphia, and Los Angeles. I no longer had many close relatives in my home town, Baltimore, nor had Betsy any old friends still living in New England. On reflection it seemed to us that Rochester, our first really settled place of residence together, where our children had grown up, had more associations with our married life than any other place, so we held our party there. George, Jr., his wife Betty and our grandsons came from Sayre. The other guests were Rochester medical friends, Wallace and Clara Fenn, John and Nancy Morton, Karl and Mildred Wilson. George Whipple was ill at the time; he and Katherine could not be with us. The dinner, at Town House, a supermotel near the medical school, with the traditional appurtenances, a wedding cake and champagne, was a happy time for all of us, rich in friendship and affection.

My agreement with Henry Allen Moe, president of the American Philosophical Society when I became executive officer, included the assurance that I should have time to write, just as if I were still a university professor. For a few years free time was fairly easy to find, but somehow my executive and editorial duties gradually increased until only weekends remained. Quite soon after our move to Philadelphia in 1960 a call came from the Rochester medical alumni with the request that I write a biography of the well-loved dean of the school, George Hoyt Whipple, who had retired in 1953 after thirty-one years of service to the University of Rochester. My affection for George Whipple and my continuing interest in the great professional school I had helped him to found, drew me irresistibly to the proffered task. The alumni association provided funds for the necessary travel to New England, Baltimore, and San Francisco to talk with George's sister and to consult Johns Hopkins and Hooper Foundation records and for several trips to Rochester, one of them a month long, in the summer of 1963. I spent many an hour in the dusty storerooms in the dome of the Rush Rhees Library on the River Campus studying correspondence regarding the foundation of the school. George was happy to have me write about him and patiently bore what must have sometimes seemed searching questions. Once when I showed some hesitation about discussing an episode for which he might possibly be criticized, he said, "Look here, if you were an artist painting my portrait in oil instead of ink, and you saw a wrinkle on my face, you'd have to show it, wouldn't you?" He read every chapter as I drafted it, never once offering a correction. Katherine, his wife, was more critical. She complained that I made him too good; why didn't I tell more about his faults? The Rochester alumni subsidized publication of the book in 1963 by Lippincott of Philadelphia. Because George's friendships were a key to his character, I entitled the book *George Hoyt Whipple and His Friends.*

In 1965 the medical school of the University of Pennsylvania, oldest in the United States, was about to celebrate its 200th anniversary. The committee planning the celebration, wishing to publish a history of the school, offered to commission my colleague, Richard H. Shryock, to write it, but he had other work in hand. Hearing of this, I volunteered to take it on. I knew that Shryock, not a physician but an experienced professional historian, could have done better than I with the general background of the story, but perhaps I, medically trained and having had the experience of helping to organize and conduct a medical school, might contribute a professional tone to the narrative. The committee agreed and put me to work with the promise of a modest honorarium and a salary for an assistant.

Materials were plentiful. The faculty records were complete from the beginning; those compiled before 1776 had during the

Revolution been stored somewhere in the country to save them from the British invaders. There was an excellent centennial history of the school. I had already learned much about the earliest years from Betsy's study of William Shippen, Jr., one of the founders, and from my own work on Benjamin Rush's autobiography. Roy Nichols, professor of American history in the University of Pennsylvania, a member of the bicentennial committee, read each chapter as I completed the draft. His bright smile and sparkling eyes as he approved the first chapter told me that I was on the right track. With a little burning of midnight oil I got the book ready for Lippincott to edit and publish in time for the celebration. It received very good reviews. At commencement 1965, the University of Pennsylvania conferred upon me the honorary degree of doctor of letters, which I assume attests to the literary quality of my book; at any rate it is a reassuring credential for my daily work as an editor. If an M.D. looks after sick people, a Litt.D. should be specially qualified to care for poor English.

We spent the honorarium the next year on a forty-day cruise to Australia. Crossing the continent by rail—the last time we traveled in a sleeping car—we spent two or three days in Berkeley for old times' sake, then sailed aboard the S.S. *Mariposa* of the Moore-McCormack line for Sydney by way of Bora-Bora, Tahiti, and New Zealand, and back by Fiji and Honolulu. Betsy was bright and happy and totally carefree every day of the enchanting voyage, as indeed she always was when the daily routine of life did not weigh upon her.

Betsy had been writing as busily as I. After fifteen years of intermittent work transcribing the Fothergill letters, doing library research, and conferring with her collaborator on each of our trips to England, she had drafted her biographical introduction and the numerous notes to the letters. She had herself written practically all of this mass of comment and explanation. Christopher Booth had of course contributed much to her understanding of the Fothergill correspondence and had supplied the contents of a few notes. I too had furnished two or three notes on medical subjects. The wording was all Betsy's—a considerable feat for an author whose formal education had included only one year at college. Her clear, smooth English style reflected a literate home and superior secondary education at Robinson Seminary at Exeter, New Hampshire, plus wide reading and a lifetime spent among educated people.

She sent the manuscript, as nearly as I can remember, early in 1967 to Harvard University Press. Several months later a letter from Cambridge told her that two experienced reviewers, a historian and a botanist, had recommended it for publication. The syndics of the press had accepted it, subject to some shortening of the introduction and a few overlong notes. Editorial care had been assigned to Mrs. L. J. Kewer, the press's chief editor for special projects.

We drove to Cambridge, where Mrs. Kewer went over the editorial stipulations with Betsy. These, I thought, were reasonable, but Betsy found it hard to cut her introduction and notes. At home she began the task, but without the drive that had enabled her to accomplish the long years of research and writing. It should have taken only a week or two to make the changes, but I would come home from work and find her sitting in her bedroom with a tablet of paper on her work table and, on the floor, a layer of sheets on each of which she had written a sentence or two before helplessly tossing it away and beginning again.

Yet her pride in doing the writing herself persisted. I dared not offer to help. I did what I could to lighten her housework. We had a housemaid coming to the apartment to sweep and dust. I had often prepared our breakfasts; now I also cooked our simple dinners, if it may be called cooking to heat up a can of consommé and a package of frozen food or to make a sandwich and serve ice cream or fruit for dessert. I took her for long Saturday afternoon drives in the beautiful country about Philadelphia. She would brighten up from time to time, but the writing did not progress. Slowly it dawned upon me that the trouble was more than mere fatigue or depleted energy; it was a loss of mentality. At the age of seventy-seven Betsy was succumbing to senile dementia.

I have no heart to inflict upon those who read this book the distressing details of our calamity, but my wife's illness was for more than nine years part of the pattern of my life and I cannot black it out of my story. The process of deterioration went on slowly. Betsy knew that she was failing. At last, one day in the late spring of 1967, beside me on the sofa of our sitting room, she spoke of her difficulty in writing and said that it had occurred to her that the help she needed was close at hand. I was an experienced editor; would I aid her to make the changes that Harvard University Press had requested? Seeing at least a chance that I could get her to fulfill her obligation to the press and to Christopher Booth, I gladly agreed to her request, putting aside a book on which I was working, which I shall mention later. Thinking that a change of scene would help, I proposed that we should go to New York for six weeks, June to August. The Rockefeller Institute would let us have a couple of rooms in its student dormitory during the summer. Betsy always liked to travel; the plan pleased her. We hired a young man typist for whom the institute provided a room by the day and lent us a typewriter. Meals were available in the institute's dining room. We worked every day except Sundays, with a daily nap for Betsy. I fed the necessary work to her, seeing to it that she did not overdo the revisions. After dinner we sat outdoors watching the traffic on the East River and occasionally went to a movie. On Saturdays we took long drives in the country.

This was a relatively happy time. We got most of the cutting done, though not as much as Mrs. Kewer wanted. I restored the whole manuscript to correct order, which Betsy had disarranged in her futile efforts at home. In mid-July I had to go to London for five days to attend a conference at CIBA House. Betsy was well enough oriented still to get her meals, and no harm came from my absence. We resumed work together, but two things happened just before it was time to return to Philadelphia that changed the picture. Betsy entered a phase of depression and irritability that often characterizes her type of brain disease. She had, one evening, a spell of acute depression, lying on a couch and wailing over and over again, for no obvious reason, "I want to die! I want to die!" The next morning she was in good spirits again.

To complicate matters I suddenly developed an acutely painful knee which an orthopedist friend of mine in the neighborhood diagnosed as osteoarthritis. Obviously I could not drive our car to Philadelphia. One of my grandsons offered to come to New York to drive us home, but I, remembering that my mother had been seriously crippled by arthritis in her old age, feared that I would never be able to drive again. I sold the car in New York and hired a car and driver for the journey to Philadelphia. At home our regular physician, Dr. Paul Havens, was away; his associate Dr. Theodore G. Duncan prescribed a drug that much relieved my pain, although this attack proved to be the beginning of a mild arthritic condition that has persisted, though it has not crippled me.

Betsy, on the other hand, worsened. I hired an experienced young black woman as nurse-companion for her during my daily absence at the office. Another frequent symptom of the disease developed, suspicion of me even though she was consciously dependent upon me. She was still fiddling with her manuscript, for I had not yet obtained her consent to send it to Harvard University Press. One night the first hundred typed pages (most of the introduction) were missing, and she spent several hours declaring that I had secreted it out of jealousy because she had written a book. To see a once fine intellect deteriorate is grievous enough; to be accused of such evil was worse. She slept badly and in spite of my supposed misdeeds wanted me to sit by her bed until she dropped off to sleep. She rather unwillingly let me take her to a psychiatrist who advised hospital care for a time. Our son came to Philadelphia to help me take her to an excellent sanitarium in the suburbs. While she was there I found the missing pages of her typescript under the seat cushions of the sitting-room davenport, where she had hidden them.

After a few weeks at the sanitarium, treatment by electroconvulsive shock (under anesthesia) brought a blessed relief of depression and disorientation. I took her home, and during the next few months four more shock treatments headed off the depressive phase, but her ability to care for her person deteriorated. To have round-the-clock nursing at our apartment was out of the question. George, Jr., devoted as always to his parents' welfare, came to Philadelphia again and helped me find a good nursing home, fortunately only about fifteen minutes' walk from our home. There Betsy spent the rest of her life, not unhappy and always glad to see me on my frequent visits. The precision of the New England speech she had never lost, and a line of light banter revived from her childhood made her a pet of the black attendants of the nursing home. During the next seven years I visited her twice a week except when I was on vacation, taking her flowers weekly. She always welcomed me, but conversation gradually diminished to mere greetings. She could not believe that she was in Philadelphia. At almost every visit she asked me how old she was, and when I said "eighty-three," or "eighty-five," she laughingly cried, "Are you kidding me?"

While she was first in the sanitarium, I went to Cambridge to assure Mrs. Kewer that I would see the Fothergill book through the press. Feeling a bit like a traitor to Betsy I completed the cutting of the introduction and a few still overlong notes. Mrs. Kewer asked that the long series of letters be broken into something like chapters. I divided it into eight sections, each headed by an apt quotation from one of the letters. As the book passed through the press I read the galley proofs and page proofs. A set of galleys was sent to Christopher Booth in London. Finally I compiled the index. In 1971 the first copy arrived, *Chain of Friendship: Selected Letters of Dr. John Fothergill*, beautifully printed, handsomely bound, and clad in a sturdy jacket of blue paper showing Dr. Fothergill's bewigged Quaker face above the names of Betsy Copping Corner and Christopher C. Booth. I took it to the nursing home and handed it to Betsy. She clasped it to her breast with a happy smile and looked at a few pages but soon tired and laid it aside. Lying on the dresser in her room it attracted much attention from the nurses and ward attendants. This, I think, was the first time that a patient in Town Court Nursing Home had ever published a scholarly book.

As soon as the index to *Chain of Friendship* was off my hands, I resumed the work begun some years before, a biography of Elisha Kent Kane (1820–57). Kane, a young Philadelphia physician who became the first American Arctic explorer of note, had been a hero of my childhood. His lavishly illustrated book, *Arctic Explorations in the Years 1853, '54, '55*, had stood on my grandfather Corner's shelves, and before I could read I was permitted, on the long Methodist Sunday afternoons, to turn its pages and marvel at the brave little doctor and his men lost in a maze of Arctic ice. When I grew up and found that he had lived in the city next to ours, had belonged to my own profession, and had bought supplies for his expedition from my grandfather Evans, I began to collect information about him and resolved some day to write the story of his life.

Moving to Philadelphia in 1960 I found much source material. Kane had been a member of the American Philosophical Society. His portrait and that of his father, Judge Kane, hang in Philosophical Hall, and I found that some of his grandnephews and grandnieces live in Pennsylvania. I made friends with his namesake, E. Kent Kane, and Betsy and I made the journey of 250 miles from Philadelphia to Kane, Pennsylvania, for a few days' stay to learn from Kent Kane about his celebrated granduncle. Because of my interest, other members of the Kane family gave the American Philosophical Society a large collection of family papers, among them letters and notebooks of the explorer. The Historical Society of Pennsylvania had numerous Kane documents. I visited the Stefansson Arctic Collection at Dartmouth College and during my brief visit to England in 1967 spent a day at the Scott Polar Research Institute at Cambridge reading the correspondence of Lady Franklin. At other libraries in New York, Baltimore, and Washington I ran down details of Dr. Kane's brief career and often reckless adventures. When the manuscript was ready I sent it to the recently started Temple University Press in Philadelphia. Its director, the poet-editor Maurice English, was enthusiastic about *Doctor Kane of the Arctic Seas* and brought it out in 1972 in a handsome format with beautiful typography. This was my fourteenth book. Meanwhile I kept busy writing obituary notices about friends and acquaintances of the scientific world. Such is the responsibility imposed by a long life; it becomes a duty to record the lives of those who have taught us or worked with us. Between 1960 and 1979 I wrote more than forty such articles. Five of these were thirty- to forty-page essays for the *Biographical Memoirs* of the National Academy of Sciences (on Herbert M. Evans, Warren H. Lewis, Oscar Riddle, George L. Streeter, and John D. Rockefeller, Jr.). A dozen were briefer accounts for the *Year Book of the American Philosophical Society;* the rest were short articles for the *Dictionary of American Biography* (DAB), the *Dictionary of Scientific Biography,* and *Notable American Women.*

In 1967 Frederick Burkhardt, president of the American Council of Learned Societies, asked me to join the editorial committee of DAB, whose chairman was then Walter Whitehill, the genial sage of the Boston Athenaeum. It has been a joy to meet for a day or two each year with these dozen learned and humane scholars who plan the successive supplement volumes of the great reference work.

I have been fortunate, in my old age, in having sufficient health and opportunity for travel. In 1971 my son and his wife and boys took me along with them on a trip by car from their home to Nova Scotia and Cape Breton Island. In 1972 I took my grandsons Thomas and Christopher to England with me, my excuse for the trip being an international congress of medical historians in London. We crossed the Atlantic aboard *Queen Elizabeth II* to give the young men a voyage on one of the grand passenger liners that were disappearing from the seas. We hired a car for Tom to drive, since I was too old and Chris too young for a British driving license. We had a companionable time visiting some of the famous places—Winchester, Oxford, Canterbury, Stonehenge, Salisbury.

In 1973 their parents accompanied me on a similar brief visit to England and Wales, the occasion being a meeting of the British Society for the Study of Fertility, held at Bangor. That organization of leading workers in the physiology of reproduction—physicians and veterinarians, biochemists, physiologists, and geneticists—awarded me their Marshall Medal, struck in honor of Francis H. A. Marshall of Cambridge University, whose work had been an inspiration to me when I began research in the physiology of reproduction. Another reminder of a great leader came to me in 1975, the William H. Welch Medal of the American Association for the History of Medicine, doubly valued because its bas-relief likeness of Dr. Welch in bronze was modeled by my late friend, the anthropologist Adolf W. Schultz.

The early fall of 1975 took me to one of the most beautiful places of all my travels, Lake Como in northern Italy, where I was the guest at Menaggio of the sculptor Joy Buba and her husband. For two weeks I sat for two or three hours daily while Joy worked up her life-sized plasticine model of my head, brightly chatting to keep an animated look on my countenance. In the evenings we walked in the lakeside gardens of the Bubas' home, Villa Evelyn, or Joy showed me her albums full of sketches of places she had visited and people she had known. On a couple of evenings the Bubas were a kind audience for me as

I read some of the narrative poems, reminiscent of my youth, that I have written in recent years, too slight and intimate for any but special friends.

A medical history club in San Francisco invited me in the fall of 1975 to present a lecture at its meeting of January 11, 1976. I had no recent historical studies suitable for such an occasion, but the prospect of seeing San Francisco once more was so tempting that I offered to give for the twenty-first time my still unpublished lecture on medicine in the poems of Chaucer. Two serious difficulties arose between my acceptance of the invitation and the trip to California. When I was about eighty years old, cataracts in both eyes began to cloud my vision. My ophthalmologist, Dr. Thomas R. Hedges of the Pennsylvania Hospital, thought it advisable to operate, and in November 1975 he removed the lens from my left eye. By the time of my scheduled lecture in January 1976, I was not yet fully accustomed to the new eyeglass lens, and the right eye was too cloudy to read signs in the airports. Worse yet, my lecture was illustrated with lantern slides of passages from Chaucer's poems. A test in Philosophical Hall showed that I could not read them from the screen. At Thanksgiving at Sayre, grandson Tom solved both problems. He would go with me to San Francisco, and by incredible good luck he had a friend there, John Schanck, who was teaching Chaucer in a local college. A long distance call was sufficient to enlist John's willing help. I made reservations for the two of us to fly to San Francisco on January 9.

Wednesday, January 8, was the day for my regular midweek visit to my wife at the nursing home. When late in the afternoon I entered her room, expecting the usual bright exclamation of welcome, I found her slumped, unconscious, in her chair at her little bedside table on which her dinner tray lay barely touched. She had taken her soup but that was all. Her face was pallid, her breathing somewhat rapid, her pulse rapid and irregular. Unable to wake her, I got the head nurse and one of her aides, who lifted Betsy's helpless body into her bed. When they had her lying on her back and had tucked in the bedclothes around her, with her arms lying outside the cover, I saw her right arm, slightly flexed at the elbow, rise slowly from the bed until her hand was higher than her recumbent head; then it slowly dropped and lay motionless at her side. I knew that this strange movement was a mechanical response to some stimulus to the left motor cortex of her brain, probably from leakage from a broken blood vessel, but it seemed like a gesture of farewell.

While we waited for a physician to arrive my head was spinning with the problems that faced me. Tom was due from Sayre the next morning. Our plane to San Francisco was to depart soon after. It was too late to call off the scheduled trip. The rule "the show must go on" applies to a scholar-lecturer as much as to an actor. I could do nothing whatever for Betsy. At least she was living and might recover from the stroke, if that was what it was. I wrote out a page of instructions in case she should die during my absence—to call my son in Sayre and Miss Noonan at my office—and went home to pack my suitcase. Before going to bed I walked back to the nursing home and found that Betsy was still unconscious, with regular respiration and a good pulse.

The flight across the continent was uneventful. Tom was a helpful guide through the airport and to our hotel. His friend John Schanck came the next morning to go over the Chaucer slides. I found him a self-confident chap; he read the verses with a good Middle English accent. In the afternoon he offered to take us for a drive in his station wagon. I asked to go over the Golden Gate bridge to Muir Woods. I wanted to revisit the grand red-wood grove where Betsy and I had often strolled together in 1915–19.

The meeting on Saturday evening, held at a downtown club, was preceded by an excellent dinner. A projector was ready for my slides. A young man who had been assigned to operate it seemed unfamiliar with its use, but grandson Tom, an engineer by training, got it working and sat by the operator in case of trouble, which developed when I was about two-thirds of the way through my lecture. The lamp bulb in the projector suddenly imploded with a loud bang. There was no fresh lamp to replace it. John Schanck had been reading the slides with good effect from the screen; now there was nothing on the screen to read. Again Tom came to the rescue. These were the large, old-fashioned glass slides. He promptly obtained somehow a pocket flashlight and held the slides one by one in front of John to read from them directly. Nobody thought to turn on the lights in the room; the sound of John's voice coming from the darkness gave an uncanny impression that Chaucer himself was speaking to us from the fourteenth century. We finished the lecture in triumph over our difficulties.

There had been no message from Philadelphia. After a smooth return flight Tom and I went to the baggage claim area to pick up our bags. There, standing by the side of the luggage carousel, were George, Jr., and Betty. The look on his face told me what had happened. "Bad news?" I asked. "Yes," said George, "early this morning. We were called and caught the morning plane from Elmira." Betsy and I had been married sixty years and two weeks. I was glad that she could leave us without suffering, but her departure left a vacancy in my life.

So I go on living on Rittenhouse Square and working at the American Philosophical Society. People remember as I approach the end of my ninth decade that I am about and at work. The Johns Hopkins University in 1975 gave me the honorary degree of doctor of laws. Coming from my alma mater this was a heart-warming honor. In 1979 the American Association of Anatomists conferred on me the Henry Gray Award "in recognition of substantial and meritorious service to the entire scientific community through scholarly accomplishments in original investigation, teaching, and writing in the field of anatomy."

I had begun, however, to think some years ago that it was high time for me to resign my post with the American Philosophical Society; I said so more than once to our wise and kindly president, Jonathan Rhoads. In 1977 at a quiet dinner for two at the Rittenhouse Club, Jonathan said that he wanted me to continue, with lightened duties. My colleague and friend, our librarian Whitfield J. Bell, Jr., would take my place as executive officer, but Jonathan wanted him to continue as librarian. To make it possible for him to conduct both positions Jonathan wanted me to lighten Bell's executive duties by retaining my work as editor and also chairman of the committee on research, which conducts the Society's grants.

So Bell and I have exchanged offices, he moving into Philosophical Hall and I to the library. Miss Julia Noonan, who has served the Society longer than Bell and I put together, has also been given somewhat lightened duties; she carries on the arduous work of correspondence and record-keeping concerning the grants. She and I come to work at ten o'clock and leave at four five days a week, she often and I occasionally taking office work home for the evenings just as we both always did.

At home I have some lonesome hours but am not lonely. My affectionate and ever-thoughtful son, now professor of obstetrics and gynecology at the University of Alabama's school of medicine at Huntsville, and his wife, Betty, who has become a real daughter to me, are often on the telephone, and I go to them at Thanksgiving and Christmas. My grandsons, both of whom are married now and busy with domestic life, call me now and then. I have nephews and nieces, their children and their children's children, now scattered from Maine to Texas, who seem to enjoy a chat with the old professor when they come my way. There are old friends with whom I keep in touch, people whom I have known for years with whom I can communicate familiarly —the Belts in Los Angeles, the Richters in Baltimore, Arpad Csapo in St. Louis, Christopher Booth in London, Graham Weddell at Oxford, Inés de Allende in Córdoba. There is a gracious lady of eighty years in Baltimore, childhood playmate of my late sister, who for love of old times often sends me clippings from her newspaper that tell me what is going on in my native city.

At Philadelphia I find companionship, of course, at Philosophical Hall and in the Wistar Association, an inner circle of the Philosophical Society whose members dine together several times a year. Among these local associates I find new friends. At the Franklin Inn Club I meet the city's artists and writers. Edgar Preston Richardson, who has returned to his native city after a fine career as art historian and art museum director, and his artist wife, Constance Coleman Richardson, have become friends as faithful and understanding as if I had known them all my life instead of only a decade. They ask me often to dine with them at their art-filled home on Society Hill in old Philadelphia. Ted is an accomplished scholar, Constance an expert cook and raconteur. An evening of high-level conversation with them passes all too quickly and leaves me with gratitude for their warm and humane friendliness.

I once had a correspondent who held that the universe is no good and should not exist. I disagree with him. I think highly of the universe. The buffets it gives us, we must take as they come; the benefits we can often help to arrange. I am proud to have been a member of the universe these ninety years past. One accepts, of course, the regulations for enrollment, pays his annual assessment of hard work, and aims to be a useful citizen of the local galaxy. In return, he receives the friendship of other members and the love of those who are near and dear to him.

PUBLICATIONS OF
GEORGE W. CORNER

BOOKS

1927   Anatomical texts of the earlier Middle Ages: A study in the transmission of culture. Washington, D.C.: Carnegie Institution of Washington.

1930   Anatomy. Clio Medica. New York: Hoeber. (A brief history.)

1938   Attaining manhood: A doctor talks to boys about sex. New York: Harper.

1939   Attaining womanhood: A doctor talks to girls about sex. New York: Harper.

1941   Ourselves unborn: An embryologist's essay on man. Terry Lecture. New Haven: Yale University Press.

1942   The hormones in human reproduction. Vanuxem Lecture. Princeton, N.J.: Princeton University Press.

1948   The autobiography of Benjamin Rush. Princeton, N.J.: published for the American Philosophical Society by Princeton University Press.

1950   Cytology of the human vagina. Trans. from the Spanish of Inés L. C. de Allende and Oscar Orias. New York: Hoeber.

1953   With Sophie D. Aberle. Twenty-five years of sex research: History of the National Research Committee for Research in the Problems of Sex. Philadelphia: Saunders.

1958   Anatomist at large: Selected essays. New York: Basic Books.

1963   George Hoyt Whipple and his friends: The life story of a Nobel Prize pathologist. Philadelphia: Lippincott.

1964   A history of the Rockefeller Institute, 1901–1953: Origins and growth. New York: Rockefeller University Press.

1965 Two centuries of medicine: A history of the school of medicine, University of Pennsylvania. Philadelphia: Lippincott.

1972 Doctor Kane of the Arctic Seas. Philadelphia: Temple University Press.

ARTICLES

From more than 200 articles published in scientific and scholarly journals, the following have been selected as representative.

1914 The structural unit and growth of the pancreas of the pig. *American Journal of Anatomy* 16: 207–36.

1915 Mithridatium and theriac, the most famous remedies of old medicine. *Johns Hopkins Hospital Bulletin* 26: 222–26.

1915 The corpus luteum of pregnancy as it is in swine. Publications of the Carnegie Institution of Washington, no. 222 (Contributions to Embryology, no. 5), pp. 69–94.

1919 Anatomists in search of the soul. *Annals of Medical History* 2: 1–7.

1919 On the origin of the corpus luteum of the sow from both granulosa and theca interna. *American Journal of Anatomy* 26: 117–83.

1921 Cyclic changes in the ovaries and uterus of the sow, and their relation to the mechanism of implantation. Publications of the Carnegie Institution of Washington, no. 276 (Contributions to Embryology, no. 64), pp. 117–46.

1923 The problem of embryonic pathology in mammals, with observations upon intrauterine mortality in the pig. *American Journal of Anatomy* 31: 523–45.

1923 Ovulation and menstruation in Macacus rhesus. Publications of the Carnegie Institution of Washington, no. 332 (Contributions to Embryology, no. 75), pp. 75–101.

1927 The relation between menstruation and ovulation in the monkey: Its possible significance for man. *Journal of the American Medical Association* 89: 1838–40.

1928 Physiology of the corpus luteum: 1. The effect of very early ablation of the corpus luteum upon embryos and uterus. *American Journal of Physiology* 86: 74–81.

1929 With Willard M. Allen. Physiology of the corpus luteum: 2. Production of a special uterine reaction (progestational proliferation) by extracts of the corpus luteum. *American Journal of Physiology* 88: 326–39.

1929 With Willard M. Allen. Physiology of the corpus luteum: 3. Normal growth and implantation of embryos after very early ablation of the ovaries, under the influence of extracts of the corpus luteum. *American Journal of Physiology* 88: 340–46.

1930   The hormonal control of lactation: 1. Non-effect of the corpus luteum. 2. Positive action of extracts of the hypophysis. *American Journal of Physiology* 95: 43–55.

1935   Influence of the ovarian hormones, oestrin and progestin, upon the menstrual cycle of the monkey. *American Journal of Physiology* 113: 238–50.

1936   With A. W. Makepeace and Willard M. Allen. The effect of progestin on the in vitro response of the rabbit's uterus to pituitrin. *American Journal of Physiology* 115: 376–85.

1937   Salernitan surgery in the twelfth century. *British Journal of Surgery* 25: 84–99.

1937   The rate of secretion of progestin by the corpus luteum. Cold Spring Harbor Symposia on Quantitative Biology 5: 62–65.

1945   Development, organization, and breakdown of the corpus luteum in the rhesus monkey. Publications of the Carnegie Institution of Washington, no. 557 (Contributions to Embryology, no. 31), pp. 117–46.

1954   A glimpse of incomprehensibles. (Address given at Swarthmore College, February 11, 1954.) *American Scholar* 23: 321–31.

1955   The observed embryology of human single-ovum twins and other multiple births. (Joseph L. Baer Lecture of the Chicago Gynecological Society, delivered October 15, 1954.) *American Journal of Obstetrics and Gynecology* 70: 933–51.

INDEX

Freiburg im Breisgau, 53, 55
French, C. Stacey, 295
French, John C., 23
Full-time professors, 228–29

Gage, Simon H., 264–65
Gale, Arthur F., 201, 219, 220
Galen, 225, 266
Garden party, royal, 348
Gardner, Arthur, 324
Garrison, Fielding H., 101
Gasser, Herbert S., 357
Gates, Frederick L., 41, 42
Gault, Matthew, 12
Gaunt, Robert, 260
Genesee fever, 226
Gerdine, Linton, 41, 307
Gergen, J. J., 229
Gibbons, James Cardinal, 28
Gilbert, Walter A., 296
Gilchrist, Donald, 224
Gilchrist, Mina, 67
Gilchrist, T. Caspar, 59, 60
Gildersleeve, Basil L., 21
Gilfillan, Jessica, 130
Gilman, Daniel Coit, 21
Gleason, Harold, 204
Glencoe, Md., 17, 145
Gloucester, Duke and Duchess of, 348, 349
Gödel, Kurt, 376
Goldman, Carl, 102
Goldstein, Jacob, 212
Goldstein, Louis, 246
Goler, George W., 174, 202, 204, 210, 211, 217, 229, 263
Goodhart, Arthur, 324, 346
Gordon, Robert, 87
Gorsuch, Dickinson, 17, 18, 145
Grant, Emma, 14, 77
Green, Fitzhugh, 92
Greene, Herbert E., 23, 26
Greenman, Milton J., 276
Gregg, Alan, 316
Grenfell, Sir Wilfred T., 63, 93, 94, 99
Grenfell Association, 62, 94
Grieve, John, 65, 66, 67, 70–73, 83, 88
Gudger, 32
Guggenheim, Simon, 320
Guggenheim Foundation, 320, 321

Guild, Stacy R., 107, 325
Guttmacher, Alan, 167, 168, 212, 213
Guttmacher, Manfred, 167

Hale, Edward Everett, 63
Halsted, William S., 60, 61, 84, 118, 149, 169, 170
Hamburger, Louis, 59, 79
Hammond, John, 193
Hampstead Garden Suburb, 183, 184
Harris, Reginald, 259, 261
Harrison, Ross G., 213, 214
Hartman, Carl, 168, 240, 250, 284, 292
Harvard University, 67, 273
Harvey, William, 105, 324
Harvey Lecture, 308
Haskins, Caryl P., 325, 328
Haskins, Edna, 328, 329
Haswell, Alice, 105
Havens, Paul, 388
Health service, British, 344, 345
Heape, Walter, 187, 192, 206, 296
Heard, Osborne, 288
Hedges, Thomas R., 392
Heisenberg, Werner, 368
Henry Gray Award, 394
Hepburn, Rebecca, 288
Hermann, 234
Hertig, Arthur T., 195, 285, 290, 355
Heuser, Chester, 284–86, 290, 291
Hickman, Kenneth, 239
Hill, A. V., 184, 186
Hill, Christopher, 336
Hill, Eben C., 140
Hill, J. P., 187
Hisaw, Frederick L., 238, 240, 251, 313
Histology course, 100, 101, 215–17
History-taking, gynecological, 110–11
Hoag, Mrs., 107–9
Hoffman, B., 229
Hoffman, Malvina, 180
Hoh-Königsburg, 55, 198
Holman, Emil, 169, 170
Holmes, Walter, 110, 114–16
Hooker, Davenport, 107
Hooker, Donald, 45
Hoover, Herbert, 49, 295, 376
Horne, Herman H., 17
Horrax, Gilbert, 41, 96
Hough, Theodore, 140
Houssay, Bernard, 364, 380
Howard, Eugene H., 204

FEB 1982